AGING IN ASIA

FINDINGS FROM NEW AND EMERGING DATA INITIATIVES

Panel on Policy Research and Data Needs to
Meet the Challenge of Aging in Asia

James P. Smith and Malay Majmundar, *Editors*

Committee on Population

Division of Behavioral and Social Sciences and Education

NATIONAL RESEARCH COUNCIL
OF THE NATIONAL ACADEMIES

THE NATIONAL ACADEMIES PRESS
Washington, D.C.
www.nap.edu

THE NATIONAL ACADEMIES PRESS   500 Fifth Street, NW   Washington, DC 20001

NOTICE: The project that is the subject of this report was approved by the Governing Board of the National Research Council, whose members are drawn from the councils of the National Academy of Sciences, the National Academy of Engineering, and the Institute of Medicine. The members of the committee responsible for the report were chosen for their special competences and with regard for appropriate balance.

This study was supported by the National Institute on Aging's Division of Behavioral and Social Research through Contract No. NO1-OD-4-2139, Task Order Numbers 92, 226, and 260 between the National Academy of Sciences and the U.S. Department of Health and Human Services. Any opinions, findings, conclusions, or recommendations expressed in this publication are those of the author(s) and do not necessarily reflect the views of the organizations or agencies that provided support for the project.

International Standard Book Number-13: 978-0-309-25406-9
International Standard Book Number-10: 0-309-25406-X

Additional copies of this report are available from the National Academies Press, 500 Fifth Street, NW, Keck 360, Washington, DC 20001; (800) 624-6242 or (202) 334-3313; http://www.nap.edu.

Suggested citation: National Research Council. (2012). *Aging in Asia: Findings from New and Emerging Data Initiatives.* J.P. Smith and M. Majmundar, Eds. Panel on Policy Research and Data Needs to Meet the Challenge of Aging in Asia. Committee on Population, Division of Behavioral and Social Sciences and Education. Washington, DC: The National Academies Press.

THE NATIONAL ACADEMIES
Advisers to the Nation on Science, Engineering, and Medicine

The **National Academy of Sciences** is a private, nonprofit, self-perpetuating society of distinguished scholars engaged in scientific and engineering research, dedicated to the furtherance of science and technology and to their use for the general welfare. Upon the authority of the charter granted to it by the Congress in 1863, the Academy has a mandate that requires it to advise the federal government on scientific and technical matters. Dr. Ralph J. Cicerone is president of the National Academy of Sciences.

The **National Academy of Engineering** was established in 1964, under the charter of the National Academy of Sciences, as a parallel organization of outstanding engineers. It is autonomous in its administration and in the selection of its members, sharing with the National Academy of Sciences the responsibility for advising the federal government. The National Academy of Engineering also sponsors engineering programs aimed at meeting national needs, encourages education and research, and recognizes the superior achievements of engineers. Dr. Charles M. Vest is president of the National Academy of Engineering.

The **Institute of Medicine** was established in 1970 by the National Academy of Sciences to secure the services of eminent members of appropriate professions in the examination of policy matters pertaining to the health of the public. The Institute acts under the responsibility given to the National Academy of Sciences by its congressional charter to be an adviser to the federal government and, upon its own initiative, to identify issues of medical care, research, and education. Dr. Harvey V. Fineberg is president of the Institute of Medicine.

The **National Research Council** was organized by the National Academy of Sciences in 1916 to associate the broad community of science and technology with the Academy's purposes of furthering knowledge and advising the federal government. Functioning in accordance with general policies determined by the Academy, the Council has become the principal operating agency of both the National Academy of Sciences and the National Academy of Engineering in providing services to the government, the public, and the scientific and engineering communities. The Council is administered jointly by both Academies and the Institute of Medicine. Dr. Ralph J. Cicerone and Dr. Charles M. Vest are chair and vice chair, respectively, of the National Research Council.

www.national-academies.org

Preface

The population of Asia is growing both larger and older. Demographically the most important continent in the world, Asia's population, currently estimated (by the Population Division of the United Nations) to be 4.2 billion, is expected to increase to about 5.9 billion by 2050. At that time, the number of Asians aged 65 and older will have grown fourfold, from about 250,000,000 today to about 1 billion by 2050. Rapid declines in fertility, together with rising life expectancy, are altering the age structure of the population so that in 2050, for the first time in history, there will be roughly as many people in Asia over the age of 65 as under the age of 15.

This demographic transformation, from a youthful to a more mature society, is occurring far more rapidly in Asia than in today's more industrially advanced countries. Changes in the population age structure that played out over more than 140 years in Western Europe are occurring in countries such as China in less than 25 years. And while some Asian countries are experiencing rapid economic development, reflecting their integration in the world's economy, other countries are developing considerably more slowly.

Although population aging can be considered a triumph of social and economic development, public health, and modern medicine, it also creates major challenges for Asian governments that strive to provide social and economic security for their older populations. The projected growth in the proportion of the population aged 65 and older also has significant implications for families and kinship networks in Asia, given that the responsibility for economic support for older persons still rests almost entirely with their immediate and extended family members. All too often, older people represent a population that is vulnerable and invisible, missed by interventions to eliminate poverty or improve health and well-being.

The Committee on Population's interest in aging issues goes back at least to the early 1990s, when it published the report *Demography of Aging*.[1] Since then, the committee has taken up many issues relating to international demography and the challenges associated with population aging that have led to several reports, including *Preparing for an Aging World: The Case for Cross-National Research*,[2] *Aging in Sub-Sahara Africa: Recommendations for Furthering Research*,[3] *International Differences in Mortality at Older Ages*,[4] and *Explaining Divergent Levels of Longevity in High-Income Countries*.[5]

It is against this backdrop that the Division of Behavioral and Social Research at the U.S. National Institute on Aging (NIA) asked the National Research Council (NRC), through the Committee on Population, to undertake a project on advancing behavioral and social research on aging in Asia. The Panel on Policy Research and Data Needs to Meet the Challenge of Aging in Asia was appointed to carry out this project.

The first of the project's two activities was a collaborative effort with the Chinese Academy of Social Sciences, the Indian National Science Academy, the Indonesian Academy of Sciences, and the Science Council of Japan to develop a report on strengthening the scientific basis for developing policies to meet the challenges of population aging in Asia. That effort—the first ever collaboration between all five organizations—resulted in *Preparing for the Challenges of Population Aging in Asia: Strengthening the Scientific Basis of Policy Development,* published in 2011.[6]

The second part of the project included two conferences and this publication. Following a planning meeting that was hosted by the Indian National Science Academy in New Delhi on May 3-4, 2010, the first conference was in Beijing, hosted by the Chinese Academy of Social Sciences, on December 9-10, 2010; the second was in New Delhi, hosted by the Indian National Science Academy, on March 14-15, 2011. These conferences provided an opportunity for Asian and other researchers to discuss important data collection initiatives (at different stages of evolution and development) taking place throughout the region, exchange knowledge, share common experiences, and engage with policy makers.

---

[1] Available: http://www.nap.edu/catalog.php?record_id=4553 [February 2012].
[2] Available: http://www.nap.edu/catalog.php?record_id=10120 [February 2012].
[3] Available: http://www.nap.edu/catalog.php?record_id=11708 [February 2012].
[4] Available: http://www.nap.edu/catalog.php?record_id=12945 [February 2012].
[5] Available: http://www.nap.edu/catalog.php?record_id=13089 [February 2012].
[6] Available: http://www.nap.edu/catalog.php?record_id=12977 [February 2012].

Subsequently, selected papers from the conferences were reviewed and revised for inclusion in this volume.

This project would not have been possible without a great deal of effort, good will, and cooperation on the part of a large number of people. Particular thanks go to Dr. Richard Suzman of NIA for providing intellectual support and encouragement for the project. We are also especially grateful to members of the organizing committees appointed by our sister academies in Asia for their assistance in planning the two conferences: see Box P-1.

This project also would not have been possible without financial support from many organizations. First and foremost, we gratefully acknowledge the Division of Behavioral and Social Research at NIA for providing the principal source of financial support for the project. Thanks also go to the Carnegie Foundation, for providing funding for the 2010 planning meeting in New Delhi; to the Chinese Academy of Social Sciences, for

---

BOX P-1

CHINESE ACADEMY OF SOCIAL SCIENCES

Zhenzhen Zheng *(Chair)*, Institute of Population and Labor Economics
Fang Cai, Institute of Population and Labor Economics
Yang Du, Institute of Population and Labor Economics
Guangzhou Wang, Institute of Population and Labor Economics

INDIAN NATIONAL SCIENCE ACADEMY

P.N. Tandon *(Chair)*, National Brain Research Centre, Haryana
Moneer Alam, Population Research Centre, Institute of Economic Growth, New Delhi
P. Arokiasamy, Department of Development Studies, International Institute for Population Sciences, Mumbai
A.B. Dey, All India Institute of Medical Sciences, New Delhi

INDONESIAN ACADEMY OF SCIENCES

Mayling Oey-Gardiner *(Chair)*, Faculty of Economics, University of Indonesia
R. Sjamsuhidajat, School of Medicine, University of Indonesia

SCIENCE COUNCIL OF JAPAN

Hiroko Akiyama, Institute of Gerontology, University of Tokyo

hosting and cofunding the Beijing conference; to the Indian National Science Academy, for hosting and cofunding the New Delhi conference; and to the United Nations Population Fund, for supporting the participation of a number of researchers from around India to attend the New Delhi conference.

Special thanks are also due to James P. Smith, chair of the panel that helped organize the Beijing and New Delhi conferences and that oversaw this volume, and to Malay Majmundar, who provided key staff support for the panel's work. Thanks are also due to other NRC staff—to Danielle Johnson for her help in preparing the report for production, Jacqui Sovde for providing administrative support, and to Yvonne Wise for overseeing the production process. Thanks, too, to Paula Whitacre for her skillful editing. This project was carried out under the general direction of Barney Cohen, director of the Committee on Population.

The papers in this volume have been reviewed in draft form by individuals chosen for their diverse perspectives and technical expertise, in accordance with procedures approved by the Report Review Committee of the NRC. The purpose of this independent review is to provide candid and critical comments that will assist the institution in making its published volume as sound as possible and to ensure that the volume meets institutional standards for objectivity, evidence, and responsiveness to the study charge.

We thank the following individuals for their review of these papers: Yukiko Abe, Graduate School of Economics and Business Administration, Hokkaido University; Emily Agree, Department of Population, Family, and Reproductive Health, Johns Hopkins University; Kathleen Beegle, Development Research Group, World Bank; Charles C. Brown, Department of Economics, University of Michigan; Lisa Cameron, Department of Econometrics, Monash University; Angelique Chan, Department of Sociology, National University of Singapore; Amitabh Chandra, John F. Kennedy School of Government, Harvard University; Courtney Coile, Department of Economics, Wellesley College; Donald Cox, Department of Economics, Boston College; Eileen Crimmins, Davis School of Gerontology, University of Southern California; Sonalde Desai, Department of Sociology, University of Maryland; William H. Dow, School of Public Health, University of California, Berkeley; Andrew Foster, Department of Economics, Brown University; Peter Gardiner, consultant; John Giles, Development Research Group, World Bank; Dana Glei, Center for Population and Health, Georgetown University; Noreen Goldman, Woodrow Wilson School, Princeton University; Tara Gruenewald, Department of Medicine, University of California, Los Angeles; Mark Hayward, Department of Sociology, University of Texas at Austin; Charles Hirschman, Department of Sociology, University of Washington; Charles Yuji Horioka, Institute of Social and Economic

Research, Osaka University; Arun Karlamangla, School of Medicine, University of California, Los Angeles; Cynthia Kinnan, Department of Economics, Northwestern University; Ronald Lee, Center on the Economics and Demography of Aging, University of California, Berkeley; Xiaoyan Lei, China Center for Economic Research, Peking University; Ajay Mahal, Faculty of Medicine, Nursing, and Health Sciences, Monash University; Manoj Mohanan, Global Health Institute, Duke University; Xin Meng, College of Business and Economics, Australian National University; Olivia Mitchell, Wharton School, University of Pennsylvania; Mayling Oey-Gardiner, Faculty of Economics, University of Indonesia, Jakarta; Mary Beth Ofstedal, Institute for Social Research, University of Michigan; Albert Park, School of Humanities and Social Science, Hong Kong University of Science and Technology; Krislert Samphantharak, Department of Economics, University of California, San Diego; Sam Schulhofer-Wohl, Federal Reserve Bank of Minnesota; Grant Scobie, New Zealand Treasury; Alessandro Tarozzi, Department of Economics, Duke University; Barbara Torrey, consultant: Emily E. Wiemers, Department of Economics, University of Massachusetts Boston; Richard Wight, School of Public Health, University of California, Los Angeles; Jean Yeung, Department of Sociology, National University of Singapore; Julie Zissimopoulous, Department of Clinical and Pharmaceutical Economics and Policy, University of Southern California; and Xuejin Zuo, Shanghai Academy of Social Sciences.

Although the reviewers listed above have provided many constructive comments and suggestions, they were not asked to endorse the content of any of the papers, nor did they see the final version of any paper before this publication. The review of this volume was overseen by Duncan Thomas, Department of Economics, Duke University. Appointed by the NRC, he was responsible for making certain that an independent examination of the papers was carried out in accordance with institutional procedures and that all review comments were carefully considered. Responsibility for the final content of this report rests entirely with the authors.

Linda J. Waite, *Chair*
Committee on Population

Foreword

Science academies are in a unique position to draw on the expertise of scholars from a variety of disciplines and to help lay a solid evidentiary foundation for policy. Science academies can synthesize relevant research results in nontechnical language and can use rigorous, apolitical procedures to produce objective and unbiased analysis. Consequently, science academies can generate authoritative, credible, evidence-based findings and recommendations for policy makers.

Most countries around the world are experiencing a rapid increase in the proportion of their populations who are over the age of 65, because people are living longer and because many couples are choosing to have smaller families than their parents had. The world's population aging reflects great social, economic, and medical progress over the last 100 years, but it raises major challenges for governments in almost all areas, most especially related to health, pension, and employment policies.

Perhaps nowhere in the world is this demographic transition as stark as in parts of Asia, where rapid population aging is occurring at the same time as a dramatic economic transformation. In the face of these rapid social, economic, and demographic changes, there is a clear need to enhance our understanding of how they will affect the well-being of older people and, particularly, how they will influence long-standing societal and familial arrangements that have been a vital part of the economic support of older people in the region.

Although the scientific basis for formulating evidence-based policy to address population aging is relatively underdeveloped in many Asian countries, there is still time for them to mobilize resources and make investments in research and data collection that can have long-term benefits. The countries in Asia can learn from the experiences of countries in other parts of the world, and cross-national collaboration and coordination can further multiply the returns on investment in scientific infrastructure made by individual countries.

To contribute to that understanding, the national science academies of China, Japan, India, Indonesia, and the United States sponsored two conferences on policy research and data needs to meet the challenges of population aging in Asia. The first, hosted by the Chinese Academy of Social Sciences, was held in Beijing on December 9-10, 2010; the second, hosted by the Indian National Science Academy, took place in New Delhi on March 14-15, 2011. A third conference, organized independently by the Indonesian Academy of Sciences, took place in Bali on October 11-12, 2011. The current volume contains selected papers from the first two of these conferences. Papers from the third conference will be published separately.

We hope that this volume of papers and the intellectual ferment they represent can contribute to the long-term well-being of older people in Asia.

Chen Jiagui
Former Vice President
Chinese Academy of Social Sciences

Krishan Lal
President
Indian National Science Academy

Sangkot Marzuki
President
Indonesian Academy of Sciences

Ichiro Kanazawa
President
Science Council of Japan

Ralph J. Cicerone
President
U.S. National Academy of Sciences

Contents

1

Introduction and Overview

James P. Smith and *Malay Majmundar*

The 17 chapters in this volume have their origins in two "sister" conferences on the challenges and opportunities of population aging in Asia, one of which was hosted by the Chinese Academy of Social Sciences in Beijing and the other by the Indian National Science Academy in New Delhi.[1] The chapters, which include contributions from China, India, Indonesia, Japan, and Thailand, cover the major subject areas relevant to population aging and can be grouped into four categories: (1) new and emerging data initiatives, (2) economic growth, labor markets, and consumption, (3) family roles and responsibilities, and (4) health and well-being (see Table 1-1).[2] While we separate the chapters into these categories for summary purposes, it is important to note that a central point of new and emerging international data initiatives is that research and analysis should not be conducted solely within individual topic domains.

The need for integration is addressed by James P. Smith in "Preparing for Population Aging in Asia: Strengthening the Infrastructure for Science and Policy," which describes the historical demographic and economic forces at work that made the development of data infrastructure projects to prepare for population aging so compelling in many countries. These surveys were all built on the recognition that the main domains of life—health, income, work, family, and cognition—had to be integrated into the

---

[1]See "Preface" for further details.

[2]The chapters are meant to be stand-alone and may, for the convenience of the reader, repeat some background information (e.g., where and how surveys were conducted).

TABLE 1-1 Papers Organized by Subject Area

Author(s)	Title
NEW AND EMERGING DATA INITIATIVES	
James P. Smith	Preparing for Population Aging in Asia: Strengthening the Infrastructure for Science and Policy
P. Arokiasamy, David Bloom, Jinkook Lee, Kevin Feeney, and Marija Ozolins	Longitudinal Aging Study in India: Vision, Design, Implementation, and Preliminary Findings
ECONOMIC GROWTH, LABOR MARKETS, AND CONSUMPTION	
Ronald Lee and Andrew Mason	Population Aging, Intergenerational Transfers, and Economic Growth: Asia in a Global Context
David Wise	Facilitating Longer Working Lives: The Need, the Rationale, the How
John Giles, Dewen Wang, and Wei Cai	The Labor Supply and Retirement Behavior of China's Older Workers and Elderly in Comparative Perspective
Albert Park, Yan Shen, John Strauss, and Yaohui Zhao	Relying on Whom? Poverty and Consumption Financing of China's Elderly
Hidehiko Ichimura and Satoshi Shimizutani	Retirement Process in Japan: New Evidence from the Japanese Study on Aging and Retirement (JSTAR)
FAMILY ROLES AND RESPONSIBILITIES	
Xiaoyan Lei, John Giles, Yuqing Hu, Albert Park, John Strauss, and Yaohui Zhao	Patterns and Correlates of Intergenerational Nontime Transfers: Evidence from CHARLS
Firman Witoelar	Household Dynamics and Living Arrangements of the Elderly in Indonesia: Evidence from a Longitudinal Survey
Lisa F. Berkman, T.V. Sekher, Benjamin Capistrant, and Yuhui Zheng	Social Networks, Family, and Care Giving Among Older Adults in India
Yuqing Hu, Xiaoyan Lei, James P. Smith, and Yaohui Zhao	Effects of Social Activities on Cognitive Functions: Evidence from CHARLS

TABLE 1-1 Continued

Author(s)	Title
HEALTH AND WELL-BEING	
Firman Witoelar, John Strauss, and Bondan Sikoki	Socioeconomic Success and Health in Later Life: Evidence from the Indonesia Family Life Survey
John Strauss, Hao Hong, Xiaoyan Lei, Lin Li, Albert Park, Li Yang, and Yaohui Zhao	Healthcare and Insurance Among the Elderly in China: Evidence from the CHARLS Pilot
Subhojit Dey, Devaki Nambiar, J.K. Lakshmi, Kabir Sheikh, and K. Srinath Reddy	Health of the Elderly in India: Challenges of Access and Affordability
Jinkook Lee, P. Arokiasamy, Amitabh Chandra, Peifeng Hu, Jenny Liu, and Kevin Feeney	Markers and Drivers: Cardiovascular Health of Middle-Aged and Older Indians
Paul Kowal, Sharon Williams, Yong Jiang, Wu Fan, P. Arokiasamy, and Somnath Chatterji	Aging, Health, and Chronic Conditions in China and India: Results from the Multinational Study on Global AGEing and Adult Health (SAGE)
Dararatt Anantanasuwong and Udomsak Seenprachawong	Life Satisfaction of the Older Thai: Findings from the Pilot HART

same survey platform in order to understand and prepare for successful population aging. Smith's essay also describes the history of international sister studies of the U.S. Health and Retirement Study (HRS), with special attention paid to the status and unique attributes of the six Asian countries that have adapted the HRS model—South Korea, Japan, China, India, Thailand, and Indonesia.

One key new Asian aging survey is the Longitudinal Aging Study in India (LASI), which had finished its fieldwork for its pilot study shortly before we held our second meeting in New Delhi. In their paper "Longitudinal Aging Study in India: Vision, Design, Implementation, and Preliminary Findings," P. Arokiasamy, David Bloom, Jinkook Lee, Kevin Feeney, and Marija Ozolins summarize the main protocols of the field work and the development of the questionnaire content. As with the other Asian HRS surveys, the field results were uniformly encouraging, with very high response rates, a good understanding of the questions by respondents, and a set of results that highlighted the diversity of health and economic outcomes for the Indian elderly living in a very heterogeneous country.

Five of the chapters in this volume deal with issues related to economic resources and work in Asia. In their conceptual background paper "Population Aging, Intergenerational Transfers, and Economic Growth: Asia in a Global Context," Ronald Lee and Andrew Mason develop a set of conceptually consistent National Transfer Accounts for many countries with aging populations, including those in Asia. These National Accounts are put through past and future country-, year-, and age-specific fertility and mortality distributions in order to evaluate the implications, magnitude, and directions of private and public transfers. Their simulations not only serve as a useful guide on what the advantages and disadvantages of population aging really are, but also highlight the timing of the main transitions that warrant a policy response.

David Wise's paper "Facilitating Longer Working Lives: The Need, the Rationale, the How" also provides an important conceptual framework for how countries need to adjust to the important bounty of longer lives in terms of the length of their working lives. In the past 50 years, most of the countries of Europe and Asia gained an extra 5 to 10 years of life at age 65. In spite of those extra years, the labor force trends over the same period showed declining participation rates largely induced by high implicit taxes on work. In his essay, Wise makes a persuasive case that some of the bounty of longer lives must be allocated to prolonging the labor force participation of older workers.

The other three chapters in this section on work and income are case studies of work and retirement behaviors in China and Japan using the new HRS surveys in those countries. In their paper using data from the China Health and Retirement Longitudinal Study (CHARLS), "The Labor Supply and Retirement Behavior of China's Older Workers and Elderly in Comparative Perspective," John Giles, Dewen Wang, and Wei Cai emphasize the distinction between workers in the formal labor market where pensions are often quite generous and lead to relatively early retirement, and the informal (often rural) labor market where individuals work to very old age and rely primarily on their families for income and health support. In another paper in the Chinese context using the CHARLS data, "Relying on Whom? Poverty and Consumption Financing of China's Elderly," Albert Park, Yan Shen, John Strauss, and Yaohui Zhao examine how the Chinese elderly finance their consumption. One innovation of CHARLS is that it follows the lead of the Indonesia Family Life Survey (IFLS) and includes a detailed consumption module. In these settings, consumption by the elderly is well above their private income, and the authors show that the difference is largely due to transfers from family and government.

In "Retirement Process in Japan: New Evidence from the Japanese Study on Aging and Retirement (JSTAR)," Hidehiko Ichimura and Satoshi

Shimizutani, two of the principal investigators of the Japanese HRS, use the panel aspects of the JSTAR survey to model work transitions. Until JSTAR, publicly available panel data on labor market transitions simply have not been available in Japan to either Japanese or foreign scholars. The authors report a sharp decline in the probability of remaining employed at age 60 for men, reflecting eligibility due to existing pension rules and a high degree of correspondence in spousal retirement decisions.

Four chapters in this volume deal with family roles and responsibilities—set in China, Indonesia, and India. "Patterns and Correlates of Inter-generational Nontime Transfers: Evidence from CHARLS," by Xiaoyan Lei, John Giles, Yuqing Hu, Albert Park, John Strauss, and Yaohui Zhao, studies intergenerational transfers between adult children and their elderly parents. The authors report that the direction of transfers is decidedly upward in age—from children to their parents—and that these transfers form an important part of the economic resources of the parents. While all children tend to contribute to this support, married and better-off children are more likely to give financial support to their parents. The red flag for the future, of course, is the dwindling numbers of children of the future elderly, implying a higher per child cost or fewer total resources going to parents.

In his paper "Household Dynamics and Living Arrangements of the Elderly in Indonesia: Evidence from a Longitudinal Survey," based on the longitudinal waves of the IFLS from 1993 to 2007, Firman Witoelar documents patterns of living arrangements of the elderly in Indonesia from the early 1990s to the late 2000s. In Indonesia, the percentage of those 55 and older living alone or as a couple in a household did not change much between 1993 and 2007. While these patterns in Indonesia have been stable, future demographic pressures will likely affect living arrangement as populations age further. This observation is important since, given lags in fertility, most of the challenging demographic changes centered around the family will occur in the next few decades.

"Social Networks, Family, and Care Giving Among Older Adults in India," by Lisa F. Berkman, T.V. Sekher, Benjamin Capistrant, and Yuhui Zheng, describes the basic social networks and relationships of older Indian men and women across four states from the LASI pilot study. The authors report that the vast majority of both men and women are well connected in terms of their intimate family ties as well as more extended, weaker social networks. While only about 5% of participants lived alone and about 24% of women were widowed, it will be critical to monitor the ways in which informal social networks from both family and friends continue to support Indians well into old age as India continues to experience demographic and health transitions.

One of the primary concerns of older populations everywhere is how to delay, and then deal with, the consequences of cognitive decline at older ages. In "Effects of Social Activities on Cognitive Functions: Evidence from CHARLS," Yuqing Hu, Xiaoyan Lei, James P. Smith, and Yaohui Zhao investigate the relationship between cognitive abilities and social activities for people aged 45 and older. Social activities are defined as participating in certain common activities in China such as playing chess, card games, or Mahjong; interacting with friends; and other social activities. There appear to be strong associations of memory with engagement in social activities. While the authors do not present causal estimates, they also report that having an activity center in the community is significantly related to higher episodic memory.

The final life domains covered by the chapters in this volume are health and overall well-being. Long life and better health during old age are relatively new phenomena in Asian countries and represent great improvements in human welfare. However, these successes come with a challenge—maintaining good health of, and providing medical care for, a population that was previously small and whose health needs were largely ignored. Reflecting the importance of health, six chapters in this volume deal with the health of the elderly in Asian countries.

In "Socioeconomic Success and Health in Later Life: Evidence from the Indonesia Family Life Survey," Firman Witoelar, John Strauss, and Bondan Sikoki document long-term trends in the health of the Indonesian elderly using the IFLS. Many of the changes they find represent improvements in health, such as lower under-nutrition and communicable disease. Yet there are some disturbing signs as well—the increase in overweight and waist circumference, especially among women, and continuing high levels of hypertension. In addition, low hemoglobin, low HDL cholesterol, and high rates of undiagnosed hypertension seem to be inadequately addressed by the health system, and smoking among male Indonesians has continued unabated. These results raise serious questions regarding the ability of the health system in Indonesia to cope with the rapid aging of the population and the transition from infectious to chronic diseases.

In developing Asian countries, the availability of health insurance and access to healthcare for older populations has been very problematic. This situation, however, is in a rapid state of flux, with new programs being introduced to extend health insurance into rural areas. In "Healthcare and Insurance Among the Elderly in China: Evidence from the CHARLS Pilot," John Strauss, Hao Hong, Xiaoyan Lei, Lin Li, Albert Park, Li Yang, and Yaohui Zhao take advantage of the CHARLS pilot data to model the probability of having health insurance and receiving care. Those with a lower probability of having health insurance (even with these new programs) are the poor, older women, and migrants. Reimbursement rates vary significantly by type of care and place of residence, reflecting the important role of communities in China in financing and organizing healthcare.

The Indian case is addressed in "Health of the Elderly in India: Challenges of Access and Affordability," by Subhojit Dey, Devaki Nambiar, J.K. Lakshmi, Kabir Sheikh, and K. Srinath Reddy. As in other Asian countries, the Indian elderly face a unique set of health-related challenges owing to the dual burden of chronic and degenerative noncommunicable diseases and communicable diseases. Key challenges to access to health for this population include social barriers shaped by gender and other dimensions of social inequality (e.g., religion, caste, socioeconomic status, and stigma); physical barriers such as reduced mobility; declining social engagement; and the limited reach of the health system. Even as India aspires to move forward on a path towards universal health coverage, this chapter points out that stark data gaps persist for policy measures to improve access.

Two common attributes about health status in developing Asian countries are high rates of undiagnosed disease and great regional heterogeneity in health outcomes. In their paper "Markers and Drivers: Cardiovascular Health of Middle-Aged and Older Indians," Jinkook Lee, P. Arokiasamy, Amitabh Chandra, Peifeng Hu, Jenny Liu, and Kevin Feeney report similar findings for India based on LASI pilot data. These findings are made even more compelling by the fact that they combine self-reports of health status with biomarkers. Given the high rates of undiagnosed disease in these developing Asian countries, these findings confirm that biomarkers are absolutely necessary in surveys of the elderly in Asia.

In "Aging, Health and Chronic Conditions in China and India: Results from the Multinational Study on Global AGEing and Adult Health (SAGE)," Paul Kowal, Sharon Williams, Yong Jiang, Wu Fan, P. Arokiasamy, and Somnath Chatterji compare health outcomes of the elderly in India and China. The authors report that 80% of cardiovascular disease deaths occur in lower- and middle-income countries, including China and India. There are important similarities between the two countries, including considerable underreporting of chronic diseases associated with older ages and high levels of disease co-morbidity. The detection of underdiagnosis was possible by comparing self-reports and symptom-reporting, both of which are part of the SAGE survey protocols. China's levels of treatment for chronic health conditions were generally higher than India's, with the highest levels of treatment for angina and diabetes. Overall, though, and in particular for depression, healthcare coverage for patients with noncommunicable diseases is strikingly low in both countries.

In the final chapter in this volume, "Life Satisfaction of the Older Thai: Findings from the Pilot HART," Dararatt Anantanasuwong and Udomsak Seenprachawong investigate the determinants of life satisfaction using the Thai version of the HRS, the Panel Survey and Study on Health, Aging, and Retirement in Thailand (HART). They report large urban and rural differences in life satisfaction in Thailand, with rural Thais being significantly less satisfied with their lives. Physical health has the strongest association with life satisfaction compared to other domains, and having friends and being engaged in social activities are also strongly positively associated with life satisfaction.

STRENGTHENING INSTITUTIONAL CAPACITY FOR AGING RESEARCH IN ASIA

The broad range of topics covered by the chapters in this volume exemplify the way in which investments in high-quality data and research can produce information and insights that may prove valuable to policymakers as they confront the challenges of aging populations. One important prerequisite to the production of useful scientific knowledge is to have in place well-designed institutions that facilitate innovation and collaboration.[3]

In the United States, government funding of social science research is relatively decentralized and generally uncoordinated (Calhoun, 2010). Within this pluralistic environment, the National Institute on Aging (NIA), which is one of 27 institutes and centers within the National Institutes of Health (NIH), plays a primary and pivotal role in supporting aging research. NIA conducts on-site "intramural" research and funds off-site "extramural" research on genetic, biological, clinical, behavioral, social, and economic topics related to aging processes, diseases, and conditions.[4] NIA is also primarily responsible for funding the Health and Retirement Study (HRS), a nationally representative longitudinal survey of Americans over the age of 50 that collects information every two years about income, work, assets, pension plans, health insurance, disability, physical health and functioning, cognitive functioning, and healthcare expenditures.

Even though NIA is the main sponsor of the HRS, the study itself is designed, administered, and conducted by researchers in the academic community rather than by government statisticians (Juster and Suzman, 1995; National Institute on Aging, 2007). Such cooperative arrangements have proven to be fundamental to the success of studies that are longitudinal and model-based (as distinguished from cross-sectional surveys that may be more descriptive in nature). It is also important that such studies

---

[3]The discussion that follows is based in part on Majmundar (2011).

[4]Grants to individual researchers, usually for three to five years, are the extramural grant type most commonly used by NIH. Other extramural grant types include grants to research centers and multi-project research projects, as well as exploratory grants and small grants.

be sponsored by agencies—such as NIA—that are sufficiently involved in aging research across different scientific disciplines so as to be able to bring together the different kinds of expertise necessary for the design and management of those studies (Juster and Suzman, 1995).

HRS-type studies in Asia are, to an extent, beginning to develop along just such institutional lines. CHARLS and LASI, for example, are designed and managed by networks of academics (CHARLS by the China Center for Economic Research at Peking University; and LASI by the International Institute for Population Studies, Mumbai, and the School of Public Health at Harvard University). What remains to be seen in the longer term, however, is whether and how these surveys will find appropriate institutional support from their own national governments, comparable to that provided by NIA to the HRS. If, for example, the governments of China and India decided to lend their full support to CHARLS and LASI, the question as to which government agencies would actually fund and oversee those surveys is something that would require careful consideration.

These institutional issues are relevant not only to the future of HRS-type surveys in Asia, but also more generally to the overall quality of aging research in those countries. After all, a government agency that does not have the resources and expertise to support a sophisticated longitudinal survey is, by definition, an agency that will find it difficult to play a lead role in promoting high-quality aging research. This raises a number of additional questions about research infrastructures in Asian countries, the lessons that may be learned from the U.S. experience, and the variety of approaches (and the potential tradeoffs among them) that should be taken into account when thinking about institutional design. At least four issues are worth considering in more detail: (1) finding the optimal degree of centralization and coordination, (2) managing peer review, (3) facilitating interdisciplinary research, and (4) diversifying funding streams.

Finding the Optimal Degree of Centralization and Coordination

One fundamental issue is the extent of centralization within public institutions and the degree of coordination between them. The 27 institutes that make up NIH, for example, are organized around (among other things) specific diseases, life stages, and disciplines. These institutes generally enjoy considerable amounts of budgetary and operational autonomy, so much so that they have been characterized as "largely independent fiefdoms" (Cohen, 1993:1,675; Varmus, 2001). NIH can benefit politically and financially when the enthusiasm of supporters and advocacy groups is reflected in the creation of new institutes to which those constituency groups feel especially loyal. The drawback of the "proliferation of institutes," however, is that they may result in "less flexibility, less managerial capacity, less coordination, and more administrative burden" for NIH as a whole (Varmus, 2001:1,905).

These political and bureaucratic dynamics can also have significant implications for relationships between different government agencies. In the United States, early supporters of the National Science Foundation (NSF) envisioned a strong central role for NSF as the major supporter of basic research. By the time NSF came into existence in 1950, however, NIH had already gained sizeable appropriations from Congress and had begun to establish enduring political constituencies for itself. NSF therefore had to coexist with the "extensive though disjointed" government-sponsored research system that was already in place (Mazuzan, 1994:5). The question of how these forces and factors will unfold across the different countries of Asia is an important one. (See Box 1-1 for an overview of some of the major scientific institutions in China, India, Indonesia, and Japan.)

Managing Peer Review

Asian countries that are interested in expanding their investments in aging research may want to give some consideration to peer review processes. NIH has an elaborate peer review mechanism in place for funding extramural research. Peer review allows the quality of funding proposals to be evaluated rigorously and independently, and it makes NIH accountable for how funds are used (National Research Council, 2003). Peer review may also provide funding agencies with a measure of protection against politically motivated attacks on controversial research (Kaiser, 2003). One of the limitations of peer review when it becomes too conservative and establishment-oriented in its evaluation of science is that it may discriminate against novel, high-risk proposals and create a bias against young investigators and researchers (National Research Council, 2003). Striking an appropriate balance with peer review can sometimes be a challenge.

In China, the use of peer review for funding social science research has become increasingly common since the early 1980s. Since 2000, in response to perceived deficiencies in the peer review process, several measures have been taken, such as including more experts in the pool of referees and making their selection more standardized; making the evaluation process more anonymous and putting into place regulations to supervise panel meetings and make the project approval and evaluation systems more accountable; and making it easier for projects that are interdisciplinary, multidisciplinary, experimental, or controversial to be submitted to special panels of experts who are drawn from different fields of research (Lili, 2010). In Japan, similarly, there has been an

---

BOX 1-1
Scientific Institutions in China, India, Indonesia, and Japan

The management and organization of research funding can vary greatly across different Asian countries. In China, the major government agencies in the field of science and technology are the Ministry of Science and Technology, which formulates development plans and implements policy guidelines; the Ministry of Education, which manages education funds for higher and postgraduate education; the National Natural Science Foundation, which provides funding for basic research and some applied research; and the National Social Science Foundation, which allocates resources for social science researchers at universities and to research institutes (Ping, 2010).

In India, major promoters of social science research include the University Grants Commission, which is the main body administering universities and is responsible for providing funds and coordinating, determining, and maintaining standards; and the Indian Council of Social Science Research, which sponsors autonomous research institutes in different parts of the country (Krishna and Krishna, 2010). Social science research is also funded by agencies such as the Ministry of Health and Family Welfare, Ministry of Social Justice and Empowerment, Ministry of Women and Child Development, Ministry of Statistics and Programme Implementation, and the Reserve Bank of India.

In Indonesia, the Ministry of Research and Technology, which has seven research and development agencies under its direct authority, is primarily responsible for driving science and technology policy (Turpin et al., 2010). One of these institutes, the National Institute for Scientific Research (LIPI), contains a Division of Social Sciences and Humanities that is responsible for conducting and promoting social science research. The division has five research centers, including a Center for Economic Research and a Population Research Center. As in India, a number of other ministries (such as the Ministry of National Education) also support social science research.

In Japan, the Ministry of Education, Culture, Sports, Science, and Technology (MEXT) administers Grants-in-Aid for Academic Research, which is the largest competitive fund allocated on the basis of merit and may be regarded as the closest equivalent in Japan to the U.S. National Science Foundation. The Ministry of Health, Labor, and Welfare administers the Health and Labor Sciences Research Grants, which focus on health and medical research as well as social science research related to health policy; this fund may be regarded as the closest equivalent in Japan to the U.S. National Institutes of Health.

Japan also has a number of government-funded institutes on the social sciences. The Research Institute of Economy, Trade, and Industry is funded by the Ministry of Economy, Trade, and Industry and is the largest contributor to the Japanese Study on Aging and Retirement. Other examples include the National Institute of Population and Social Security Research, which was established by the Ministry of Health, Labor, and Welfare; and the National Institute of Science and Technology Policy, which falls under the jurisdiction of MEXT. As in India and Indonesia, many other ministries in Japan also have some funds with which to pursue policy-related research.

increased emphasis on competitive funds allocated on the basis of merit (Sato, 2010).

Facilitating Interdisciplinary Research

The aging process is multifaceted and multidimensional, and it touches upon a broad range of biological and social issues. Aging research ought to span multiple disciplines and approach questions from a variety of perspectives. Therefore, Asian countries may want to think about the best ways of incorporating interdisciplinary principles into the design of public institutions. The research components of NIA, for example, include the Division of Aging Biology, Division of Behavioral and Social Research, Division of Neuroscience, and Division of Geriatrics and Clinical Gerontology. This organizational structure reflects the multidisciplinary and interdisciplinary mission of NIA, with the social and behavioral sciences housed in the same place as the biomedical and other sciences.

It is worth noting that the social and behavioral sciences have often had to struggle for equitable footing with the "hard" sciences. In the late 1950s, for example, the incorporation of the social sciences into NSF's formal mandate was met with resistance (Mazuzan, 1994). In 2005, research expenditures on "social science and humanities" constituted 5.5% of "gross expenditure on R&D" in the United States, 4.6% in Japan, and 1.4% in China (Kahn, 2010).[5]

Diversifying Funding Streams

Although governmental institutions play a key role in supporting research and setting broad scientific priorities, their resources are also limited—perhaps now more than ever. In 2002, for example, around 30% of researchers submitting grant applications to NIA were successful (for any single deadline) in obtaining funding; by 2010, that figure had fallen to 8% (Wadman, 2010). Consequently, Asian countries may want to consider the role that could be played by private foundations in filling this gap. In India, for example, the Tata Trust, Birla Trust, and Ford Foundation have been longtime supporters of social science research, and a number of new foundations supporting social science research have been established by corporate firms (Krishna and Krishna, 2010). In Japan, similarly, academic research is supported by private organizations such as the Toyota Foundation and Mitsubishi Foundation.

---

[5]In 2005, gross expenditure on all research and development constituted 2.6% of gross domestic product in the United States, 3.3% in Japan, and 1.3% in China (Kahn, 2010).

In the United States, the research priorities and decision processes of private foundations are diverse and often idiosyncratic, and the research support that they provide may be less consistent and predictable than the support provided by governmental institutions. For example, of the 10 wealthiest foundations in the United States,[6] only the MacArthur Foundation, with its Research Network on an Aging Society, has an organized research program that is explicitly focused on aging. As Asian countries strengthen their institutional capacity for aging research, they may want to think about ways of designing public institutions and forging public-private partnerships so that private resources are more likely to be mobilized and, subsequent to that, allocated in ways that are systematic, coordinated, and consistent with good science.

THE PATH FORWARD

Policymakers cannot address the challenges and opportunities of population aging without a strong evidentiary base. Science academies in China, India, Indonesia, Japan, and the United States have recognized the importance of data collection efforts that are nationally representative, internationally comparable, interdisciplinary, and publicly available (Chinese Academy of Social Sciences et al., 2010). The chapters in this volume are the product of new and emerging data initiatives that can facilitate informed decision-making well into the future. In order to derive maximal benefit from these efforts, national governments in Asia will need to support and invest in these data infrastructures and, more generally, ensure that appropriate institutional mechanisms are in place for encouraging high-quality research. The papers that follow provide new information on various social and economic aspects of population aging in Asia, and they are promising examples of the kinds of research and analysis that could help inform policy development in those countries.

REFERENCES

Calhoun, C. (2010). Social sciences in North America. In *World Social Science Report: Knowledge Divides*. Paris: United Nations Educational, Scientific and Cultural Organization and International Social Science Council.

---

[6]In 2009, the 10 largest U.S. foundations by asset size were the Bill and Melinda Gates Foundation, Ford Foundation, J. Paul Getty Foundation, Robert Wood Johnson Foundation, William and Flora Hewlett Foundation, W.K. Kellogg Foundation, David and Lucille Packard Foundation, John D. and Catherine T. MacArthur Foundation, John and Betty Moore Foundation, and the Lilly Endowment (Foundation Center, 2010).

Chinese Academy of Social Sciences, Indian National Science Academy, Indonesian Academy of Sciences, National Research Council of the U.S. National Academies, and Science Council of Japan. (2010). *Preparing for the Challenges of Population Aging in Asia: Strengthening the Scientific Basis of Policy Development.* Washington, DC: The National Academies Press.

Cohen, J. (1993). Conflicting agendas shape NIH. *Science 261*:1,674-1,679.

Foundation Center. (2010). *50 Largest Foundations by Assets, 2008.* Available: http://foundationcenter.org/findfunders/statistics/pdf/11_topfdn_type/2008/top50_aa_all_08.pdf.

Juster, F.T., and R. Suzman. (1995). An overview of the Health and Retirement Study. *The Journal of Human Resources 30*:S7-S56.

Kahn, M. (2010). Measure for measure: Quantifying the social sciences. In *World Social Science Report: Knowledge Divides.* Paris: United Nations Educational, Scientific and Cultural Organization and International Social Science Council.

Kaiser, J. (2003). NIH roiled by inquiries over grants hit list. *Science 302*:758.

Krishna, V.V., and U. Krishna. (2010). In *World Social Science Report: Knowledge Divides.* Paris: United Nations Educational, Scientific and Cultural Organization and International Social Science Council.

Lili, W. (2010). Funding and assessment of humanities and social science in China. In *World Social Science Report: Knowledge Divides.* Paris: United Nations Educational, Scientific and Cultural Organization and International Social Science Council.

Majmundar, M. (2011). *Roundtable Discussion on Strengthening Scientific Capacity for Aging Research—Background and Context.* Presented at the Indian National Science Academy, New Delhi, March 15. Available: http://nationalacademies.org/AgingInAsia/Presentations/Majmundar.pdf.

Mazuzan, G.T. (1994). *The National Science Foundation: A Brief History.* NSF 88-16. Available: http://www.nsf.gov/about/history/nsf50/nsf8816.jsp.

National Institute on Aging. (2007). *Growing Older in America: The Health and Retirement Study.* NIH Publication No. 07-5757. Bethesda, MD: U.S. Department of Health and Human Services.

National Research Council. (2003). *Enhancing the Vitality of the National Institutes of Health: Organizational Change to Meet New Challenges.* Committee on the Organizational Structure of the National Institutes of Health. Washington, DC: The National Academies Press.

Ping, H. (2010). The status of the social sciences in China. In *World Social Science Report: Knowledge Divides.* Paris: United Nations Educational, Scientific and Cultural Organization and International Social Science Council.

Sato, Y. (2010). Japan. In *UNESCO Science Report 2010: The Current Status of Science around the World.* Paris: United Nations Educational, Scientific and Cultural Organization.

Turpin, T., R. Woolley, P. Intarakumnerd, and W. Amaradasa. (2010). Southeast Asia and Oceania. In *UNESCO Science Report 2010: The Current Status of Science around the World.* Paris: United Nations Educational, Scientific and Cultural Organization.

Varmus, H. (2001). Proliferation of National Institutes of Health. *Science 291*:1,903-1,905.

Wadman, M. (2010). Funding crisis hits US ageing research. *Nature 468*:148.

New and Emerging Data Initiatives

2

Preparing for Population Aging in Asia: Strengthening the Infrastructure for Science and Policy[1]

James P. Smith

Throughout most of the developed and developing world, one of the most daunting issues deals with the challenges raised by population aging. Rapid increases in life expectancy, especially at older ages, alongside unprecedented declines in fertility will soon lead throughout North America, Europe, and Asia to never before seen rates of population aging. The "problem" of population aging is easy to state—to provide income and health security at older ages and to do so at affordable budgets. All rapidly aging countries face similar risks, but Asian countries have some advantages and disadvantages. The disadvantages are that compared to Europe and North America, Asian countries are now aging more rapidly at lower incomes with weak nonfamilial income and health security systems in place. The big advantage is that it is much easier to change public systems in Asia than in Europe and America where the vested interest around the status quo has proven to be a major impediment to any policy adjustment.

Until recently, the one shared disadvantage throughout America, Europe, and Asia is that a scientific data infrastructure was not available that would inform simultaneously in one common platform about the status of key life domains at older ages—work, economic resources, health status and healthcare, the role of the family, and cognition. With-

[1]A presentation based on this paper was presented in New Delhi, India, in March 2011. This research was supported by grants from the National Institute on Aging in the United States.

17

out that type of data infrastructure, we would not be able to monitor the key simultaneous transitions in these domains as people age and, even more importantly, how the various life domains mutually influence each other. The implication is that we would be unable to anticipate unforeseen consequences of policies centered on one domain in isolation on major life outcomes in the other domains. The absence of a common data infrastructure platform also implies that countries would not learn from the successes and failures of other countries in their attempts to deal with population aging.

Fortunately, this situation is rapidly changing for the better. Starting in the United States with the Health and Retirement Study (HRS), a data infrastructure platform has emerged that has spread throughout Europe and Asia centered on issues of population aging. In this chapter, I describe the origins and world-wide spread of this data infrastructure, its common elements, and its potential to inform policy and enhance the science.

This chapter is organized into three sections. The next section describes the primary demographic trends driving aging in several Asian countries over the next century. Section 2 summarizes the new aging data sets that are based on the U.S. HRS, with discussion on the European and Asian comparable surveys that have emerged to provide a scientific and policy infrastructure to study population aging around the world. Section 3 provides illustrations of the way these surveys can be used to study population aging. The final section also highlights the chapter's main conclusions.

DEMOGRAPHIC TRENDS IN ASIA

There are several fundamental demographic trends that are rapidly changing population aging throughout the world, and Asia is no exception. Figure 2-1 highlights one of the forces contributing to the aging of the Asian population by plotting changing life expectancies for four large Asian countries—China, India, Indonesia, and Japan—over a 100-year period from 1950 to 2050. In 1950, average life expectancy was around 30 years in China, India, and Indonesia, but over the subsequent 60 years until the present time, life expectancy in all three countries improved dramatically—to around age 70 in China and Indonesia and over age 60 in India. While Japan started at a higher base with more than a 60-year life expectancy in 1950, Japan, too, experienced large drops in mortality, reaching a life expectancy in the mid-80s by 2010, one of the highest life expectancies in the world. Nor is there any sign of much abatement in these trends. The best demographic projections foresee additional added years of life in all four countries in the future, with China and Indonesia both reaching life expectancies of about 80 years, double the level that existed 100 years earlier.

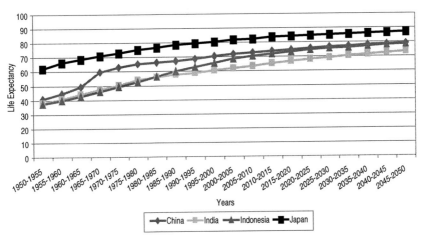

FIGURE 2-1 Average life expectancy at birth in four Asian countries, 1950–2050. SOURCE: Chinese Academy of Sciences et al. (2010).

The second and far more important driving demographic force in Asian population aging is trends in fertility, which are plotted in Figure 2-2. Using 1950 once again as the starting point, average fertility in China, India, and Indonesia was around six children per woman. The subsequent fertility declines in all three countries were so dramatic that they are now below replacement levels in all three. The speed of the decline was more rapid in China, no doubt due to the one-child policy in that country, although the endpoint suggests that this decline would have happened there anyway, even if not at the same speed. As the most developed of the four countries at the start of the comparisons, the size of change in fertility in Japan was smaller than the others, but even there, fertility has been cut in half.

While declining mortality and especially fertility contribute to population aging by making populations on average "older," it is important to keep in mind that both of these fundamental causes of population aging represent enormous progress in the human condition in these Asian countries. The extension of life and the decline in fertility are very beneficial trends driving population aging around the world and especially in Asia that lead to significant improvements in the human condition.

At the same time, population aging raises some important challenges in maintaining a good life for older people in these countries as they attempt to maintain income security and lower health risk at older ages. Our first look at the underlying demographics of these challenges is provided in Figure 2-3, which lists the changing fractions of the population in the four countries who are at least 65 years old. In 1950, this fraction

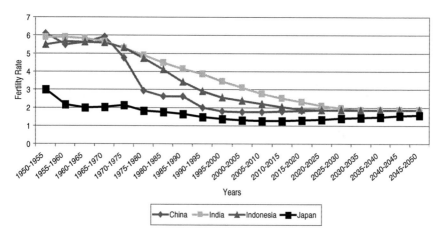

FIGURE 2-2 Changing total fertility rate per woman, 1950–2050.
SOURCE: Chinese Academy of Sciences et al. (2010).

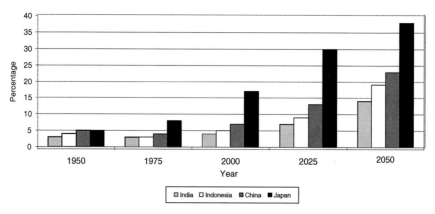

FIGURE 2-3 Percentage of population aged 65 and older, 1950–2050.
SOURCE: Chinese Academy of Sciences et al. (2010).

was 5% or lower in all four Asian countries. Using this metric, change was slow until the end of the 20th century in all countries except Japan, where the fraction rose to about 18 percent. In the first half of the 21st century, the pace of change will be dramatic with about one-third of the Japanese population over age 65 and with rates of about one in five in Indonesia and China. Population aging is slower in India over this time period, but this is mostly due to using the other three countries as the comparison group.

Figure 2-4 expresses the consequences of population age in terms of aging support ratios. For each country for the years 2000 and 2050, this figure measures the number of workers (those in the age groups 25–64) relative to the number of people aged 65 and older. Taking China as the first example, the dramatic change across a relatively short 50-year time period is evident. At the turn of this century, there were more than 12 potential Chinese workers for every person over age 64. By the year 2050, the ratio will be about two to one. Similar trends are evident in Indonesia and India. While Japan was already well into the population aging process in 2000, the subsequent change still gives one pause, as Japan reaches a position in the year 2050 where there is about one worker for every retired person.

One potential avenue of adjustment to population aging is to delay retirement and to work to older ages. However, the data on male labor force participation rates in Figure 2-5 indicate that many men are already

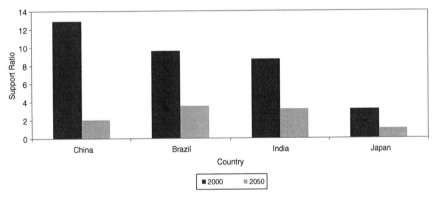

FIGURE 2-4 Support ratios (people aged 25–64/65 and older).
SOURCE: Data from United Nations (2008).

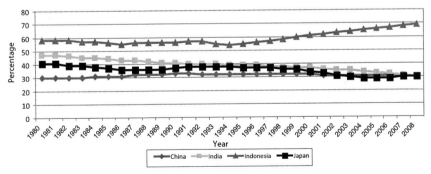

FIGURE 2-5 Percentage of labor force participation among men aged 65 and older, 1980–2008.
SOURCE: Chinese Academy of Sciences et al. (2010).

working at these ages (more than 60% in Indonesia), and with the exception of Indonesia, trends over time are either stagnant or show declining male labor force participation rates.

THE NEW DATA INFRASTRUCTURE FOR POPULATION AGING

The world will continue its rapid rate of population aging, which raises challenges for many countries. New institutions and new programs must be implemented and evaluated to determine whether the dual goals of providing income and health security at older ages can be achieved at affordable budgets. In response to that challenge, a set of harmonized data sets have evolved in the last 20 years to document in detail the changing health, economic status, and family relations of older populations. This set of surveys also is now in place to attempt to monitor the impacts of any new health and retirement programs and policies that may affect incentives of the older population on whether they continue to work, how they obtain their health care and whether it is effective, and whether they are able to achieve adequate incomes.

The Health and Retirement Study

The first of these studies was the Health and Retirement Study in the United States. The HRS was originally conceived as a panel study of those 51–61 years old in 1991 using a two-year periodicity to monitor the economic (especially retirement) and health transitions (especially into poorer health) in the subsequent years and the manner in which these economic and health domains mutually influence each other at older ages.[2] The scope of the study has expanded significantly in the subsequent 20 years, in part by adding older and younger birth cohorts so that the HRS now attempts to be continuously population representative of Americans at least 50 years old.[3]

The key innovation of the HRS, which has been adopted in HRS-type surveys in the rest of the world, is that it broke with the tradition of other surveys that focused almost entirely on the concerns of a single domain of life and were run by a single academic discipline. For example, many countries had good economic surveys dealing with work and income, other excellent surveys specializing in health outcomes and/or healthcare

---

[2]The HRS has been primarily funded by the Division of Behavioral and Social Research (BSR) at the National Institute on Aging, with significant supplemental funding from the Social Security Administration.

[3]See Juster and Suzman (1995).

utilization, and demographic surveys concentrating on the role of the family. These are all key life domains and worthy of study.

But this separation is based on an implicit and false premise that these life domains are independent of each other and that understanding behavior in one domain can be achieved without knowing very much about the others. This is not how people organize their lives anywhere around the world. Health can affect the ability to work and earn income; economic resources can help families deal more effectively with illness, especially of the old; and the family is a primary resource in many countries for ensuring the well-being of the elderly. The rigid separation of life domains of family, economics, and health was often reinforced by the equally rigid separation and ownership of domains and surveys claimed by the academic disciplines. This was no easy issue to resolve, but from the very beginning the HRS was governed and implemented as a multi-domain and multidisciplinary survey.

By now, the substantive content of HRS covers the following broad range of topics—*health* (physical/psychological self-report, conditions, disabilities; cognitive testing, health behaviors [smoking, drinking, exercise]); *health services* (utilization, expenditure, insurance, out-of-pocket spending); *labor force activity* (employment status/history, earnings, disability, retirement, type of work); *economic status* (income, wealth, consumption); and *family structure* (extended family, proximity, transfers to/from of money, time, housing). In addition to personal interviews, linkages are also provided to pension, Social Security earnings/benefit histories, and Medicare usage and expenditures. Interviews were conducted with both partners/spouses in a household about their own lives and with the more knowledgeable of the two about their joint lives. This substantive template served as the model for all the other international aging surveys to follow.

One marker of the HRS's eventual success and its adoption in other countries is its exponential growth in scientific productivity. By June 2010, there were about 1,700 papers written using the HRS—932 published in academic journals, 127 book chapters, 193 dissertations, and 445 working papers. The number of papers based on the HRS has more than doubled since the HRS's 10th birthday in 2001, with a 45% growth in HRS papers since 2005.[4] These publications were written by scholars from many disciplines and were published in the leading journals in health, economic, and demographic journals.

---

[4] I thank David Weir of the University of Michigan and the current principal investigator of the HRS for these numbers.

The International Landscape in Comparable Data Collection—
Before Asia

Another metric of its success is that the HRS has spawned 24 other international surveys that share a common scientific and policy mission with a mutual desire to harmonize some of their main survey content. HRS sister surveys currently include the Mexican Health and Aging Study (MHAS) in Mexico, English Longitudinal Survey of Ageing (ELSA) in England, the Irish Longitudinal Study of Ageing (TILDA) in Ireland, 15 countries in the Survey of Health, Ageing and Retirement in Europe (SHARE) network, and six surveys in Asia—Indonesian Family Life Survey (IFLS) in Indonesia, Korean Longitudinal Study of Ageing (KLoSA) in South Korea, Chinese Health and Retirement Longitudinal Study (CHARLS) in China, Longitudinal Aging Study in India (LASI) in India, Survey of Health, Ageing and Retirement in Thailand (HART) in Thailand, and Japanese Study on Aging and Retirement (JSTAR) in Japan. Below, I first briefly describe the Mexican and European surveys in the network, followed by those in Asia.

The first country follow-up to the HRS was the Mexican Health and Aging Study, which was fielded in 2001 with a follow-up in 2003. MHAS is a prospective panel study of health and aging in Mexico. The baseline survey includes a nationally representative sample of Mexicans aged 50 and older and their spouse/partners regardless of their age. Areas covered include health behavior and health status, childhood and family background, migration history, sources and amounts of income, and housing environment. The MHAS was suspended after its second round due to lack of funding, but new funding was obtained in 2011 and a third round of the panel and a new baseline are in the planning stages.

A decade after the HRS started, the second country to follow up on the HRS model was England with the English Longitudinal Survey of Ageing. ELSA was designed to collect longitudinal data on health, disability, economic circumstances, social participation, and well-being, from a representative sample of the English population aged 50 and older (http://www.ifs.org.uk/elsa/). The initial sample for ELSA in 2002 was drawn from three years of the Health Survey for England (HSE): 1998, 1999, and 2001. Interviews were carried out with 11,391 individuals, and new cohorts have been subsequently added to keep it representative of the English population aged 50 and older. Operating on a two-year periodicity like the HRS, ELSA has now completed five waves of data collection.[5]

In most respects, ELSA's measurement of socioeconomic status (SES)

---

[5]For more details on ELSA, see Marmot et al. (2003).

and health closely parallels that in the HRS, and ELSA also links to administrative records. The major ELSA innovation was to take biological measures from venous blood in every second wave. These biological measures included markers such as fibrinogen (which controls blood clotting and is a risk factor for cardiovascular disease [CVD]), HbA1c (a test for diabetes), C-reactive protein (CRPC—measuring the concentration of a protein in serum that indicates acute inflammation and possible arthritis), and cholesterol. Such measures can be used to validate respondents' self-reports and to monitor overall health. They also can inform about pre-clinical levels of disease of which respondents may not have been aware and to which they have not yet able to react behaviorally. The power of this innovation is probably best documented by the adoption of biomarkers in subsequent waves of the HRS. This attribute within the HRS network of allowing scientific innovation at the country level and having others within the network adopt the more successful innovations is one of the gains from the network's close partnerships.

The Survey of Health Ageing and Retirement in Europe is a multi-disciplinary and cross-national panel interview survey on health, SES, and social and family networks of individuals aged 50 and older in continental Europe. The original 2004/2005 SHARE baseline included nationally representative samples in 11 European countries (Austria, Belgium, Denmark, France, Germany, Greece, Italy, Netherlands, Spain, Sweden, and Switzerland) (http://www.share-project.org/). For these countries, a second wave of data collection took place in 2006, and a third wave collecting a retrospective wave documenting prior life experiences took place in 2008. The fourth wave of data collection was scheduled for completion in 2011. Once again, the SHARE instruments are similar to those in the HRS and ELSA. SHARE's big innovation is an insistence on very strict comparability of survey instruments within the SHARE countries.

The latest addition in the European network of aging surveys is The Irish Longitudinal Study of Ageing, which completed its baseline field work in spring 2011 (http://www.tilda.tcd.ie). Like the other surveys in the North American-European network, TILDA was meant to be population representative of the Irish population aged 50 and older, and has a two-year periodicity for its follow-up rounds to chart health, social, and economic circumstances of the Irish population.

Like other surveys in this network, TILDA includes its own version of scientific innovation. In addition to completing a computer-assisted personal interview, most TILDA respondents agreed to visit a Health Assessment Centre in one of two cities—Dublin and Cork—where appropriate medical measurement facilities are available to take detailed physical measurements especially related to disability and functioning (gait assessment and balance), cognition, macular degeneration, and cardiovascular health (heart rate variability, pulse wave velocity, phasic blood pressure) and to provide biomedical samples. It remains to be seen how many of these TILDA innovative measures will be judged to be sufficiently cost-effective to transfer to some of the other studies in the network.

The International Landscape in Comparable Data Collection—On to Asia

The successful implementation of the HRS model in Western Europe was soon followed by similar efforts in six Asian countries—China, India, Indonesia, Japan, South Korea, and Thailand. While overall comparability with the HRS model was maintained, several changes were made to reflect the reality of the Asian context. This reflects the general principle in this network that while it is important to have significant comparable content so that cross-national studies can be conducted, the content has to reflect the reality and policies of each country.

One of those changes was that in many of the Asian countries, the age cutoff for participation in the survey was moved down five years to age 45. The reason for this was two-fold—in developing countries such as China, India, Indonesia, and Thailand, the transition into poorer health starts at younger ages than in Western Europe and the United States. Second, in some of these countries, such as China, at least in the formal wage and government sectors, rules for mandatory retirement often take place at younger ages than in Western Europe and the United States. Third, due to the central importance of local communities in many Asian countries not only in providing healthcare and income security but also in organizing social life, many of the Asian countries appended community surveys to the respondent interviews. Another change discussed in more detail below is that in order to accurately measure the economic domain in countries with sectors where economic activity is largely nonmonetarized, it is necessary to take a broader view by including modules that measure income, assets, and consumption.

The Korean Longitudinal Study of Ageing is a longitudinal survey of the Korean population aged 45 and older who reside in a community. The baseline survey instrument was modeled after the HRS, using an internationally harmonized baseline survey instrument with the following core content: demographics; family and social networks; physical, mental, and functional health; health care utilization; employment and retirement; and income and assets. The baseline wave was collected in 2006, and two subsequent follow-ups have been conducted.

The China Health and Retirement Longitudinal Study (CHARLS) is conducted by the China Center for Economic Research (CCER) at Peking University. It is a survey of households with members aged 45 years and older, plus their spouses. Given the complexity of doing a survey at the national level in China, a pilot was conducted in 2008 in two provinces, Gansu and Zhejiang (Zhao et al., 2009). Zhejiang, located in the developed coastal region, is one of the most dynamic provinces in terms of its fast economic growth, private sector, small-scale industrialization, and export orientation. Gansu, located in the less developed western region, is one of the poorest, most rural provinces in China.

The pilot survey collected data from 95 communities/villages in 32 counties/districts, covering 2,685 individuals living in 1,570 households. The CHARLS pilot survey experience was very positive. The overall response rate was 85%, with 79% in urban areas and 90% in rural areas. Given the importance of community in the everyday life of older Chinese people, the community questionnaire focuses on important infrastructure available in the community, plus the availability of health facilities used by the elderly and on prices of goods and services often used by the elderly. The 2008 pilot data are now available publicly (http://charls.ccer. edu.cn). The baseline national wave of CHARLS was fielded from June 2011 to March 2012, with a second wave fielded in 2013. This national survey will include about 10,000 households and 17,500 individuals.

The Panel Survey and Study on Health, Aging, and Retirement in Thailand was developed in 2008. The first stage was a pilot baseline survey of 1,500 household samples, which was conducted during August–October 2009 by interviewing, face-to-face, one member aged 45 and older from each household. HART was conducted in two sampled areas: Bangkok and its vicinity, and Khon Kaen Province. A second pilot panel survey of the same households was conducted in 2011 with research funding from the Thailand National Higher Education Commission. The survey instrument was an adaptation of that of KLoSA with some adjustments to fit local conditions. The principal investigators have applied for a grant for a national longitudinal study on aging with the first baseline survey in 2012.

The Japanese Study on Aging and Retirement is a panel of community-residing older Japanese adults. The baseline sample includes more than 4,200 Japanese aged 50 to 75. JSTAR was designed to capture the same key concepts of the HRS, and particularly those similar to SHARE. JSTAR added a self-completion questionnaire to collect data on food intake. JSTAR's sampling design is distinct from that of the others in the HRS survey network in that it represents selected municipalities and not the nation as a whole. This design was chosen because many key policy decisions about the Japanese elderly (healthcare and retirement) are set at the municipal level. This design facilitates an examination of policy differences across municipalities, and these municipalities granted permission for links with very good administrative data. The first JSTAR wave, conducted in 2007, used a sample of five municipalities with linkage to health expenditure records. Two municipalities were added in the second wave, and more municipalities will be added in the future.

LASI is an internationally harmonized panel survey representing the elderly population in India. The LASI pilot study sample of about 1,500 persons was drawn from four states (Karnataka, Kerala, Punjab, and Rajasthan) and was successfully completed in the spring of 2011. A full-scale, biennial survey of 30,000 Indians aged 45 and older is planned for 2012, with follow-ups every two years. The survey instrument includes the same core contents as the HRS. Other innovations of LASI include collecting data on physical environment and new questions on health utilization behaviors relevant to a developing country context, ranging from hospitalization to traditional healers, as well as new methods to measure social connections and expectations.

The first wave of the Indonesia Family Life Survey (IFLS1) was conducted in 1993–1994 covering about 83% of the Indonesian population living in 13 of the country's 26 provinces. IFLS2 followed up with the same sample four years later, in 1997–1998. One year after IFLS2, a 25% subsample was surveyed to provide information about the impact of Indonesia's economic crisis. IFLS3 was fielded on the full sample in 2000/2001 and IFLS4 in 2007/2008.

Originally, IFLS covered the full age distribution of the Indonesian population, but by following the same individuals over time, it has become another aging survey. For example, by IFLS4, 40% of the original IFLS1 household population were 40 years old and older.[6] In addition, as the population of the sample aged, the content of IFLS changed so that it was comparable with the other Asian aging surveys. In combination, the four waves of IFLS span a 14-year period of dramatic social and economic change in Indonesia and provide detailed longitudinal data on individuals, households, and communities that will greatly enhance the study of adults 45 years and older.

Figure 2-6 shows the worldwide spread of the HRS model of aging surveys around the world. Many countries on three continents—North America, Europe, and Asia—now have HRS-type international surveys.[7] What accounts for this spectacular success in the HRS network of surveys, including their Asian counterparts? One reason, of course, was that the time was ripe given its central motivating issue—population aging. The world is getting older, and new institutions and policies are needed

---

[6]Details of sampling and field procedures can be found in User's Guides, which are publicly available at http://www.rand.org/labor/FLS/IFLS.

[7]This year, an HRS-type survey has been funded in Brazil, and a pilot is planned for early 2012, so a fourth continent is about to be added.

29

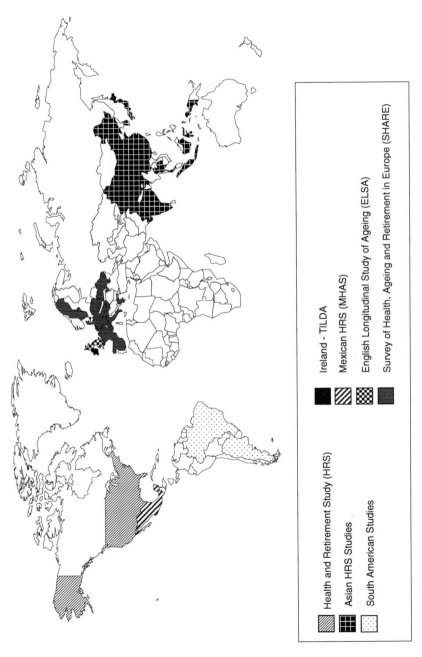

FIGURE 2-6 HRS-type surveys around the world.

to continue to provide income security and protection from increasing health risk and to do so at sustainable budgets—a long way from the current situation. While the scientific moment was seized, that is often not enough. Competence in execution certainly played a role, and the research teams leading all these studies deserve a lot of credit.

While all these factors were important, they were not enough. I believe that a central reason for success is the network's model of inclusion and openness, especially when it comes to cooperation, listening to, and implementing good scientific ideas. Openness is reflected most directly by the public release of all data in the network of surveys. Its openness also deeply reflects the perspective of the primary funding agency for these HRS surveys—the Division of Behavioral and Social Research (BSR) at the National Institute on Aging and, in particular, its leader, Dr. Richard Suzman. BSR has also provided critical start-up funding for many international surveys and continues to co-fund many of them. While the HRS international network has maintained its core focus on the domains of economics and health, its scientific scope has steadily expanded with significantly improved measurement of cognition, psychosocial risk factors, biomarker-based measures of health, and relevant dimensions of the community These domains were seen not only as important in older populations around the world, but also central in understanding the critical health and economic decisions that older people must make.

MEASUREMENT IN ASIA

Measuring Health Domains in Asia

One of the great difficulties in measuring health status in most Asian countries is that one cannot rely only on self-reports of respondents. As mentioned before, even some of the HRS surveys in North America and Europe have moved to including biomarkers in their measurement protocols. This is even more critical in developing Asian countries that are characterized by widespread undiagnosed diseases, including hypertension and diabetes, and low awareness of health problems. For example, in Indonesia, 71% of men who are hypertensive are undiagnosed. Similar rates apply in China, India, and Thailand for both hypertension and diabetes. In addition, biomarkers such as blood pressure and cholesterol level may indicate preclinical levels of disease that may not be known to respondents.

Because of this, many of the Asian surveys have included both biomarkers and performance tests in their survey protocols. The value of collecting biomarkers related to these health outcomes in population surveys has become widely recognized (Crimmins and Seeman, 2004). If we use CHARLS as an example, its biomarkers will now include systolic and diastolic blood pressure (measured three times) and pulse rate, all indicators of cardiovascular disease. Venous blood samples will be taken to measure HbA1c (a test for diabetes), total and HDL cholesterol, hemoglobin (low hemoglobin is a measure of anemia), and C-reactive protein (a measure of inflammation).

In addition to body mass index (BMI), CHARLS collects data on height, lower leg length and arm length (from the shoulder to the wrist), waist circumference, grip strength, lung capacity measured by a peak flow meter, and a timed sit to stand. Waist circumference can be used to indicate weight and adiposity. Researchers have argued that it is not obesity per se but the distribution of adipose tissue that is related to increased risk (Banks et al., 2011).

Measuring Economic Domains in Asia

Unlike many HRS-type surveys in industrialized countries, the measurement of economic resources in developing countries, where a good deal of productive economic activity is not monetized, is more complex. Many people in these countries work in family shops or farms where their labor is not directly compensated but shows up instead in the shared consumption of the household. Relying on the HRS-ELSA-SHARE-TILDA economic modules, which are based almost entirely on the receipt of money for work, would result in a substantial mischaracterization of the economic resources available and especially their distribution across households.

Fortunately, the IFLS had already pioneered the development of household consumption modules that appear to work very well and do not take inordinate amounts of survey time. Following this model, both CHARLS and LASI in their economic modules measured income, wealth, and consumption expenditures.

The importance of this comprehensive measurement of economic resources is seen in Table 2-1 using data from the 2008 CHARLS pilot survey.[8] This table displays the distribution of household income, household wealth, and household consumption of CHARLS individuals. The final two rows display two measures of inequality in the distribution of resources among CHARLS pilot respondents. If conventional income measure is used, inequality appears to be enormous—those in the 90th percentile have 334 times as much income as those at the 10th income percentile. Inequality appears to be even more widespread if household

---

[8]I am grateful to Professor Shen Yan of CCER at Peking University for providing this data. For more details on these issues, see Park et al. (2012).

TABLE 2-1 Comparisons of Distributions of Income, Wealth, and Consumption in China

Percentile	Household Income	Household New Wealth	Household Expenditure
90	25,182	230,745	15,607
75	14,704	77,569	10,559
50	5,626	30,469	5,781
25	1,289	4,792	3,314
10	75	26	1,747
90/10	334.3	8,963.1	8.9
75/25	11.4	16.2	3.2

SOURCE: Data from CHARLS pilot.

assets are used instead—almost 9,000 as many assets at the 90th wealth percentile compared to the 10th. However, when the most comprehensive and appropriate measure of availability of economic resources is used— household consumption—the ratio of the 90th to the 10th percentile is only 8.9. Nine-to-one still indicates considerable inequality within the Chinese population, but income and wealth measures significantly distort the amount of economic inequality. They may also distort trends over time when economic development is typically associated with monetizing economic activity, especially among the less well-to-do, so that inequality based on either income or assets will appear to be falling only due to monetization.

These surveys are also unique in separately measuring income and assets at the individual level (for respondents and spouse) as well as at the household level. The advantage of doing so is that who in the household controls the economic resources may matter in how those resources are used. For example, in an analysis of the Indonesian economic crisis of the late 1990s, Frankenberg, Smith, and Thomas (2003) showed using the IFLS that women's unique ownership of certain assets, including jewelry, smoothed consumption and protected the welfare of children.

Monitoring Change over Time

One of the benefits from these new sets of aging surveys is that they will provide a platform to monitor on a comparable basis the changes that take place in the future in this set of Asian countries. Given how dynamic the countries are, change will be the order of the day, but all changes may not be positive. CHARLS, HART, KLoSA, and LASI are too new to see that benefit, but the 20-year-old IFLS can illustrate the potential. For example, based on research using IFLS, it can be shown that smoking behavior among adult men has scarcely changed over those 20 years. Similarly, while the fraction of men who were undernourished (BMI < 18.5) was almost cut in half between 1993 and 2007 (from 17.5% to 9.5%), conferring a health benefit to the Indonesian population, the fraction of men who were overweight rose sharply over the same time period (from 6.5% to 10.4%), raising a signal of an impending health risk.[9]

Perhaps, the future use of these aging surveys is best illustrated by their ability to monitor the impacts of the Asian financial crisis in Indonesia. When IFLS began in the early 1990s, there was little talk of a financial crisis in the future. The second wave of IFLS was fielded in 1997, a year before the still-unanticipated financial crisis. Then, decades of economic growth in Indonesia were abruptly interrupted in 1998. In early 1998 the currency collapsed, falling four-fold in just a few days, while real wages declined by some 40% in the formal wage sector.

The immediate effects of the Asian crisis on the well-being of Indonesians are examined using IFLS. Frankenberg, Smith, and Thomas (2003) showed that families adopted several mechanisms in response to the crisis. Some families consolidated their living arrangements by moving in with relatives in low-cost locations, labor supply increased, spending on semi-durables fell while spending was maintained on food, and, especially in rural areas, wealth, particularly gold, the price of which was rising, was used to smooth consumption. The impact of the crisis was not widely reported as most severe on the poor, but rather on the more well-to-do who worked in the formal sector. This episode highlights the value of ongoing longitudinal surveys that can be put into the field very rapidly and provide basic scientific evidence to help understand the effects of major innovations on well-being and behaviors in society.

CONCLUSIONS AND LESSONS LEARNED FROM THE INTERNATIONAL HRS SET OF AGING SURVEYS

There is by now sufficient time to assess the primary lessons learned from these aging surveys and why they have been so successful. First, and perhaps most importantly, the data must be placed into the public domain in a reasonable time frame, usually less than a year. The full set of HRS international surveys have adhered to that principle, with the Asian surveys often among the most exemplary. Before this, the tradition in many of the Asian countries in this network was very much the opposite, with negative consequences for the advancement of science and policy for social scientists within these countries. Data were tightly guarded and not

---

[9]For more details on these issues, see Witoelar et al. (2012).

distributed even to host country scientists. Most of the scholars in these Asian countries had little data to analyze at all and turned instead to the more readily available American or European data. In the end, breaking the tradition of hoarding data and making the default option widespread public release may be the most important scientific impact of the HRS international aging surveys in Asia.

Second, the most common and most important studies will be conducted within a single country, dealing with the key scientific and policy issues within each country separately. Policies on population aging will be made on a country-by-country basis. Understanding patterns of behavior on retirement, healthcare, and the role of the family within countries is a prerequisite for learning from good comparative work. But there will be an important role for comparative studies, since it is much easier to step out of the conventional wisdom box constrained by country specific policy and science.

Third, the network of researchers around the world who have become an integral part of the development and diffusion of these HRS sets of international surveys is in many ways as important a scientific development as the creation of the data. This network of scholars starts with the survey developers and founders, but it has quickly spread to their students and collaborators within these countries. It now numbers in the thousands, spawning collaboration among scientists around the world who barely knew each other five years ago.

Fourth, while it is critical to maintain core principles, these studies must also be willing to evolve and grow with the science. The HRS is an excellent example. The core principles of merging the main health, family, and economic domains of life into a single platform remain, but the HRS is a very different study today than it was in 1992. Significant substantive additions have been made in cognition, key biomarkers, and the potential to do genetic studies, measuring well-being and dimensions of personality. The HRS has also responded to some of the major policy initiatives in the United States by introducing modules that have enabled the monitoring of the impact of key policy changes in healthcare use and expenditures. As new policy initiatives emerge in the Asian countries in this network—which happens at much greater frequency than in the United States—the Asian surveys should respond and become a major platform for monitoring and evaluating the impacts.

REFERENCES

Banks, J., M. Kumari, J.P. Smith, and P. Zaninotto. (2011). What explains the American disadvantage in health? The case of diabetes. *Journal of Epidemiology and Community Health* 66(3):259-264.

Chinese Academy of Social Sciences, Indian National Science Academy, Indonesian Academy of Sciences, National Research Council of the U.S. National Academies, and Science Council of Japan. (2010). *Preparing for the Challenges of Population Aging in Asia: Strengthening the Scientific Basis of Policy Development.* Washington, DC: The National Academies Press.

Crimmins, E.M., and T.E. Seeman. (2004). Integrating biology into the study of health disparities. *Population and Development Review* 30:89-107.

Frankenberg, E., J.P. Smith, and D. Thomas. (2003). Economic shocks, wealth, and welfare. *The Journal of Human Resources 38(2)*:280-321

Juster, F.T., and R. Suzman. (1995). An overview of the Health and Retirement Study. *The Journal of Human Resources, Special Issue on the Health and Retirement Study: Data Quality and Early Results 30*:S7-S56.

Marmot, M., J. Banks, R. Blundell, C. Lessof, and J. Nazroo. (Eds.). (2003). *Health, Wealth, and Lifestyles of the Older Population in England: ELSA 2002.* London, England: Institute for Fiscal Studies.

Park, A., Y. Shen, J. Strauss, and Y. Zhao. (2012). Relying on whom? Analyzing how Chinese elderly finance their consumption. Chapter 7 in *Aging in Asia: Findings from New and Emerging Data Initiatives.* J.P. Smith and M. Majmundar, Eds. Panel on Policy Research and Data Needs to Meet the Challenge of Aging in Asia. Committee on Population, Division of Behavioral and Social Sciences and Education. Washington, DC: The National Academies Press.

United Nations. (2008). *World Population Prospects: The 2008 Revision.* New York: United Nations Department of Economic and Social Affairs, Population Division.

Witoelar, F., J. Strauss, and B. Sikoki. (2012). Socioeconomic success and health in later life: Evidence from the Indonesia Family Life Survey. Chapter 13 in *Aging in Asia: Findings from New and Emerging Data Initiatives.* J.P. Smith and M. Majmundar, Eds. Panel on Policy Research and Data Needs to Meet the Challenge of Aging in Asia. Committee on Population, Division of Behavioral and Social Sciences and Education. Washington, DC: The National Academies Press.

Zhao, Y., J. Strauss, A. Park, Y. Shen, and Y. Sun. (2009). *Chinese Health and Retirement Longitudinal Study, Pilot. Users Guide.* National School of Development, Peking University.

3

Longitudinal Aging Study in India: Vision, Design, Implementation, and Preliminary Findings

P. Arokiasamy, David Bloom, Jinkook Lee,
Kevin Feeney, and *Marija Ozolins*

FOUNDATIONS FOR THE LONGITUDINAL AGING STUDY IN INDIA[1]

The Context: Global Population Aging

Population aging is a global phenomenon that all countries face, but global averages can mask considerable heterogeneity both across and within regions (Bloom, 2011a). Countries are at various stages of the process: The share of the 60+ population ranges from under 5% in a number of African and Gulf countries to more than 20% in several European and East Asian countries.[2] However, there is much less heterogeneity with respect to time trends; population aging will take place in all regions and countries going forward.

These trends have given rise to increased public thinking and dialogue on the issue of population aging. Some researchers suggest that population aging has substantial capacity to diminish the productive

[1]An early version of this chapter was presented as a paper in March 2011 at the Indian National Science Academy in New Delhi, India, at a conference on "Aging in Asia." The authors are indebted to the conference participants and to Paul Kowal and Larry Rosenberg for helpful comments. A more detailed analysis of these data is available at http://www.hsph.harvard.edu/pgda/WorkingPapers/2011/PGDA_WP_82.pdf. This research has been supported by NIA Grants R21AG032572 and P30AG024409 and by a grant from the Weatherhead Center for International Affairs at Harvard University..

[2]Except where stated otherwise, international demographic data in this report are derived from United Nations (2011).

capacities of national economies. Other studies suggest that any negative effects on economic growth are likely to be no more than modest (Bloom, Canning, and Fink, 2010; Boersch-Supan and Ludwig, 2010). Regardless of the effect on the economy as a whole, population aging will lead to increased need for elder care and support, at a time when, in developing societies, traditional family-based care is becoming less the norm than in the past. In addition, a higher share of older people will affect budget expenditures (less for education, but more for healthcare) and may affect tax rates.

Population Aging in India: Trends and Challenges

With 1.21 billion inhabitants counted in its 2011 census (Registrar General of India, Census of India, 2011), India is the second most populous country in the world. Currently, the 60+ population accounts for 8% of India's population, translating into roughly 93 million people. By 2050, the share of the 60+ population is projected to climb to 19%, or approximately 323 million people. The elderly dependency ratio (the number of people aged 60 and older per person aged 15 to 59) will rise dramatically from 0.12 to 0.31. At the same time, India's older population will be subject to a higher rate of noncommunicable diseases, a higher share of women in the workforce (thus less able to care for the elderly), children who are less likely to live near their parents, and a lack of policies and institutions to deal effectively with these issues (Bloom, 2011b).[3]

Several forces are driving India's changing age structure, including an upward trend in life expectancy and falling fertility. An Indian born in 1950 could expect to live for 37 years, whereas today India's life expectancy at birth has risen to 65 years; by 2050 it is projected to increase to 74 years. Fertility rates in India have declined sharply, from nearly 6 children per woman in 1950 to 2.6 children per woman in 2010. India has also been experiencing a breakdown of the traditional extended family structure; currently, India's older people are largely cared for privately, but these family networks are coming under stress from a variety of sources (Bloom et al., 2010; Pal, 2007).

India is in the early stages of establishing government programs to support its aging population. At the current burden of disease levels, rising numbers of older people will likely increase demands on the health system (Yip and Mahal, 2008). Less than 10% of the population has health insurance (either public or private), and roughly 72% of healthcare spending is

---

[3]James (2011) points out that the history of long-term population predictions for India has been marked by major inaccuracies.

out-of-pocket. The aging population is particularly at risk, as the health insurance scheme for the poor covers only those aged 65 or younger.

Older Indians also face economic insecurity; 90% of them have no pension. According to official statistics, labor force participation remains high (39%) among those aged 60 and older and is especially high (45%) in rural areas (see Alam, 2004, and Registrar General, 2001). These high participation rates reflect an overwhelming reliance on the agriculture and informal sectors, which account for more than 90% of all employment in India. They also reflect the inadequacy of existing social safety nets for older people (Bloom et al., 2010). In addition, more than two-thirds of India's elderly live in rural areas, limiting their access to modern financial institutions and instruments such as banks and insurance schemes.

With India in the early stages of a transition to an older society, little is known about the economic, social, and public health implications. Data on the status of older people are needed to analyze population aging and formulate mid- and long-term policies. The Longitudinal Aging Study in India (LASI) is an effort to fill this gap through a large-scale, nationally representative, longitudinal survey on aging, health, and retirement. LASI's longitudinal character is key: Over an extended period, researchers can assemble a data set that shows the changes in India's older population and, at the same time, have access to up-to-date data. The survey results and subsequent data analyses will be disseminated to the research community and policymakers.

LASI joins several existing sister surveys of the seminal Health and Retirement Study (HRS), a longitudinal survey of Americans aged 50 and older conducted by the Institute for Social Research (ISR) at the University of Michigan and supported by the National Institute on Aging (NIA). HRS has inspired similar studies outside the United States; current and planned HRS-type studies cover more than 25 countries on four continents (Lee, 2010). One striking feature of the HRS-type surveys is the possibility of pooling data from different countries to assess the effects of differing institutions on behavior and outcomes. Taken as a whole, the HRS family offers many opportunities to widen and deepen research on the nature and implications of aging.[4]

---

[4]Another source of valuable micro-data on older populations is the Study on Global AGEing and Adult Health, or SAGE, developed by the World Health Organization Multi-Country Studies Unit. SAGE covers six countries (China, Ghana, India, Mexico, Russian Federation, and South Africa), and while focused on those aged 50+, includes a small sample of adults aged 18-49 years. It has more focus on health and less on economic and financial data than the HRS family of surveys.

LONGITUDINAL AGING STUDY IN INDIA (LASI)

Design and Vision

In this section of the chapter, we discuss the design and sampling frame for the LASI pilot, highlighting features that allow researchers to begin to identify and answer important questions about population aging in India. We also evaluate the validity of the fieldwork by comparing the LASI pilot sample to that of other surveys in India.

India, like other countries in which HRS-style surveys have been conducted, presents a unique set of challenges. Income and assets, for example, are difficult to measure due to lack of written documentation and the fact that a significant portion of income and production does not take place in market contexts. In addition, people may be disinclined to reveal certain information (e.g., some women may be reluctant to reveal that they have savings balances for fear that their husbands or sons-in-law will claim them).

To capture India's demographic, economic, health, and cultural diversity, the LASI pilot focused on two northern states (Punjab and Rajasthan) and two southern states (Karnataka and Kerala). Rajasthan and Karnataka provide some overlap with the World Health Organization's Study on Global AGEing and Adult Health (SAGE). Punjab is an economically developed state, while Rajasthan is relatively poor. Kerala, known for its relatively developed healthcare system, has undergone rapid social development and is a potential harbinger of how other Indian states might evolve (Pal and Palacios, 2008). The LASI instrument was developed in English and translated into the dominant local languages: Hindi (Punjab and Rajasthan), Kannada (Karnataka), and Malayalam (Kerala).

The LASI questionnaire was also designed to collect information conceptually comparable to related HRS surveys and SAGE.[5] The instrument consists of a household survey, collected once per household by interviewing a selected key informant about household finances and living conditions for those in the household; an individual survey, collected for each age-eligible respondent at least 45 years of age and their spouse (regardless of age); and a biomarker module, collected for each consenting age-eligible respondent and spouse.

The household interview consists of five sections: a roster detailing basic demographic information about each household member; a ques-

---

[5]These include the Health and Retirement Study (HRS) in the United States, the English Longitudinal Survey of Ageing (ELSA), the Chinese Health and Retirement Longitudinal Survey (CHARLS), the Indonesian Family Life Survey (IFLS), the Korean Longitudinal Study of Ageing (KLoSA), the Japanese Study of Aging and Retirement (JSTAR), and the Study of Health, Ageing and Retirement in Europe (SHARE), which covers 15 European countries.

tionnaire about the housing and neighborhood environment, including questions about access to water, neighborhood conditions, and other attributes; income of all family members from labor and nonlabor sources; assets and debts of the household; and consumption and expenditure of the household on food and nonfood items, including items that were exchanged in-kind, gifted, or home-grown.

The individual interview consists of seven sections: demographics, family and social networks, health, healthcare utilization, work and employment, pension and retirement, and one experimental section.[6]An important component of the health section is a biomarker module collected by the interview team. Given the lack of healthcare services, biological markers (e.g., anthropometrics, blood pressure, and dried blood spots) and performance measures (e.g., gait speed, grip strength, balance, lung function, and vision) allow researchers to assess the health of LASI's sample population. The dried blood spot collection, for example, allows for up to 35 different assays, including four that the LASI team initially plans to test: C-reactive protein (CRP, a marker of inflammation), glycosylated hemoglobin (HbA1c, a marker of glucose metabolism), hemoglobin (Hb, a marker of anemia), and Epstein-Barr virus (EBV) antibodies (a marker of cell-mediated immune function).

Sampling Plan, Fieldwork, and Administration

Funded by the National Institute on Aging, LASI is a partnership between the Harvard School of Public Health, the International Institute for Population Sciences in Mumbai, India, and the RAND Corporation. Also involved in LASI are two other Indian institutions, the National AIDS Research Institute (NARI) and the Indian Academy of Geriatrics (IAG). The University of California Los Angeles (UCLA) School of Medicine is also a participant in LASI.

The fieldwork was carried out by a network of Population Research Centers (see Table 3-1). Fieldwork lasted from October to December 2010. The rapid turnaround from data collection to the analysis of the data was possible through use of state-of-the-art technology in data management and computer-assisted personal interviewing (CAPI).

Using the 2001 Indian Census,[7] we drew a representative sample from the four states. Age-qualifying individuals were drawn from a stratified,

---

[6]The experimental section consists of a module of questions on one of the following three topics, randomly assigned: economic expectations, anchoring vignettes, and social connectedness.

[7]The Indian Census is conducted every 10 years. The 2011 wave was recently released, so the first full LASI wave will be able to utilize the latest population sample during fieldwork.

TABLE 3-1 Administration of the 2010 LASI Pilot Survey

	Karnataka	Kerala	Punjab	Rajasthan
Timeline				
From	29 October	1 November	14 November	14 November
To	3 December	14 December	12 December	18 December
Organization				
	Population Research Centre, Institute for Social and Economic Change, Bangalore	Population Research Centre, Department of Demography, University of Kerala, Thiruvananthapuram	Population Research Centre, Department of Economics, Himachal Pradesh University, Shimla	Population Research Centre, Department of Economics, University of Lucknow, Lucknow

NOTE: LASI fieldwork was planned in order to avoid monsoon season, which typically lasts from June to September.

multistage, area probability sampling design, beginning with census community tracts. From each state, two districts were selected at random from Census districts for 2001; eight primary sampling units (PSUs) were randomly selected from each district. PSUs were chosen to match the urban/rural share of the population. Twenty-five residential households were then selected through systematic random sampling from each PSU, from which an average of 16 households contained at least one age-eligible individual.

The LASI pilot achieved a household response rate of 88.5%, calculated as the ratio of consenting to eligible households (as further adjusted for cases of no contact, missing eligibility information, or refusal to give eligibility information; see Table 3-2). The individual response rate (90.9%) and biomarker module response rate (89%) were calculated conditional on belonging to a household that consented to participate in the LASI interview. Eligible households were defined as those with at least one member 45 years of age and older, and eligible individuals were those who were 45 years of age and older or married to an individual who was.[8]

[8]Eligible age for response rates was determined from the coverscreen household roster, which was reported by the household respondent, who was not always an individual respondent. The respondent who consented to the individual interview did self-report age in the demographics component of the module, effectively creating two possible age variables. On occasion, some individuals who were listed as 45 years of age and older reported they were not or vice versa in the individual interview. For consistency, we calculate the response rates using ages reported in the coverscreen, though for the remaining analysis presented in the paper we rely on self-reported age. The results of all models were not sensitive to the age variable used.

TABLE 3-2 LASI Pilot Study, Response Rate

	Urban	Rural	Punjab	Rajasthan	Kerala	Karnataka	Total
Household Survey							
Sampled	485	1,062	375	371	395	406	1,547
Unable to contact	10	13	0	0	17	6	23
Contact established	475	1049	375	371	378	400	1,524
Age eligible	325	756	254	255	297	275	1,081
Not eligible	140	284	120	114	70	120	424
Unknown eligibility	10	9	1	2	11	5	19
Did not start interview	31	56	28	13	24	22	87
Started interview	294	700	226	242	273	253	994
Completed interview	281	669	222	230	261	237	950
Household Response Rate (%)	85.2	90.0	88.6	94.2	84.0	88.5	88.5
Individual Survey							
Total eligible	567	1,359	419	485	559	463	1,926
Age eligible	505	1,201	385	423	506	392	1,706
Spouse eligible	62	158	35	61	53	71	220
Started individual interview	492	1,259	410	436	483	422	1,751
Age eligible	439	1,109	375	380	436	357	1,548
Spouse eligible	53	150	35	56	47	65	203
Completed individual interview	472	1,211	402	417	462	402	1,683
Age eligible	419	1,067	368	363	418	337	1,486
Spouse eligible	53	144	34	54	44	65	197
Individual Response Rate (%)	86.8	92.6	97.9	89.9	86.4	91.1	90.9
Biomarker Module							
Total eligible	567	1359	419	485	559	463	1,926
Consented to start biomarker module	474	1241	398	436	480	401	1,715
Biomarker Response Rate (%)	83.6	91.3	95.0	89.9	85.9	86.6	89.0

Response Rates for Selected Questions (%)							
Dried blood spot collection (biomarker module)	64.6	77.5	76.4	75.8	69.6	76.5	74.3
Satisfaction with spousal relationship (family and social networks)	93.4	93.9	97.3	90.6	89.0	99.7	93.8
Income (household questionnaire)	77.2	79.2	77.9	73.5	85.1	77.2	78.6
Consumption (household questionnaire)	79.4	82.8	92.3	73.9	80.8	80.6	81.8
"Probability" respondent will die in one year (expectations module)	87.3	88.0	94.7	89.1	71.6	98.5	87.8

NOTES: Response rates are calculated by dividing the total number of individuals or households who consented to the interview by the total number of contacted, eligible individuals (including spouses under 45 years of age) or households as reported in the coverscreen household component of the interview. Households that were not contacted indicate cases when the interviewing team was unable to speak with an individual residing at the house either because no one was home, the family has moved, or for some other reason. Five contact attempts were suggested before classifying a household as "no contact." The **household response rate** across all states is thus calculated by dividing 994 households that initially consented to the interview by the sum of the number of no contacts (23), the contacted eligible households (1,081), and the 19 households with missing or refused age eligibility. Note that this reflects a conservative estimate to the response rate. The **individual response rate across all states** is calculated by dividing the 1,751 individuals who consented to start the individual interview by the 1,926 eligible household members listed in the coverscreen of the household roster once the survey began. **Response rates for select questions** pertain to respondents who were asked that specific question, not the total eligible persons listed in the coverscreen. This approach was chosen to best capture the effects of the sensitive nature of the questions. Thus the **dried blood spot collection response rate** captures the share of respondents who specifically agreed to participate. **Response rates for income and consumption** are among households and are the share of households that did not require imputation and had no missing income components queried about during the household module. The **probability respondents will die in one year** is a question from the expectations module, one of three experimental modules that was randomly assigned to respondents at the end of the individual interview. The question asked respondents to select a number of beans from a pile of 10 beans to indicate how likely they were to die in the next year. Response rates for more standard survey questions were 98% and above; response rates of selected questions were chosen to showcase survey items with lower response rates.

SOURCE: Data from Longitudinal Aging Study in India (LASI) Pilot Wave.

Among households and individuals who consented to start the LASI interview, not all individual or household modules were completed after initial consent was given. Table 3-2 tabulates the number of respondents and households that completed an individual or household interview; these 950 households and 1,683 individuals constitute the complete LASI pilot sample. Of the 1,683 individuals who completed an individual interview, 1,486 respondents[9] were aged 45 years and older. The 197 who were not age-eligible were female spouses of age-qualifying participants.

Table 3-2 also shows relatively high response rates to selected potentially sensitive questions.

We observed significant heterogeneity in the length of time to complete the survey across states, from a total time of 137 minutes in Rajasthan and Karnataka to a high of 215 minutes in Punjab (see Table 3-3). Some interviews were split over time: about 15% of the interviews occurred over a span of two or more days.[10]

The average duration of the household module was 33 minutes. For the individual interview, including the biomarker module, the mean duration was 78 minutes. Households had a mean of 1.8 respondents who completed individual interviews.

Profile of LASI Respondents

The LASI design and implementation was successful in creating a sample comparable to other nationally representative surveys conducted in India. In Table 3-4, we present the initial results of the fieldwork through a comparison of the basic demographic indicators of LASI respondents to those of respondents from other surveys conducted in India: the National Sample Survey (NSS), India Human Development Survey (IHDS), World Health Survey (WHS), and SAGE. As the other surveys have broader age inclusion categories, we restrict the comparison to individuals aged 45 and older only.

We compare the distribution of demographic characteristics for those aged 45 and older across the four surveys, looking specifically at age, sex, urban-rural residence, marital status, and education. We expect some differences across these metrics, given the different sets of states surveyed. For example, LASI has a comparatively small sample size from four

---

[9]Of the 1,486 respondents who were identified in the coverscreen as being aged 45 and older, 1,451 confirmed that status in the individual interview. We use these 1,451 as our analysis sample. The remaining 232 respondents consists of 230 who self-reported their age as less than 45 (of which 181 were also identified as less than age 45 in the coverscreen), and 2 who did not report an age. These 232 individuals were not included in the analysis sample.

[10]Such a span took place when at some point during the interview, the interview team was asked to leave and come back on a different day.

TABLE 3-3 Average Survey Duration by State of Key Survey Components (in minutes)

	Punjab	Rajasthan	Kerala	Karnataka	All States
Total Time at Household (HH)	215.2	137.3	205.2	137.4	174.7
Household Module					
Total	41.9	29.1	37.6	24.6	33.4
Housing and environment	9.2	7.6	7.0	5.3	7.2
Consumption	12.3	7.6	13.1	7.3	10.1
Income	7.9	5.0	7.4	5.2	6.4
Agricultural income and assets	3.9	4.0	1.7	2.1	2.9
Financial assets and real estate	8.6	5.0	8.5	4.8	6.8
Number of interviews	222	230	261	237	950
Individual Module					
Total	93.9	57.8	92.5	66.5	78.1
Demographics	9.5	5.7	6.7	5.6	6.9
Family and social network	15.0	11.2	13.1	8.9	12.1
Health	27.4	17.2	30.5	15.9	23.0
Healthcare utilization	4.7	2.7	4.8	3.0	3.8
Employment	7.2	2.5	7.3	4.8	5.5
Pension	4.2	1.1	2.7	2.0	2.5
Experimental: social connectedness	11.3	4.9	10.0	7.6	8.4
Experimental: expectations	5.9	3.5	6.2	3.0	4.7
Experimental: vignettes	4.8	1.5	4.1	1.7	3.1
Biomarker	18.9	14.2	21.0	22.3	19.1
Number of interviews	402	417	462	402	1,683
Number of individual interviews per HH	1.8	1.8	1.8	1.7	1.8
Duration of Interviews					
One day (n)	298	338	390	380	1,406
Multiple days (n)	103	74	61	20	258
Interviews lasting multiple days (%)	25.7	18.0	13.5	5.0	15.5

NOTE: Total time at HH is the average time spent at a household, including the time spent conducting the household module and all individual modules (including the biomarker module).
SOURCE: Data from Longitudinal Aging Study in India (LASI) Pilot Wave.

TABLE 3-4 External Validity: Comparison of LASI to Other Surveys on Select Demographic Indicators

	All States in Sample					Rajasthan		Karnataka	
	LASI	NSS	IHDS	WHS	SAGE	LASI	SAGE	LASI	SAGE
Survey year(s)	2010	2004	2004–05	2003	2007–08	2010	2007–08	2010	2007–08
Total number of individuals	1,683	383,338	215,754	10,750	12,198	417	2,374	402	1,744
Number of individuals aged 45+	1,451	81,146	45,074	3,706	7,841	358	1,587	315	1,139
Age structure (%) Among Respondents 45 Years and Older									
Age 45–54	44.3	44.1	44.9	41.7	48.7	43.1	49.9	49.5	52.3
Age 55–64	28.4	32.7	29.7	26.1	28.3	23.4	26.9	31.8	25.8
Age 65–74	17.8	17.4	17.9	18.1	16.4	21.8	16.3	14.0	15.2
Age 75+	9.5	5.9	7.6	14.1	6.7	11.8	6.8	4.8	6.8
Sex (%) Among Respondents 45 Years and Older									
Male	48.7	50.5	51.4	50.7	55.2	51.5	53.7	47.6	56.6
Female	51.3	49.5	48.6	49.4	44.8	48.5	46.3	52.4	43.5
Residence (%) Among Respondents 45 Years and Older									
Urban	27.1	26.3	26.9	11.1	26.8	19.2	20.5	35.7	32.3
Rural	72.9	73.8	73.1	88.9	73.2	80.8	79.5	64.3	67.7
Marital Status (%) Among Respondents 45 Years and Older									
Married	78.0	75.8	78.2	80.7	81.5	81.0	81.5	75.3	82.4
Never married	1.8	1.1	0.7	1.3	0.6	0.9	0.3	2.2	0.4
Divorced	1.2	0.6	0.5	0.7	0.6	1.4	0.7	0.6	0.5
Widowed	19.1	22.5	20.6	17.3	17.3	16.8	17.5	21.9	16.7

Education (%) Among Respondents 45 Years and Older

No education	48.2	58.6	53.2	63.4	47.6	79.1	62.7	42.6	48.1
< 5 years	8.1	8.6	10.7	11.2	13.2	3.3	9.3	12.9	14.2
5–9 years	22.0	19.5	21.0	15.0	19.8	8.3	15.2	23.6	17.5
10+ years	21.7	13.4	15.1	10.5	19.4	9.2	12.7	20.9	20.2

NOTES: For this table, we use the 1,451 respondents who self-reported age of at least 45 years in the individual interview. LASI is the Longitudinal Study of Aging in India, NSS is the National Sample Survey, IHDS is the Indian Human Development Survey, WHS is the World Health Survey, and SAGE is the Study on Global AGEing and Adult Health. SAGE states include Assam, Karnataka, Maharashtra, Rajasthan, Uttar Pradesh, and West Bengal. **NSS** is a nationally representative, cross-sectional survey of all Indian states conducted by the Indian government's Ministry of Statistics and Programme Implementation. **IHDS** is a nationally representative survey among 33 states and territories conducted between 2004 and 2005 to assess the health of all household members, with special questions to assess children's well-being. It is conducted by the University of Maryland. **WHS** is a nationally representative survey conducted by the World Health Organization and was later reorganized as **SAGE** survey to target aging populations and produce harmonized survey data with parallel efforts in Africa, Latin America, and Eastern Europe.
SOURCES: Data from Longitudinal Aging Study in India (LASI) Pilot Wave, Ministry of Statistics and Programme Implementation (2004), Indian Human Development Survey (2005), and World Health Organization (2003, 2010).

diverse states, including Kerala, which is exceptional because of the relatively high level of educational attainment among the population. This is
reflected in Table 4-4: 22% of the LASI sample report having some high
school or more for their education, which is higher than the other data
sets. With respect to this indicator, LASI is most comparable to SAGE
(19%), which likely reflects the overlap in state coverage.

Table 3-4 takes a closer look at the LASI pilot and SAGE results.
The SAGE states of Karnataka and Rajasthan were included in the LASI
pilot in part to measure the validity of the LASI sample against a more
established survey, so we examine the validity of these states' samples
separately. In these two states we again see similar respondent populations, despite the small sample sizes in the LASI pilot. The LASI sample
in Rajasthan was slightly older than that of SAGE, while in Karnataka the
sample was slightly younger. LASI surveyed proportionally more women
from Karnataka than did SAGE. The differences in education and marital
status are negligible.

In making cross-state comparisons, it should be kept in mind that
each state's sample is drawn from a relatively small number of districts.
As such, the state comparisons referred to herein reflect district-specific
idiosyncrasies, in addition to more pervasive state characteristics. Nevertheless, most of the state-by-state comparisons accord reasonably well
with independent data and perceptions.

WHAT CAN WE LEARN FROM LASI?

Characteristics of India's Aging Population

The LASI pilot is able to provide researchers with a picture of life for
aging Indians that reflects the significant regional and social variations
within the country. Even the most basic demographic indicators—such as
education, marital status, and self-rated health—differ not only by gender
and socioeconomic status within regions, but also across regions. Table 3-5
displays demographic differences in the representative LASI sample of
those aged 45 years and older as self-reported in the demographics module. Men and women both have a mean age of 58, and there is a slightly
higher representation of men among rural populations, which make up
70% of the sample overall. Figure 3-1 shows a similar age distribution
among men and women, though there are more women than men in the
45–59 group, as well as more women among respondents 85 years and
older. Men are also more likely to be married and women more likely to
be widowed, an important demographic difference that reflects the traditional age gap between spouses in India. Educational attainment and

TABLE 3-5 Demographic Characteristics by Gender and State in LASI Sample

	Men	Women	Punjab	Rajasthan	Kerala	Karnataka
N	706	745	365	358	413	315
Age (yrs)	58.1	57.9	56.9	59.0	60.4	55.3
	[10.17]	[11.26]	[11.07]	[11.26]	[10.81]	[8.86]
Rural	75.7	71.8	70.6	82.4	75.8	63.9
	[0.41]	[0.44]	[0.46]	[0.33]	[0.40]	[0.48]
Married	91.5	64.3	80.7	80.4	75.8	74.8
	[0.28]	[0.48]	[0.39]	[0.38]	[0.42]	[0.43]
Widowed	6.3	31.9	18.4	17.2	18.9	22.6
	[0.24]	[0.46]	[0.39]	[0.36]	[0.38]	[0.42]
Household size	5.3	5.3	5.1	6.5	4.4	4.9
(no. of people)	[2.71]	[2.97]	[2.93]	[2.88]	[2.05]	[2.84]
Scheduled caste	13.8	15.1	34.5	10.0	7.0	17.0
	[0.34]	[0.36]	[0.48]	[0.28]	[0.24]	[0.38]
Scheduled tribe	15.4	13.3	0.0	36.3	0.0	8.8
	[0.36]	[0.34]	—	[0.47]	—	[0.28]
Other backward	38.4	39.4	9.7	27.9	42.5	60.6
caste	[0.48]	[0.48]	[0.30]	[0.44]	[0.49]	[0.49]
None/other caste	32.5	32.1	55.8	25.8	50.5	13.6
or tribe	[0.46]	[0.46]	[0.50]	[0.42]	[0.49]	[0.34]
Hindu	75.6	75.7	30.2	84.6	71.1	89.6
	[0.42]	[0.43]	[0.46]	[0.34]	[0.44]	[0.31]
Muslim	7.9	8.1	0.0	15.1	4.5	6.7
	[0.26]	[0.27]	—	[0.34]	[0.21]	[0.25]
Christian	6.1	7.6	1.0	0.0	24.4	2.6
	[0.24]	[0.26]	[0.10]	—	[0.41]	[0.16]
Sikh	8.2	7.4	60.2	0.0	0.0	0.0
	[0.28]	[0.26]	[0.49]	—	—	—
Other religion	1.8	1.3	8.6	0.3	0.0	1.1
	[0.13]	[0.11]	[0.28]	[0.06]	[0.00]	[0.10]
Education (yrs)	5.1	3.4	3.3	1.7	7.7	4.4
	[5.10]	[4.43]	[4.45]	[3.65]	[3.70]	[4.79]
Literate	57.4	40.7	41.4	18.7	88.3	51.4
	[0.49]	[0.49]	[0.49]	[0.37]	[0.31]	[0.50]
Labor force	71.3	26.2	47.1	55.7	32.9	53.8
participation	[0.45]	[0.44]	[0.50]	[0.48]	[0.46]	[0.50]
Per capita income	41,752	42,123	53,888	31,354	68,930	25,272
(Rs)	[92,649]	[84,883]	[85,304]	[77,059]	[125,534]	[44,460]
Self-rated health	3.3	3.2	3.5	3.4	2.8	3.5
	[0.80]	[0.80]	[0.78]	[0.85]	[0.72]	[0.64]
Poor or fair self-	12.3	15.7	12.3	14.5	24.3	5.4
rated health	[0.32]	[0.36]	[0.33]	[0.34]	[0.42]	[0.23]

NOTES: This table only considers respondents who self-reported an age of at least 45 years in the individual interview and provided an answer for each of the variables listed in the table. All numbers are reported as a percentage unless otherwise noted; standard deviations

continued

TABLE 3-5 Continued

are reported in brackets. LASI used a stratified sampling design that sampled respondents independently by state, rural-urban areas, and district. Means are weighted using either the pooled-state weight or the state-specific weight, and the standard errors have been corrected for design effects of stratification. Labor force participation is a dummy variable for having worked in the past 12 months. It includes self-employment, employment by another, or agricultural work both paid and unpaid as reported in the household income module by a household financial respondent or as self-reported in the individual interview. Self-rated health asks respondents whether they feel their health in general is excellent (scored 5), very good (4), good (3), fair (2), or poor (1).
SOURCE: Longitudinal Aging Study in India (LASI) Pilot Wave.

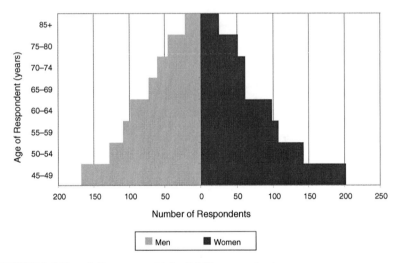

FIGURE 3-1 Population pyramid for LASI respondents.
NOTE: Among respondents aged 45 years and older only.
SOURCE: Data from Longitudinal Aging Study in India (LASI) Pilot Wave.

literacy are also higher for men than women, although with considerable heterogeneity across states.

Economic activity also differs by gender; 69% of men report working in the past year in either agricultural labor, for an employer, or self-employed work, compared to less than one-quarter of women. Men tended also to have better self-rated health than women, and women were more likely to report poor or fair self-rated health. Generally, women in the sample were more likely to be widowed, less educated, have lower self-rated health, and to be not working, which is consistent with literature on India and other surveys.

Table 3-5 also shows some important interstate differences across the LASI sample. Kerala has an older sample, with a mean age of 60, while Karnataka, the other southern state in the LASI sample, has a comparatively young population (with a mean age of 56) compared to the other three states. Rajasthan tends to be more rural than the other states and Karnataka the least rural. Family demographics, such as household size and marital status, vary as well.

The distribution of caste, tribe, and religion across the four states reflects the regional and sociocultural variation that LASI has been able to capture. About one-third of the Rajasthan sample identifies itself as members of a scheduled tribe, while in Punjab, almost 60% of the population does not identify itself as a scheduled tribe, scheduled caste, or other backward caste. Each state also reflects the diversity in religious belief systems in India—the large Sikh population in Punjab and the sizable Christian population in Kerala, in addition to Hindus and Muslims that make up most of Karnataka and Rajasthan.

These four states reflect different patterns of social and economic well-being. For example, Kerala's population has comparatively high educational attainment, attributable to a legacy of social development programs. Respondents from Kerala are older and report relatively low labor force participation and worse health than respondents from the other states. The higher prevalence of poor or fair self-rated health may indeed reflect high morbidity in the population, but high literacy rates and better access to healthcare services than in other Indian states also contribute to a more health-literate population (Bloom, 2005). Conversely, Rajasthan, the poorest state in the sample, has the lowest mean years of education, at just below two years, yet the highest labor force participation, at 56%. This reflects the rural-based subsistence economy that requires all household members to engage in some work, even at older ages.

Basic Living Conditions of Older People in India

While economic growth has been rapid, basic living conditions for many Indians, especially the aging, are still poor (Husain and Ghosh, 2011; Pal and Palacios, 2008). Table 3-6 reports indicators of hardship and vulnerability among the LASI pilot sample aged 45 and older, looking specifically at such indicators as drinking water, sanitation, basic household utilities, health, and food security. These are common markers used in the development literature to assess quality of life (Ahmed et al., 1991; Clark and Ning, 2007).

Table 3-6 shows that almost 80% of LASI respondents live in households that do not have access to running water in the home, and 45% do not have access to an "improved water source." Sixty percent live in

TABLE 3-6 Select Indicators of Hardship and Vulnerability by State Among Individuals 45 Years and Older

	Punjab	Rajasthan	Kerala	Karnataka	All States
Household					
N	222	230	261	237	950
Basic utilities					
No electricity in home	3.5	42.6	1.5	2.8	15.0
No running water in home	40.7	86.3	94.8	74.3	78.6
No access to improved water source	2.2	68.9	79.8	10.7	44.5
No private toilet facility	10.1	67.8	0.3	42.0	35.8
No access to improved sewerage disposal	48.7	88.1	5.7	75.2	59.0
Does not use good quality cooking fuel	31.0	88.0	52.4	43.5	57.9
No refrigerator in home	33.7	93.2	48.0	87.1	72.6
Individual					
N	365	358	413	315	1,451
Living alone	10.8	6.4	17.3	16.7	12.8
Illiterate	61.4	79.7	11.1	46.5	50.3
Health insurance*	0.5	0.8	12.2	6.8	5.7
Difficulty with at least 1 ADL	9.5	7.0	20.1	14.1	12.7
Undiagnosed hypertension	39.5	40.9	19.4	27.6	31.3
Urban	37.1	39.1	19.3	36.4	33.4
Rural	40.2	41.1	19.8	22.6	30.6
Men	46.0	38.5	19.7	26.1	31.5
Women	32.7	43.0	19.6	28.8	31.2
Under age 60	39.4	39.6	20.0	20.4	28.6
Age 60 and older	39.2	42.1	19.3	42.1	35.2
Food insecurity (past 12 months)	4.2	3.9	1.4	2.4	2.9
Underweight (BMI < 18.5)	12.2	41.1	13.4	28.3	26.7

*Of the respondents aged 45 and older who said they did not have health insurance, 46% said they did not have it because they did not know what it is (have never heard of it); 23% said they could not afford it; 16% did not feel that they needed it; 7% did not know where to purchase it; 3% reported being denied health insurance and 5% listed some other reason for not obtaining health insurance.

NOTES: All numbers are percentages. The sample is restricted to respondents who reported they were at least 45 years old in the individual interview and provided a nonmissing answer for each of the variables listed in the table, with the exception of hypertension variables. Hypertension prevalence was calculated only among respondents in the biomarker module. Improved water source includes piped water, tube well, and protected dug well. Sources of water not considered improved are unprotected wells, water from springs/rainwater/surface water, and tanker trucks. Access to improved sewage disposal includes piped sewer system or septic tanks. Dry toilets, pit latrines, or no facility are not included. Good quality cooking fuel includes coal, charcoal, natural gas, petroleum, kerosene, or electric. Activities of daily life (ADL) include using a toilet, bathing, dressing, eating, walking across a room, and getting out of bed. Undiagnosed hypertension is among all respondents,

TABLE 3-6 Continued

whether hypertensive or not. It is a binary indicator if hypertension is indicated from the biomarker module but the respondent reports never having received a diagnosis for high blood pressure or hypertension from a health professional. Lee et al. (2012) includes an in-depth analysis of undiagnosed hypertension. Living alone is defined as living with one's self only or with one's spouse only (Dandekar, 1996). The surprisingly high figures for Kerala for lack of access to improved water sources and for not having running water in the home are consistent with other relevant reports about Kerala, e.g., International Institute for Population Sciences and Macro International (2007). Food insecurity is a binary indicator for respondents who report having lost weight due to hunger, not eaten for a whole day or gone hungry because there was not enough money to buy food, or otherwise reduced the size or frequency of meals because there was not enough money to buy food. Means are weighted using the state-specific or the pooled-state weights.
SOURCE: Data from Longitudinal Aging Study in India (LASI) Pilot Wave.

households without proper sewer systems. Nearly 60% also live in households that use poor quality cooking fuel, which can contribute to indoor air pollution (World Bank, 2002). More than 90% of households in Rajasthan use low-quality cooking fuel, compared with just 31% of households in the wealthier, more urbanized state of Punjab. Conditions vary widely across states. In Kerala and Punjab, the great majority of respondents have access to a private toilet facility, while more than 65% of respondents in Rajasthan do not.

Compounding poor living and environmental conditions are health and economic concerns. Thirteen percent reported living alone. Living alone is most common in the southern states of Kerala (17%) and Karnataka (16%) and least common in Rajasthan. An essentially nonexistent health insurance system and high rates of illiteracy also leave aging individuals vulnerable.

Measuring the Health of Aging Indians

LASI relies on a wide spectrum of health measures, ranging from self-reports of general health ("In general, would you say your health is excellent, very good, good, fair, or poor?") to queries about specific diagnoses ("Have you ever been diagnosed by a health professional with hypertension?"). Older respondents who are poor, uneducated, and lack access to healthcare may underreport health conditions that do not have severe symptoms. Self-reports by literate populations with better access to health services may more accurately reflect prevalence rates.

To understand the degree to which this bias can affect estimates, we present results in Table 3-6 from LASI's biomarker module. Specifically, we report the percentage with high blood pressure who reported never receiving a diagnosis for hypertension by a health professional. Thirty-one percent of the sample population had undiagnosed hypertension. In Rajasthan, 41% of respondents had undiagnosed hypertension, while in Kerala, only half that percentage registered undiagnosed hypertension. The high prevalence points to the sizable incidence of noncommunicable diseases, the burden of conditions that go unrecognized and untreated, as well as the wide disparity in access to health services (Alwan et al., 2010; Mahal, Karan, and Engelgau, 2010).

In addition to measuring health, LASI assessed self-reported disability rates. Disability was measured by difficulty with at least one activity of daily life (ADL) and averaged 13% across all states, with older people in Kerala reporting the most difficulty and those in Rajasthan the least. While there is some doubt about the validity of self-reported health measures (Sen, 2002), other literature has shown that ADLs and measures of disability in particular can be useful in understanding health burdens in this population along with other research that shows self-reported measures are reasonable to use in the developing country context (Subramanian et al., 2009).

Tables 3-7 and 3-8 focus on LASI's measure of difficulty with ADLs, with particular attention to a well-documented sex gradient (Sengupta and Agree, 2003). Self-reported ADLs have been shown to be good markers for the health status of Indians (Chen and Mahal, 2010). Table 3-7 shows the number of disabilities reported by men and women in LASI. Of those respondents who reported difficulty with ADLs, most reported difficulty with only one or two of the activities. Women more often reported at least one difficulty with an ADL. Among women, the most common difficulties were walking across a room and getting in and out of bed. Men also reported the most difficulty with walking across a room and getting in and out of bed, although at older ages getting dressed and walking across the room were the most common difficulties (see Table 3-8).

Stratifying the associations we observe between sex and disability by age illustrates an even stronger sex disparity in health among aging Indians in our sample. Noticeably, about 50% of women aged 75 years and older report difficulty with at least one ADL, compared to only 24% of men. This disparity begins to widen among the sample at age 65, a group that includes many widows who are often left with little familial support (Sengupta and Agree, 2003). Moreover, Table 3-8 shows that this widening disparity in self-reported difficulty with ADLs does not just occur at the aggregate across all measures, but for each of the six activities asked about in LASI.

Delving deeper, we examine the socioeconomic correlates of (1) self-reported health, (2) ADL disability, and (3) a cognitive function exam administered as part of LASI (see Table 9 at http://www.hsph.harvard.

TABLE 3-7 Distribution of Difficulty with ADLs by Gender Among Respondents Aged 45 Years and Older

Count of Difficult ADLs	0	1	2	3	4	5
Number of Respondents	1,236	95	42	19	12	14
Men (%)	88.8	5.8	2.3	0.9	0.9	1.0
Women (%)	84.2	7.0	2.9	2.1	1.0	1.2

NOTES: Among respondents with only one difficult ADL, the most common was getting in and out of bed; among respondents with two difficult ADLs, the most frequent were getting in and out bed and using a toilet; among respondents with three difficult ADLs, the most commonly reported were difficulty walking across a room, bathing, and using a toilet; among respondents who reported difficulty with four ADLs, the most frequent were walking across a room, bathing, using the toilet, and getting in and out of bed; and among those respondents with five difficult ADLs, the most common were walking across a room, bathing, getting in and out of bed, and the same number of respondents reported difficulty with the remaining ADLs. The sample for this table is restricted to respondents who self-reported an age of at least 45 years in the individual interview. Percentages are weighted using the pooled-state weight.
SOURCE: Data from Longitudinal Aging Study in India (LASI) Pilot Wave.

TABLE 3-8 Distribution of Difficulty with ADLs by Gender and Age

Difficulty with...	Gender	Age 45+	45–54	55–64	65–74	75+
Any ADL	Men	11.2	6.7	10.4	16.6	24.1
	Women	15.9	9.9	10.1	22.9	48.4
Dressing	Men	4.7	2.0	4.4	6.1	15.5
	Women	4.3	2.2	1.9	2.3	24.6
Walking across a room	Men	4.9	3.0	3.4	5.3	17.5
	Women	7.8	4.2	3.5	11.8	29.0
Bathing	Men	3.2	1.2	2.8	5.5	9.4
	Women	5.8	2.7	2.4	7.4	26.3
Eating	Men	2.2	0.9	1.4	5.1	4.3
	Women	6.5	3.1	3.7	6.5	29.8
Getting in and out of bed	Men	4.9	2.8	3.6	8.7	10.7
	Women	8.9	5.5	5.1	12.8	28.8
Toileting	Men	3.9	1.2	4.1	6.6	10.1
	Women	6.8	4.3	1.5	9.7	28.3

NOTES: Respondents were asked if "due to health or memory problem" they have difficulty dressing themselves, walking across a room, bathing, eating foods, getting in and out of bed, and using the toilet. Responses are: yes, no, can't do, and don't want to do. Respondents who answered yes or that they cannot do the task were considered to have an ADL difficulty. Percentages are weighted using the pooled-state weight among the sample of respondents that self-reported an age of at least 45 years.
SOURCE: Data from Longitudinal Aging Study in India (LASI) Pilot Wave.

edu/pgda/WorkingPapers/2011/PGDA_WP_82.pdf). We observe statistically significant differences in self-reported health by age group. Older respondents report poorer self-rated health as do widows, respondents from Kerala, and the less educated. The results for difficulty with ADLs are reasonably similar, with the additional indication that women (but not widows or more educated respondents) are more likely to report difficulty with at least one ADL. Unlike self-reported health, we do not observe a statistically significant effect for education after controlling for other factors.

Cognitive health is a growing concern among aging populations in developing countries, yet remains understudied in India[11] (Jotheeswaran, Williams, and Prince, 2010; Prince, 1997). LASI includes measures of verbal and numerical fluency, as well as episodic memory recall that have been used among low-literacy aging populations in India (Ganguli et al., 1996; Mathuranath et al., 2009). Figure 3-2 focuses on episodic word recall. LASI combines two measures of word recall— immediate and delayed— to create a summary measure used in our analysis.

Unlike in studies in the United States and the United Kingdom, women in India perform worse than men on measures of cognitive health (Lang et al., 2008; Langa et al., 2008), as shown in Figure 3-2. While women tend to be less educated and older than men in India, LASI data show the female disadvantage in cognitive health persists even after controlling for these risk factors. Similar cognitive disparity between men and women has been found in other developing countries (Zunzunegui et al., 2008). Nevertheless, the factors that account for the cognitive shortfall among women deserve further exploration (Lee et al., 2012).

Regional differences were seen in the health measures, which cover both self-reported general health and self-reported disability, and one objective measure of health: episodic memory. Respondents from Kerala report worse health, somewhat surprising given Kerala's health system, access to community insurance, low infant mortality, long life expectancy, and high levels of education. Reasons why older people from Kerala report worse health may include the following: (1) higher morbidity and disability rates; (2) higher likelihood that people with better education and awareness report their ill health; (3) prevalence of smoking and drinking; (4) an elderly population that is older than in other states; and (5) high burdens of noncommunicable and cardiovascular diseases, including, of course, among Kerala's older population (Kumar, 1993; Rajan and James,

---

[11]Current studies of cognitive and mental health in India are based on small sample sizes from single cities, ignoring sociocultural and regional variation. Moreover, many of these studies examine dementia and specific neuro-degenerative diseases, while ignoring possibly more prevalent and sub-clinical forms of cognitive health impairment.

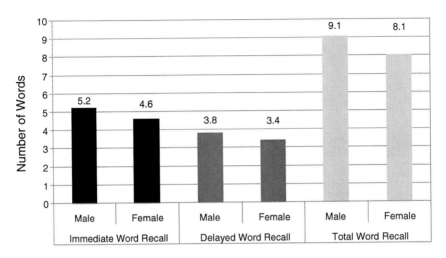

FIGURE 3-2 Cognitive performance among respondents 45 years and older by gender.
NOTES: The immediate word recall task asks respondents to recall as many words as they can from a list of 10 words immediately after the interviewer reads them aloud. Delayed word recall asks respondents to name as many words as they can after completion of a cognitive functioning questionnaire. Both delayed and immediate word recall are scored with a maximum of 10 words. Total word recall is the sum of these two. Three lists of 10 words were used, and were randomly assigned to a respondent. The standard deviation for immediate word recall pooled across both men and women was 1.9, 2.0 for delayed recall, and 3.5 for total word recall. Data for the graph are limited to respondents who self-reported an age of at least 45 years. Statistics reported in the figure are weighted by the pooled-state weight.
SOURCE: Data from Longitudinal Aging Study in India (LASI) Pilot Wave.

1993; Suryanarayana, 2008). There are also large differences between Kerala and the other states with regard to cognitive health.

As another example of health issues faced by older Indians, Table 3-6 reports the results of self-reported food insecurity among respondents. These levels may seem low for India, but they reflect substantial efforts on the part of the Indian government to reduce hunger and famine. Examining another measure, such as body mass index, illustrates that basic food provision is still a concern (see "Underweight" in Table 3-6). Body mass index has proven to be an effective marker for chronic energy deficiency in developing countries (Chaudhuri, 2009; Ferro-Luzzi et al., 2009; Nube et al., 1998). Rajasthan has the highest prevalence of underweight individuals, yet lower rates of self-reported hunger and food shortage. Com-

TABLE 3-9 Who Pays for Healthcare?

Respondent Characteristics	Relies on Family to Pay
Aged 55–64	0.112
	(1.05)
Aged 65–74	0.242*
	(2.12)
Aged 75+	0.463**
	(2.85)
Female	0.437***
	(3.94)
Education (yrs)	−0.033*
	(−2.44)
Rajasthan	−1.069***
	(−4.10)
Kerala	−0.261
	(−1.52)
Karnataka	−0.824***
	(−5.28)
Rural	−0.060
	(−0.52)
Scheduled caste	−0.299
	(−1.83)
Scheduled tribe	−0.211
	(−0.70)
Other backward caste	−0.252*
	(−2.31)
HH Consumption (middle tertile)	−0.225
	(−1.74)
HH Consumption (highest tertile)	−0.304*
	(−2.08)
Episodic memory 1	−0.662*
	(−2.23)
Episodic memory 2	−0.807*
	(−2.59)
Episodic memory 3	−0.451
	(−1.73)
Any ADL disability	−0.028
	(−0.21)
Chronic condition	−0.023
	(−0.24)
Working	−0.069
	(−0.48)
Constant	1.399***
	(3.72)
N	1,311
F-stat	6.45***
Estimator	probit

TABLE 3-9 Continued

NOTES: In this model, we create a categorical scheme for our measure of cognitive health using episodic memory recall. We derive four dummies: episodic memory 1 includes respondents (18%) who were able to recall 0 to 5 words out of 20; episodic memory 2 includes respondents with 6 to 10 words (54%); episodic memory 3 includes respondents with 11 to 15 words, and the final category (omitted) was for the 3% of respondents who could recall 16 or more of the 20 possible words. The sample is restricted to respondents who self-reported an age of at least 45. Chronic condition is self-reported diabetes, heart disease, lung disease, stroke or hypertension. Working is defined as engaging in any labor market activity in the past 12 months; and any ADL is a binary indicator for having difficulty with at least one ADL. LASI used a stratified sampling design that sampled respondents independently by state, rural-urban area, and district. All multivariate models are unweighted, and the standard errors have been corrected for design effects of stratification. Table presents coefficients with t statistics in parentheses. * denotes $p < 0.05$; ** $p < 0.01$; *** $p < 0.001$.
SOURCE: Longitudinal Aging Study in India (LASI) Pilot Wave.

paring these results to self-reported measures highlights the multiplicity of health concerns among the aging Indian population, and the difficulty in ascertaining accurate reports of disease burden.

Table 3-9 indicates that many aging Indians rely on their family networks to pay for healthcare. Although India has free, government-sponsored public healthcare, most Indians, even the poorest, opt to use private services over government facilities (Gupta and Dasgupta, 2003). However, with longer lives, an increasing chronic disease burden, rising healthcare costs, and a shortage of service facilities and healthcare workers in India, the older population's access to healthcare is increasingly tenuous. In the LASI data, more than 80% of respondents indicated that they themselves or their family would have to pay for any sort of healthcare. We focus on this set of respondents below, fitting a multivariate model to better understand the determinants of family-reliance for healthcare costs.[12]

The results reflect notable demographic and regional differences in healthcare accessibility. Older members are increasingly reliant on their family for support, as are women, perhaps because of more complex medical needs and little cash-earning potential. By contrast, respondents with more education and higher household socioeconomic status are more likely to pay out of their own pocket, suggesting that households responsible for the well-being of their aging family members are among the poorest.

---

[12]Respondents are considered to "rely on family to pay" if they wholly (48.2%) or partially (12.9%) rely on the family to finance the costs, either out of pocket or through a family member's insurance scheme (6.0%). Respondents not considered to rely on family indicated that they alone finance their healthcare out of pocket (38.9%).

In addition, these results[13] reflect the traditional intra-household support system, but they also suggest important levers for implementing policy to ensure well-being in old age. Women tend to be more reliant on family networks for access to healthcare. Older respondents also tend to rely on family members, which reflects loss of economic agency and increasing burden of age-related morbidities. Finally, there is some interesting regional variations. Respondents in Rajasthan and Kerala are much less likely to have family members who would pay for their healthcare, despite the larger household sizes. The same pattern holds in comparatively more developed Karnataka. Another salient finding is that individuals who report working in the past year are more likely to rely on themselves for healthcare. (This model excludes respondents who reported having their healthcare expenses paid by their employer or by an insurance company.) Further analysis of who provides and who pays for elder care, as well as who makes the decisions and what drives those decisions, is possible using the LASI pilot data and would be worthwhile.

Regional associations should, of course, be interpreted with caution. While respondents from both Karnataka and Rajasthan are more likely to rely on their own out-of-pocket expenditures for healthcare, the two states have vastly different socioeconomic profiles. While Karnataka is more affluent, as noted earlier, Rajasthan is one of the poorest states in India, with the aging men and women largely paying for their own medical expenses out of pocket.

Measuring Health: Innovations in LASI

State-of-the-art survey methods,[14] in addition to their diverse measures to assess the multiplicity of health concerns, are a hallmark of LASI. For example, anchoring vignettes permit refined analysis of many subjective survey responses. The World Health Organization has made

---

[13]We also present results from additional models of healthcare utilization in an earlier and more detailed version of this paper, which is available online at http://www.hsph.harvard.edu/pgda/WorkingPapers/2011/PGDA_WP_82.pdf. The models further corroborate our understanding of patterns of healthcare use among the aged in India, drawing support from a wider range of outcome variables to model visiting a doctor when ill, undiagnosed hypertension, and preventive measures such as a cholesterol check. These models reflect demographic, regional, and economic patterns that we observe in this paper.

[14]LASI also includes innovations that are not related to health. Among them are (1) some specific types of questions about assets and income; (2) use of a geographic information system database to support community-level analysis; (3) questions about water quality, sanitation, and safety in the neighborhood; and (4) questions about a broad range of psychological, social, and behavioral risk factors (e.g., measuring social connectedness in addition to traditional social network questions).

extensive use of vignettes in several of its SAGE surveys around the world (Kowal et al., 2010), as have several of LASI's sister surveys.

Anchoring vignettes allow researchers to correct for cross-person heterogeneity in the subjective nature of responses to some health questions by asking respondents to characterize a set of short hypothetical stories (vignettes) that describe fictional individuals with varying health problems. Respondents' scoring of a common set of vignettes may allow researchers to standardize answers to self-health questions that naturally require subjective answers.[15]

However, vignettes can only serve their intended purpose if respondents can understand and make reasonable assessments of them. For example, respondents should rank a vignette intended to describe someone in extreme pain as exhibiting a much higher level of pain than one intended to show very mild pain. If a respondent does not rank the vignettes in the intended order, the scoring should not be used to adjust the respondent's answers to questions about severity of pain.

In the LASI pilot, roughly one-half the respondents ranked the vignettes in an order that was different from the intended order. In these cases, it was therefore impossible to use the vignettes to adjust respondents' answers. Several studies explore the reasons for unexpected results in vignette ranking and possible means for avoiding or remedying such situations (for example, Delevande, Gine, and McKenzie, 2010; Gol-Propoczyk, 2010; Hopkins and King, 2010; Lancasr and Louviere, 2006; and Mangham, Hanson, and McPake, 2009). Because this required us to ignore a large fraction of respondents, we caution against extrapolating these results to a larger population. We did a multivariate analysis to try to find patterns that distinguish those whose answers we had to ignore from those that were usable, but no significant patterns emerged.

Using data restricted to respondents whose vignette rankings were in the expected order, Figure 3-3 shows the results of two anchoring vignettes for pain and mobility. Respondents were asked to rate the degree to which they experience bodily aches and pains and have trouble moving around. The vignettes suggest respondents who have some difficulty moving around and report some chronic pain tend to underreport the severity.[16]

---

[15]The vignettes module in LASI is randomly assigned to one-third of the sample (n = 463); it is one of three experimental modules in the survey. In addition to vignettes about pain and difficulty with mobility, other vignettes include sleep difficulty, concentration, shortness of breath, feeling sad/low/depressed, bathing, and personal relationships.

[16]Here, we are careful to distinguish between measures of disability and the questions in the vignette section, which may at first seem incongruent. The six questions about ADL ask specifically if the respondent is unable (without help) to do a series of tasks because of a "health or memory problem." However, the vignettes ask much more generally about pain and mobility: an older person, for example, may have chronic back pain, but otherwise be

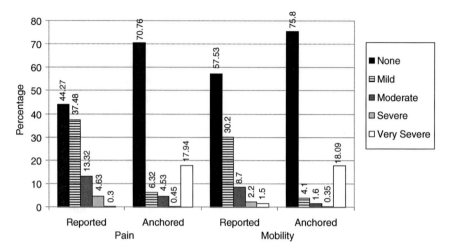

FIGURE 3-3 Pain and mobility difficulty vignettes for LASI respondents aged 45 years and older.

NOTES: The sample size is 232 for pain and 202 for mobility, among respondents who self-reported an age of at least 45 years. Responses are weighted using the pooled state-weight.

SOURCE: Data from Longitudinal Aging Study in India (LASI) Pilot Wave.

The data imply nearly one-fifth of respondents could have very severe pain or mobility problems, while less than 2% for each domain reported so originally. For both pain and mobility, the number of respondents who experience "none" is much higher than initially reported, while the number of respondents who have very severe problems within either domain increases substantially.

Social and Civic Participation among the Aged and Aging

Aside from physical and economic well-being, LASI provides a snapshot of daily life, particularly social and civic participation in local communities. The LASI pilot found that men tended to be more social than women and that the most common social activities[17] for both sexes were visiting friends/relatives, attending cultural events or performances, and

---

able to move around by him or herself, use the toilet, eat a meal, bathe, and get dressed. Among older populations, this sort of pain is likely to be more prevalent than severe disabilities that prevent someone from functioning day to day.

[17]For social activities, LASI asks about going to the cinema, eating outside the house, going to a park or beach, playing cards or games, visiting relatives/friends, attending cultural performances/shows, and attending religious functions/events.

attending religious festivals and functions. Men were more likely than women to report eating outside the home, visiting a park or beach, and playing cards or games. Sex differences in social participation are present even when stratified by age. Overall, social participation declines for both men and women in the LASI sample as respondents age. For example, prevalence of visiting friends or relatives drops from 85% among women aged 45 to 54 to 58% among women aged 75 and older.

In the LASI sample, civic participation[18] is much less common overall than social activity, but is more common among women than men (although gender differences drop out in the multivariate models below). This is likely because LASI asks about *mahila mandal*, a women's self-help and empowerment group. Evidence is limited that women participate in caste and community organizations, as well other activities. Men participate in self-help and nongovernmental organizations (NGOs)/ senior citizen clubs/farmers associations, and community and caste organizations.

In results not reported here (but included in the earlier online version of this paper), we explored the association between the demographic and socioeconomic characteristics, and civic and social participation. Because civic participation was relatively low in the LASI sample, we estimate a probit model and regress a binary indicator for any civic participation on the list of covariates. Social activities are more common than civic participation. We look at social participation by regressing the number of social activities per month on the same list of covariates using OLS estimation. We see a significant negative association with age and civic participation only among respondents at least 75 years of age. Respondents with more years of education were also more likely to participate in their community, as were respondents in the two southern states. An association between civic participation and health, as measured by difficulty with at least one ADL, is not apparent.

Social participation shows a similar association with age, with a statistically significant decrease in social participation in age only among respondents aged 75 and older. After controlling for the full set of respondent characteristics and regional indicators, we no longer see a sex difference in civic participation. We do see a statistically significant decrease in social participation among women, but this is not attributable to lower educational attainment or older age. Respondents in Rajasthan and Kerala

---

[18]LASI asks about respondents' participation in farmers' associations/environmental groups/political parties/senior citizen clubs; tenant groups, neighborhood watch, community/caste organizations; self-help group/NGO/cooperative/mahila mandal; education, arts or music groups, evening classes; social clubs, sport clubs, exercise classes, and any other organizations that we consider civic participation.

were less likely to participate in social activities compared with those in other states.

These models provide some evidence that aging Indians continue to stay involved in their communities as they age. They stop working for pay, are active outside the home, and participate in broader civic and social networks. The LASI pilot suggests research in civic and social networks in India is promising. Previous studies have supported the importance of civic and social participation for successful aging and health, and we see some evidence of that with the connection between difficulty with activities of daily life and social participation (Berkman et al., 2000; Moen, Dempster-McClain, and Williams, 1992; Seeman and Crimmins, 2006).

Economic Well-Being of the Aging

LASI provides considerable information about the economic activity and well-being of India's aging population. Workforce participation, for example, is central in a country without social security or pensions, particularly as intergenerational support—once the traditional and widespread means of old age support—becomes less common (Bloom et al., 2010). Given that less than 11% of older people in India have access to a pension or social security, economic activity is especially important. Additionally, private saving is often difficult or entirely infeasible for several reasons: earnings are low, a significant portion of the economic activity is informal and may not be tied to cash exchange, and bank accounts are often not available in rural India (Uppal and Sarma, 2007).

We examine labor force participation (defined as any employment, self-employment, or agricultural work in the past 12 months) in the LASI sample among respondents who are aged 45 and older. Table 3-10 presents five models of labor force participation. The results show older respondents are less likely to work, particularly in urban areas. Women are less likely to report having worked, as are respondents who report difficulty or disability with at least one ADL. The association between disability and economic activity points to the important relationship between health and economic well-being among the vulnerable and aging Indian population, although one cannot infer the direction of causality. These findings are consistent with results of similar studies (Bakshi and Pathak, 2010). Studies from other developing countries, such as China, have found health is a significant correlate of labor market participation among socioeconomically disadvantaged populations (Benjamin, Brandt, and Fan, 2003).

We do not see employment differences by education or caste. Respondents in Rajasthan are more likely to be working than respondents in other states. This finding is consistent with the largely agricultural economies in

Rajasthan and other rural areas, which absorb older workers more consistently in comparison with manufacturing and other types of economies in developing countries (Bakshi and Pathak, 2010; Nasir and Ali, 2000).

Education is not correlated with labor force participation among our sample aged 45 years and older, with the exception of the model for nonagricultural labor. Consistent with the literature, respondents with more education are slightly more likely to engage in nonagricultural labor than those with less, even after controlling for a variety of socioeconomic and regional indicators. However, our findings are somewhat inconsistent with results elsewhere that suggest educated individuals are more likely to accumulate savings and participate in formal labor markets, leading to earlier labor-market withdrawal. Our estimates reveal insignificant associations with education and all other forms of work across rural and urban sectors. However, the model could mask regional heterogeneity: When we estimate the models without state dummies, we find statistically significant relationships between education and labor force participation in nonagricultural sectors, work in rural areas (model 2), and agricultural work (model 4). In these three models without state dummies, more educated individuals were less likely to be working. Regional differences in availability of pension schemes, old age support, and labor markets account for the association between education and labor force participation in our sample. Given the lack of social security, pension, and health insurance available to most Indians, continued workforce participation is vital. However, working imposes a strain on aging individuals, and many often do so out of desperation or necessity. Policies can focus on the health of the aging workforce, so they may stay engaged in more productive work.

We also examine household expenditure. Among households, we analyze the demographic and regional correlates of household consumption expenditure to understand socioeconomic gradients in the LASI sample and to some extent in India as well. Figure 3-4 displays the distribution of annual household expenditure (in rupees, and including imputed amounts) per equivalent adult across LASI respondents aged 45 and older. Equivalency scales developed by the Organisation for Economic Co-operation and Development (OECD) are used to account for economies of scale in household consumption.[19]

Table 3-11 reports three regression models of household expenditure per equivalent adult among LASI respondents. Large households tend to have lower per capita expenditure. Across the pooled urban and rural sam-

---

[19]Equivalent adults are calculated counting the first person aged 18 and older as 1.0 equivalent adults, each additional person aged 18 and older as 0.7 equivalent adults, and each person under age 18 as 0.5 equivalent adults. See http://www.oecd.org/dataoecd/61/52/35411111.pdf.

TABLE 3-10 Demographic and Regional Variation in Binary Indicator for Any Employment in Past Year

	All Work, Rural and Urban Respondents	All Work, Rural Respondents	All Work, Urban Respondents	Agricultural Work, Rural Respondents	Nonagricultural Work, Urban, and Rural Respondents
Aged 55–64	-0.417***	-0.374**	-0.522*	-0.200	-0.357**
	(-4.23)	(-3.42)	(-2.23)	(-1.94)	(-3.29)
Aged 65–74	-0.689***	-0.612***	-0.966**	-0.317*	-0.542**
	(-5.69)	(-4.33)	(-4.31)	(-2.39)	(-3.37)
Aged 75+	-1.227***	-1.103***	-1.889***	-0.737***	-0.926***
	(-6.47)	(-5.31)	(-4.42)	(-3.62)	(-4.26)
Female	-1.349***	-1.282***	-1.597***	-0.858***	-1.016***
	(-14.27)	(-14.26)	(-5.66)	(-9.89)	(-7.91)
Education (yrs)	-0.007	0.002	-0.022	-0.022	0.029*
	(-0.57)	(0.14)	(-1.03)	(-1.98)	(2.45)
Rajasthan	0.427**	0.389*	0.604**	0.531**	-0.070
	(2.80)	(2.16)	(3.34)	(2.88)	(-0.47)
Kerala	-0.086	-0.286	0.341	-0.432*	0.056
	(-0.53)	(-1.59)	(1.54)	(-2.10)	(0.44)
Karnataka	0.300	0.355	0.270	0.528**	-0.047
	(1.89)	(1.88)	(1.52)	(2.97)	(-0.36)
Rural	0.312**				-0.488***
	(2.97)				(-5.41)
Scheduled caste	0.211	0.108	0.473	-0.256	0.483*
	(1.53)	(0.69)	(1.88)	(-1.69)	(3.44)
Scheduled tribe	0.093	0.071	-0.041	0.040	-0.199
	(0.51)	(0.38)	(-0.09)	(0.26)	(-0.71)
Other backward caste	0.093	0.038	0.243	-0.101	0.175
	(0.98)	(0.33)	(2.13)	(-0.94)	(1.67)
ADL disability count	-0.150**	-0.112*	-0.263**	-0.107*	-0.089
	(-3.02)	(-2.06)	(-2.67)	(-2.12)	(-1.39)

Constant	0.478*	0.772**	0.582	0.108	−0.124
	(2.62)	(3.33)	(2.15)	(0.54)	(−0.85)
N	1,428	1,023	405	1,023	1,428
F-stat	20.74***	19.84***	14.01	19.56***	11.07***
Estimator	probit	probit	probit	probit	probit

NOTES: Labor force participation is a dummy variable for having worked in the past 12 months. It includes self-employment, employment by another, or agricultural work both paid and unpaid as reported in the household income module by a household financial respondent or self-reported in the individual interview. The sample is restricted to respondents who self-reported an age of at least 45 years old; LASI used a stratified sampling design, which sampled respondents independently by state, rural-urban area, and district. All multivariate models are unweighted, and the standard errors have been corrected for design effects of stratification. 44.6% of respondents were classified as working. ADL disability count is the number of activities of daily life the respondent has some difficulty with or cannot do. Table presents coefficients with t statistics in parentheses; * denotes $p < 0.05$; ** $p < 0.01$; *** $p < 0.001$.

SOURCE: Data from Longitudinal Aging Study in India (LASI) Pilot Wave.

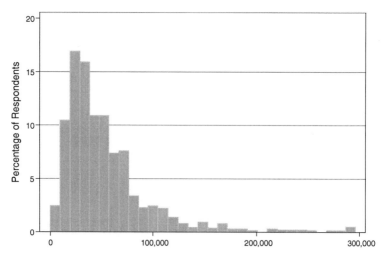

Distribution of per Equivalent Adult Expenditure Across LASI Respondents

FIGURE 3-4 Distribution of annual household expenditure per equivalent adult for age-eligible LASI respondents.
NOTES: The mean annual per equivalent adult expenditure taken across respondents (aged 45+) is 54,986 rupees, and the median is 41,993 rupees. The 3% of respondents with more than 300,000 Rs per capita were excluded from this graph.
SOURCE: Data from Longitudinal Aging Study in India (LASI) Pilot Wave.

ple, scheduled castes, especially those in rural areas, have lower per capita consumption, reflecting in part the geographic isolation of rural communities. Other affiliations are also significant: scheduled tribes in urban areas also have statistically lower per capita consumption. This reflects a continued disadvantage for these groups despite many initiatives by the Indian government to improve their well-being (Subramanian et al., 2008).

Table 3-11 also reflects geographic differences in households' per capita consumption. Households in Rajasthan have lower expenditures, especially in rural areas. To account for the effects of household composition by gender and age, we examine the percentage of women in the household and both the youth and elderly dependency ratio. The youth dependency ratio is the number of respondents under 15 years of age divided by the number of respondents of working age, which we define as ages 15 to 59. Our results show that a higher youth dependency ratio lowers per capita expenditure, presumably reflecting standard life cycle patterns of earnings and expenditure (Bloom et al., 2011).

Interestingly, we do not see significant effects of the percentage of women or older people on expenditure. This finding is somewhat puzzling

TABLE 3-11 Demographic and Regional Variation in Household Expenditure per Equivalent Adult

Household Characteristics	All	Urban	Rural
Rural HH	−0.017		
	(−0.19)		
HH size	−0.026*	−0.061	−0.012
	(−2.62)	(−1.86)	(−1.15)
Scheduled caste	−0.449***	−0.334*	−0.488***
	(−4.90)	(−2.67)	(−4.31)
Scheduled tribe	−0.352	−0.889**	−0.331
	(−1.98)	(−3.25)	(−1.72)
Other backward caste	−0.123	−0.103	−0.151
	(−1.30)	(−0.91)	(−1.30)
Rajasthan	−0.261	−0.167	−0.315
	(−1.90)	(−1.16)	(−1.79)
Kerala	−0.112	−0.023	−0.128
	(−1.04)	(−0.13)	(−0.99)
Karnataka	0.299*	0.514	0.207
	(2.28)	(1.97)	(1.48)
Youth dependency ratio	−0.167*	−0.180	−0.171*
	(−2.49)	(−0.93)	(−2.51)
Elderly dependency ratio	−0.017	−0.107	−0.006
	(−0.31)	(−0.65)	(−0.11)
Percentage of women in HH	−0.315	−0.713*	−0.164
	(−1.98)	(−2.21)	(−1.09)
Constant	11.31***	−0.167	11.19***
	(75.51)	(−1.16)	(71.08)
N	730	207	523
R sq.	0.1681	0.2300	0.1536
F-stat	6.61***	3.81	5.78***
Estimator	OLS	OLS	OLS

NOTES: Dependent variable is log of household expenditure per equivalent adult household member. The unit of observation is the household, not the individual in these models. The youth dependency ratio is the number of household members 0 to 14 years of age divided by the number of household members 15 to 59 years of age. The elderly dependency ratio is the number of household members aged 60 years and older divided by the number of household members 15 to 59 years of age. The models also exclude households where expenditure was imputed. LASI used a stratified sampling design that sampled respondents independently by state, rural-urban area, and district. All multivariate models are unweighted and the standard errors have been corrected for design effects of stratification. Standard errors are corrected for design effects and stratified on state, urban/rural residence, and district. Caste is the caste of the head of the household. Table presents coefficients with t statistics in parentheses. * denotes $p < 0.05$; ** $p < 0.01$; *** $p < 0.001$.
SOURCE: Data from Longitudinal Aging Study in India (LASI) Pilot Wave.

given the relatively low labor force participation rates of women and older household members. These two results suggest that older household members, as well as women, are contributing to the household economy in other ways not measured by labor force participation, or cash inflows. This may be especially true for rural households where much of the work is agricultural and subsistence-based, and women and older people may be contributing mostly undocumented household labor. Indeed, in urban areas where this type of household work is less common, we see that the percentage of women in the household is significant and negative, reflecting their lower earnings (either cash or in-kind).

CONCLUSION

LASI is well positioned to play a critical role in the conduct of rigorous policy-relevant research as India continues substantial transitions in the demographic, economic, and epidemiologic domains. The fact that the LASI pilot achieved high response rates and that respondent demographics are similar to those of other nationally representative surveys within India lends credibility to the survey's results concerning the well-being of aging Indians.

This chapter highlights the wide geographic variability in health, social, and economic markers across India. Even after adjusting for demographic differences, we still observe state-level variation across all three domains. Capturing the regional heterogeneity is critical for designing effective policy, and the main wave of LASI will expand on this by sampling 15 or more states and possibly two union territories as well.

Our analysis focuses on the well-being and economic status of aging Indians. While the country seeks to develop economically, basic living conditions and emerging health concerns are major problems. Our analysis (herein and in the earlier online version) reveals socioeconomic gradients across a variety of health domains, including both subjective and objective measures of self-rated health, disability, and cognitive functioning. With little institutional support, the aging population's economic activity is of particular importance given the relative absence of social security and health insurance. Our findings show that aging family members continue to be contributing members of the household economy. Improving the health of aging Indians could foster higher labor force participation as well. The social and civic lives of older Indians are also key to understanding their contributions to communities. We have found that even the oldest individuals remain socially engaged and that aging women, especially, continue to contribute to civic life in their community.

Early results from LASI suggest that older Indians are subject to a wide-ranging set of health, social, and financial insecurities, with a good deal of variation in myriad dimensions. Conduct of blood assays, expansion of the LASI sample, and collection of longitudinal data are the planned next steps in this effort. Such an evidence base should provide researchers with the raw material they need to better understand aging in India and to design policies that will improve the experience.

REFERENCES

Ahmed, A.U., H.A. Khan, and R.K. Sampath. (1991). Poverty in Bangladesh: Measurement, decomposition and intertemporal comparison. *Journal of Development Studies 27(4)*:48-63.

Alam, M. (2004). Ageing, old age income security and reforms: An exploration of Indian situation. *Economic and Political Weekly 39(33)*:731-740.

Alwan, A., D.R. MacLean, L.M. Riley, E.T. d'Espaignet, D. Mathers, G.A. Stevens, and D. Bettcher. (2010). Monitoring the surveillance of chronic non-communicable disease: Progress and capacity in high-burden countries. *The Lancet 376*:1,861-1,868.

Bakshi, S., and P. Pathak. (2010). *Who Works at Older Ages? The Correlates of Economic Activity and Temporal Changes in Their Effects: Evidence from India.* Working paper, Indian Statistical Institute, Kolkata.

Benjamin, D., L. Brandt, and J.Z. Fan. (2003). *Ceaseless Toil? Health and Labour Supply of the Elderly in Rural China.* University of Toronto manuscript. Available: http://www.princeton.edu/rpds/papers/pdfs/benjamin_ceaseless_toil.pdf.

Berkman L., T. Glass, I. Brissette, and T. Seeman. (2000). From social integration to health: Durkheim in the new millennium. *Social Science and Medicine 51*:843-857.

Bloom, D.E. (2005). Education and public health: Mutual challenges worldwide: Guest editor's overview. *Comparative Education Review 49(4)*:437-451.

Bloom, D.E. (2011a). 7 billion and counting. *Science 33*:562-569.

Bloom, D.E. (2011b). India's baby boomers: Dividend or disaster? *Current History (April)*:143-149.

Bloom, D.E., D. Canning, and G. Fink. (2010). Implications of population aging for economic growth. *Oxford Review of Economic Policy 26(4)*:583-612.

Bloom, D.E., D. Mahal, L. Rosenberg, and J. Sevilla. (2010). Economic security arrangements in the context of population aging in India. *International Social Security Review 63*:3-4.

Bloom, D.E., D. Canning, G. Fink, and J. Finlay. (2011). *Micro Foundations of the Demographic Dividend.* Paper presented at the International Union for the Scientific Study of Population Seminar on Demographics and Macroeconomic Performance, June 2010. Revision presented at the 2011 Annual Meetings of the Population Association of America.

Boersch-Supan, A., and A. Ludwig. (2010). Old Europe is aging: Reforms and reform backlashes. Pp. 169-204 in *Demography and the Economy*, J. Shoven (Ed.). Chicago: University of Chicago Press.

Chaudhuri, A. (2009). Spillover impacts of a reproductive health program on elderly women in rural Bangladesh. *Journal of Family Economic Issues 30*:113-125.

Chen, B., and A. Mahal. (2010). Measuring the health of the Indian elderly: Evidence from National Sample Survey data. *Population Health Metrics 8*:30.

Clark, T.A., and D. Ning. (2007). Towards a spatially disaggregated material-based hardship index for the cities of developing nations. *International Development Planning and Review 29(10)*:69-92.

Dandekar, K. (1996). *The Elderly in India.* New Delhi: SAGE.

Delevande, A., X. Gine, and D. McKenzie. (2010). Measuring subjective expectations in developing countries: A critical review and new evidence. *Journal of Development Economics 94*:151-163.

Ferro-Luzzi, A., S. Sette, M. Franklin, and W.P.T. James. (2009). A simplified approach of assessing adult chronic energy deficiency. *European Journal of Clinical Nutrition* 46:173-186.

Ganguli, M., G. Ratcliff, V. Chandra, S.D. Sharma, S. Gilby, R. Pandav, S. Belle, C. Ryan, C. Baker, E. Seaberg, and S. Dekosky. (1996). A Hindi version of the MMSE: The development of a cognitive screening instrument for a largely illiterate rural population in India. *International Journal of Geriatric Psychiatry* 10:367-377.

Gol-Propoczyk, H. (2010). *Age, Sex, and Race Effects in Anchoring Vignette Studies: Methodological and Empirical Contributions.* Center for Demography and Ecology, CDE working paper #2010-18, University of Wisconsin–Madison. Available: http://www.ssc.wisc.edu/cde/cdewp/2010-18.pdf.

Gupta, I., and P. Dasgupta. (2003). Health-seeking behavior in urban Delhi: An exploratory study. *World Health and Population 3(2).* Available: http://www.longwoods.com/publications/world-health-population/388.

Hopkins, D.I., and G. King. (2010). Improving anchoring vignettes: Designing surveys to correct for interpersonal incomparability. *Public Opinion Quarterly 74(2)*:201-222.

Husain, Z., and S. Ghosh. (2011). Is health status of elderly worsening in India? A comparison of successive rounds of the National Sample Survey data. *Journal of Biosocial Sciences 41(4)*:457-467.

Indian Human Development Survey. (2005). Home page. University of Maryland and National Council of Applied Economic Research, New Delhi. Available: http://ihds.umd.edu/.

International Institute for Population Sciences and Macro International. (2007). *National Family Health Survey (NFHS-3), 2005-2006: India.* Available: http://www.nfhsindia.org.

James, K.S. (2011). India's demographic change: Opportunities and challenges. *Science 333(6,042)*:576-580.

Jotheeswaran, A.T., J.D. Williams, and M.J. Prince. (2010). The predictive validity of the 10/66 dementia diagnosis in Chennai, India: A three-year follow up study of cases identifiable at baseline. *Alzheimer Disease and Associated Disorders 24(3)*:296-302.

Kowal, P., K. Kahn, N. Ng, N. Naidoo, S. Abdullah, A. Bawah, F. Binka, N. Chuc, C. Debpuur, A. Ezeh, F.X. Gomez-Olive, M. Hakimi, S. Hirve, A. Hodgson, S. Juvekar, C. Kyobutungi, J. Menken, H.V. Minh, O. Sankoh, K. Streatfield, S. Wall, S. Wliopo, P. Byass, S. Chatterji, and S.M. Tollman. (2010). Ageing and adult health status in eight lower-income countries: The in-depth WHO-SAGE collaboration. *Global Health Action Supplement, World Health Organization 3(2)*:11-22.

Kumar, B.G. (1993). Quality of life and morbidity: A reconstruction of some of the paradoxes from Kerala, India. *Population and Development Review 19(1)*:103-121.

Lancasr, E., and J. Louviere. (2006). Deleting irrational response from discrete choice experiments: A case of investigating or imposing preferences? *Health Economics* 15:797-811.

Lang, I.A., D.J. Llewellyn, K.M. Langa, R.B. Wallace, F.A. Huppert, and D. Melzer. (2008). Neighborhood deprivation, individual socioeconomic status, and cognitive functioning in older people: Analyses from the English Longitudinal Study of Aging. *Journal of the American Geriatric Society* 56:191-198.

Langa, K.M., E.B. Larson, J.H. Karlawish, D.M. Cutler, M.U. Kabeto, S.Y. Kim, and A.B. Rosen. (2008). Trends in the prevalence and mortality of cognitive impairment in the United States: Is there evidence of a compression of cognitive morbidity? *Alzheimer's & Dementia* 4:134-144.

Lee, J. (2010). Data sets on pensions and health: Data collection and sharing for policy design. *International Social Security Review 63(3-4)*:197-222.

Lee, J., R. Shih, K. Feeney, and K. Langa. (2011). *Cognitive Health of Older Indians: Individual and Geographic Determinants of Female Disadvantage.* Working paper #WR-889. Santa Monica, CA: RAND.

Lee, J., P. Arokiasamy, A. Chandra, P. Hu, J. Liu, and K. Feeney. (2012). Markers and drivers: Cardiovascular health of middle-aged and older Indians. Chapter 16 in *Aging in Asia: Findings from New and Emerging Data Initiatives*. J.P. Smith and M. Majmundar, Eds. Panel on Policy Research and Data Needs to Meet the Challenge of Aging in Asia. Committee on Population, Division of Behavioral and Social Sciences and Education. Washington, DC: The National Academies Press.

Longitudinal Aging Study in India, Pilot Wave. (2011). Harvard School of Public Health, International Institute of Population Sciences, Mumbai, India, and RAND Corporation. Available: https://mmicdata.rand.org/megametadata/?section=study&studyid=36.

Mahal, A., A. Karan, and M. Engelgau. (2010). *The Economic Implications of Non-Communicable Disease for India*. Washington, DC: World Bank.

Mangham, L.J., K. Hanson, and B. McPake. (2009). How to do (or not to do)...Designing a discrete choice experiment for application in a low income country. *Health Policy and Planning* 24:151-158.

Mathuranath, P.S., P.J. Cherian, R. Mather, S. Kumar, A. George, A. Alexander, N. Ranjith, and P.S. Sharma. (2009). Dementia in Kerala, South India: Prevalence and influence of age, education and gender. *International Journal of Geriatric Psychiatry* 25:290-297.

Ministry of Statistics and Programme Implementation. (2004). *National Sample Survey*. Government of India. Available: http://mospi.nic.in/mospi_new/site/inner. aspx?status=4&menu_id=87.

Moen, P., D. Dempster-McClain, and R.M. Williams. (1992). Successful aging: A life-course perspective on women's multiple roles and health. *American Journal of Sociology* 97:1,612-1,638.

Nasir, Z.M., and S.M. Ali. (2000). Labour market participation of the elderly. *The Pakistan Development Review* 39(4):1,075-1,086.

Nube, M., W.K. Asenso-Okyere, and G.J.M. van den Boom. (1998). Body mass index as indicator of standard of living in developing countries. *European Journal of Clinical Nutrition* 52:136-144.

Pal, S. (2007). *Intergenerational Transfers and Elderly Coresidence with Adult Children in Rural India*. IZA discussion paper #2847, University of Bonn, Germany.

Pal, S., and R. Palacios. (2008). *Understanding Poverty among the Elderly in India; Implications for Social Pension Policy*. IZA discussion paper #3431, University of Bonn, Germany.

Prince, M. (1997). The need for research on dementia in developing countries. *Tropical Medicine and International Health* 2(10):993-1,000.

Rajan, S.I., and K.S. James. (1993). Kerala's health status: Some issues. *Economic and Political Weekly* 28(36):1,889-1,892.

Registrar General, Census of India. (2001). *Socioeconomic Tables*. New Delhi: Office of the Registrar General, Government of India.

Registrar General of India, Census of India. (2011). *Census of India*. New Delhi: Office of the Registrar General, Ministry of Home Affairs, Government of India.

Seeman, T., and E. Crimmins. (2006). Social environment effects on aging and health. *Annals of the New York Academy of Sciences* 954:88-117.

Sen, A. (2002). Health: Perception versus observation. *British Medical Journal* 324(7,342):860-861.

Sengupta, M., and E. Agree. (2003). Gender, health, marriage and mobility difficulty among older adults in India. *Asia-Pacific Population Journal* 18(4):53-65.

Subramanian, S.V., L.K. Ackerson, M.A. Subramanyam, and K. Sivaramakrishnan. (2008). Health inequalities in India: The axes of stratification. *The Brown Journal of World Affairs* 14(2):127-138.

Subramanian, S.V., M.A. Subramanyam, S. Selvaraj, and I. Kawachi. (2009). Are self-reports of health and morbidities in developing countries misleading? Evidence from India. *Social Science & Medicine* 68:260-265.

Suryanarayana, M.H. (2008). *Morbidity Profiles of Kerala and All-India: An Economic Perspective.* Working paper #2008-007. Mumbia: Indira Gandhi Institute of Development Research, Mumbai. Available: http://www.igidr.ac.in/pdf/publication/WP-2008-007.pdf.

United Nations. (2011). *World Population Prospects: The 2010 Revision.* New York: United Nations Population Division.

Uppal, S., and S. Sarma. (2007). Aging, health and labour market activity: The case of India. *Journal of World Health and Population 9(4)*:79-97.

World Bank. (2002). *India: Household Energy, Indoor Air Pollution, and Health. ESMAP/South Asia Environment and Social Development Unit, November.* Washington, DC: World Bank.

World Health Organization. (2003). *World Health Survey.* Available: http://www.who.int/healthinfo/survey/en/.

World Health Organization. (2004). *WHO Medicines Strategy: Countries at the Core, 2004-2007.* Available: http://apps.who.int/medicinedocs/pdf/s5571e/s5571e.pdf.

World Health Organization. (2010). *Study on Global AGEing and Adult Health, Wave 1.* Available: http://www.who.int/healthinfo/systems/sage/en/index1.html.

Yip W., and A. Mahal. (2008). The health care systems of China and India: Performance and future challenges. *Health Affairs 27(4).*

Zunzunegui, M.V., B.E. Alvarado, F. Beland, and B. Vissandjee. (2008). Explaining health differences between men and women in later life: A cross-city comparison in Latin America and the Caribbean. *Social Science and Medicine 68*:235-242.

Economic Growth, Labor Markets, and Consumption

4

Population Aging, Intergenerational Transfers, and Economic Growth: Asia in a Global Context[1]

Ronald Lee and *Andrew Mason*

C ountries in Asia are at different points in the demographic transition. East Asian countries started earlier and are farther along, particularly Japan. The countries of South and Southeast Asia started later and are at a middle stage (Mason, Lee, and Lee, 2010). The changes in population growth rates and sizes over the transition are certainly important, but here we focus particularly on the changes in population age distributions and do not consider changes in the scale of the population.

Populations passing through the transition start with high proportions of children and low proportions of elderly and eventually move to the reverse situation: relatively few children and many elderly. In the earliest part of the transition, the proportions of children often increase because of declining infant and child mortality. In the middle of the transition, while fertility is declining, the proportions of the population in the working ages rise over a half-century or so and total dependency ratios fall. The resulting boost to per capita income growth is an important component of the "demographic dividend." However, as fertility bottoms out and the growth of the working age populations slows, the population ages as the ratio of elderly to working age rises. In the end, the proportion

[1]Research for this chapter was funded by parallel grants from the National Institutes of Health to Lee and Mason, NIA R37 AG025247 and R01 AG025488. We are grateful to Gretchen Donehower and Turro Wongkaren for their help and to all the country research teams in the National Transfer Account (NTA) project for use of their data. The researchers are identified and more detailed information is available for many countries in working papers on the NTA website: http://www.ntaccounts.org.

of the population in the working ages may be close to its level before the transition began—but with the elderly traded for dependent children.

Children and the elderly are similar from an economic perspective, because both groups have labor income that is small relative to their consumption. They must rely on sources other than their labor to provide for their material needs. However, children rely almost exclusively on public and private transfers to provide for their net consumption needs, while the elderly, in addition to these sources, may also rely on accumulated assets to fund their consumption. These assets have an important bearing on economic performance because they are a source of non-labor income and, in addition, if invested in the domestic economy, they raise its labor productivity. To the extent that the elderly rely on assets to fund their old age consumption, the burden on workers (and taxpayers) is reduced, and actual and anticipated population aging and longer life can accelerate the accumulation of capital and boost economic growth. To summarize, population aging has a negative effect on per capita consumption through increased dependency and may also have a positive effect through increased capital accumulation.

We will also suggest that lower fertility, the most important source of population aging, is associated with higher human capital investments per child. Thus, over the demographic transition, the quality and productivity of workers rise at the same time that their numbers fall. This change and the effects of population aging on physical capital provide two powerful mechanisms for maintaining or increasing standards of living despite the deterioration in the support ratio.

Estimates in this chapter are based on National Transfer Accounts (NTAs), an international project that draws on the work of research teams in 36 countries on six continents to estimate age profiles of key economic flows across age (see http://www.ntaccounts.org). We will present data for a subset of 23 countries, listed in Table 4-1, along with the dates to which the NTA estimates refer.

NATIONAL TRANSFER ACCOUNTS: DATA AND METHODS

NTAs are composed of four broad economic flows: labor income, consumption, transfers, and asset-based flows. Where appropriate, flows are distinguished by whether they are public or private and by their purpose (education, health, and other). The relationship among the flows is captured by the flow constraint: The gap between consumption and labor income must equal net transfers plus asset-based flows. Only a brief overview of methods can be provided here. They are documented fully in Lee and Mason et al. (2011) and Mason et al. (2009).

The age profiles of labor income and consumption provide a cross-

TABLE 4-1 Annual Rate of Change of Support Ratio, 2010 to 2050, Sorted by Rate

Economies (Code) Year	Annual Change (%)
Austria (AT) 2000, Germany (DE) 2003, Japan (JP) 2004, Slovenia (SL) 2004, South Korea (KR) 2000, Spain (ES) 2000, Taiwan (TW) 1998	−0.82 to −0.60
China (CN) 2002, Finland (FI) 2004, Hungary (HU) 2005, Sweden (SE) 2003, Thailand (TH) 2004, US (US) 2003	−0.42 to −0.25
Brazil (BR) 1996, Chile (CL) 1997, Costa Rica (CR) 2004, Mexico (MX) 2004, Uruguay (UY) 2006	−0.21 to −0.01
India (IN) 2004, Indonesia (ID) 2005, Philippines (PH) 1999	+0.07 to 0.31
Kenya (KE) 1994, Nigeria (NG) 2004	+0.56 to 0.76

SOURCE: Data from National Transfer Accounts database. See Lee and Mason (2011).

sectional characterization of the economic lifecycle at a point in time.[2] Labor income is a comprehensive measure that includes the pretax income of males and females, those in the labor force and those not (who enter as zeros), and unpaid family workers.[3] It includes wages, salaries, and fringe benefits, as well as two-thirds of self-employment income, with the other one-third counted as asset income. Consumption consists of private consumption that is imputed to individuals within each household,[4] as well as all public consumption including public education, publicly provided

---

[2]These age profiles are cross-sectional and do not accurately represent longitudinal life cycle profiles. For example, it is often the case that the cross-sectional age profile rises over time with productivity growth. In this case, a longitudinal age profile might continue to rise throughout life rather than turning down at older ages as it does in the cross-section. Longitudinal profiles can be approximated by introducing an assumed rate of productivity growth. When data for calculating repeated cross-sections are available, as they are in a number of countries, empirical longitudinal profiles can be estimated. Here we restrict our attention to the cross-sectional age profiles.

[3]The National Transfer Accounts are currently unisex, and all results presented here are averages across the sexes. It would be straightforward to estimate labor income separately for men and women, but because so much of women's work is in home production that falls outside National Income and Product Accounts, doing so would give a misleading picture of production differences by gender and therefore of net transfers between men and women. In order to introduce gender into the accounts, it would be necessary to draw on time use studies to estimate and monetize home production. We have begun preliminary work along these lines, but cannot address these issues here.

[4]For private consumption expenditures, the basic approach is to allocate health and education expenditures to household members using information in the survey, either directly or using regressions, while the remainder of household expenditures is allocated in proportion to equivalent adults consumption weights equal to .4 for ages 0–4, rising linearly until 1.0 at age 20, and 1.0 thereafter.

health care and long-term care, and other forms of public consumption (evaluated at cost of provision).

Transfers and asset-based reallocations are the complement of the economic lifecycle. Transfers consist of both public and private transfers. Public transfer inflows consist of cash transfers, such as pensions or family assistance, and in-kind transfers, equivalent to public consumption. Public transfer outflows are equal to the taxes paid by each age group to fund public transfer inflows. Net public transfers are the difference between public transfer inflows and outflows. Private transfers consist of inter-household transfers, including private transfers to and from the rest of the world, and intra-household transfers, in other words, transfers between co-resident household members.

Asset-based flows are defined as asset income less saving. Asset income includes the returns to capital held by corporations, partnerships, and individuals, including the return to owner-occupied dwellings. Asset income also includes property income— dividends, rent, and interest income and expense. Borrowing, lending, and repayment of loans are also included here. Saving is equivalent to net national saving. Public and private asset income and net saving are estimated, but only the combined values are presented here.

Per capita flows are calculated as population averages over all individuals at a given age, both males and females. For purposes of comparison, we divide each country's age profile of labor income and consumption by the average level of labor income for that country at ages 30–49, ages chosen to avoid masking the effects on profiles of decisions about schooling and retirement. Aggregate flows are calculated as the product of per capita flows and population at each age.

NTAs are estimated using existing cross-sectional surveys, National Income and Product Accounts (NIPAs), and public-sector administrative data. The age profiles of private flows such as consumption and transfers are estimated using nationally representative household surveys of income, consumption, and the labor force. The profiles for Japan, for example, are based on the 2004 National Survey of Family Income and Expenditure, for India on the 2004 India Human Development Survey (IHDS), and for China on the 2002 China Household Income Project (CHIP). Public flows estimates are based on a combination of household surveys and public administrative records and reports. For example, age-specific estimates for public education make use of national public education spending for primary, secondary, and tertiary levels combined with age-specific enrollment rates.

Initial estimates of per capita NTA age profiles are not necessarily consistent with their macroeconomic counterparts from NIPAs. Thus, per capita profiles are scaled, adjusted by a factor that is constant across age, to ensure that aggregate profiles are consistent with NIPAs. This procedure assumes that errors in estimates are proportionately the same at each age.

This mode of construction ensures that the general level of the NTA profiles, if not every detail of shape, will be as accurate as NIPAs. Of course, there may be quality problems with the NIPAs themselves, but it is beyond the scope of the NTA project to try to improve NIPAs. For some quantities, such as intrahousehold transfers, there is no counterpart in NIPAs, but by construction these transfers must sum to zero for each household. For interhousehold transfers, the control total is the NIPA number for net transfers with the rest of the world, which allows for remittances, for example.

We want to emphasize that these are cross-sectional profiles, and hence they are influenced by differences across cohorts, such as differences in educational attainment, wealth, and attitudes, as well as differences that can be attributed to aging per se.

ECONOMIC ACTIVITY OVER THE LIFECYCLE

The estimated profiles of consumption and labor income are shown in Figure 4-1. Panel A shows the per capita profiles for the four poorest NTA countries outside Asia and likewise for the four richest NTA countries outside Asia. Children begin productive economic activity at a younger age in the poor than in the rich countries, and their labor income is higher. At advanced ages, labor income begins to decline earlier in the poor countries. Near age 60, labor income drops precipitously in rich countries, due in part to the incentives and opportunities provided by public-sector pension programs (Costa, 1998; Gruber and Wise, 1999, 2001). Labor income is lower in the rich countries than the poor from the early 60s until age 85 or so. The greater labor income at the extremes of the age distribution is a characteristic feature of the poor countries.

There are also striking differences between the consumption age profiles in the poor and rich countries. In the rich countries, there is a characteristic bulge in consumption by children and youth, reflecting the heavy investment per child in human capital. It is equally striking that in the poor countries, consumption is quite flat from age 20 or so until the end of life. In the rich countries, by contrast, consumption rises from the early 20s on, and particularly after age 80 or so, when the costs of health and long-term care rise dramatically. Not all of this upward trend with age, however, is due to rising costs of health care and long-term care.

Putting together the age patterns of consumption and labor income, we see that population aging in rich countries is more costly than in poor ones, because the elderly in rich countries consume more and produce less than in poor countries.

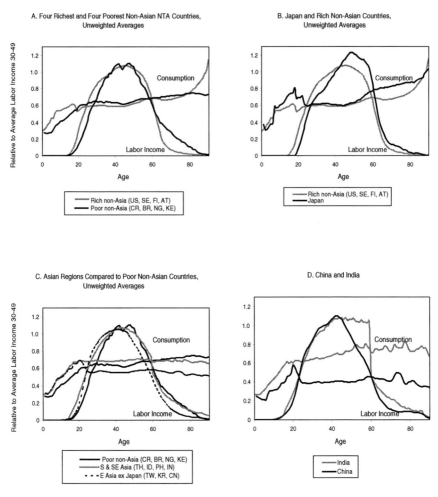

FIGURE 4-1 Age profiles of consumption and labor income for countries and regions of the world, from National Transfer Accounts.
NOTE: See Table 4-1 for country codes.
SOURCE: Calculated from the National Transfer Accounts database. See Lee and Mason (2011).

Panel B compares the age profiles of Japan to the average for the rich non-Asian countries. Investment in human capital in Japan is higher per child, particularly in late secondary and tertiary education. The broad pattern of consumption at older ages is similar, but after age 60, consumption is even higher in Japan. The age pattern of labor income in Japan is strikingly different. It begins a few years later, a gap that persists until age 40 or so. Most interestingly, the whole distribution is then pushed to the right, with earnings relatively higher from the late 40s through the early 60s, apparently reflecting the influence of the seniority system in Japan. Labor income in old age is also higher in Japan, although broadly similar in shape to the other rich countries.

Panel C shows the average age profiles for South and Southeast Asia (combined) and for East Asia excluding Japan and includes the average for the poor countries for comparison. For the moment, we set aside the difference in level of consumption, which largely reflects the situation in China. The shapes of the consumption curves are very similar above the early 20s. However, at younger ages, East Asia stands out for the high level of investment in human capital of children, which is indeed an important feature of the region. As for labor income, the profile for South and Southeast Asia looks much like that for the other poor countries. However, the age profile for East Asia starts at older ages, reflecting the greater human capital investment, and then rises more rapidly, crossing the other profiles at around age 20. Thereafter, the East Asian age profile is shifted several years to the left of the other two, to higher values up until 40 or so and then lower values after the mid-40s. This early decline in labor income is striking, and we are not sure what explains it.

Finally, Panel D compares the age profiles for India (Ladusingh and Narayana, 2011) and China (Li, Chen, and Jiang, 2011). Labor income in the two countries moves in lockstep until around age 40, but then it drops rapidly in China while continuing at a high level in India until age 60, when it drops toward the Chinese level. As for consumption, the most striking difference is that the level of consumption in China is very low relative to labor income. This reflects the extraordinarily high level of saving in China (see Li, Chen, and Jiang, 2011).

SUPPORT RATIOS

We can use these age profiles of consumption and labor income to calculate the way that changing population age distribution would affect the ratio of producers to consumers, on the hypothetical assumption that the age profiles remain the same over time or shift at the same rate, for example due to productivity growth. Given the base-year age profile of consumption, we calculate the number of "effective consumers" in a year by multiplying the population at each age by the consumption profile for that age and then summing over all ages. The number of effective producers is calculated similarly. The support ratio for a year is the ratio of effective producers to effective consumers. In the base year, the number of effective consumers equals aggregate consumption in the economy and effective producers equals aggregate labor income. In most countries, aggregate consumption exceeds aggregate labor income, so the support ratio is typically less than unity. Our interest is in the proportional changes in the support ratio, not in its level. Changes depend entirely on changing population age distributions as these interact with a country's age profiles. For easier comparison of proportional changes across countries, we set average consumption at ages 30–49 equal to 60% of average labor income at these ages in the base year. This affects the level of the support ratio in every year, but it does not affect its proportional variations over time. Without this adjustment, China would have a very, very high support ratio because it has an exceptionally high aggregate saving rate.

Support ratios calculated in this way for 1950 to 2050 are shown in Figure 4-2 based on United Nations estimates and projections (United Nations Population Division, 2009). Panel A shows regional averages for Europe, Latin America, and Africa. Europe largely achieved replacement level fertility by the 1930s, and the trajectory of its support ratio in Panel A reflects its post-World War II baby boom and baby bust more than the transition itself. Population aging will reduce Europe's support ratio to low levels starting around 2010. In Latin America, rising support ratios will boost growth rates of per capita income—an effect called "the demographic dividend"—until around 2030, after which population aging will reduce the support ratio less rapidly than in Europe. Africa, as represented here by only Kenya and Nigeria, is at the early stages of the demographic dividend phase and will benefit from it for many decades to come.

Panel B shows that China, Taiwan, and South Korea have quite similar support ratio trajectories, with deeper and more rapid variations than seen in Panel A. All three economies are about to end the dividend phase and to embark on declining support ratios, China a bit more gradually than the others. Japan's trajectory is very different from Europe's and from those of other East Asian economies.

In Panel C, Thailand's trajectory resembles that of the emerging East Asian economies in Panel B, while the other South and Southeast Asian countries' trajectories are similar to Latin America's in Panel A.

Finally, Panel D shows China, Japan, and India together for comparison purposes. They are indeed very different. Simplifying, one might say that the trajectories are similar in shape, but Japan's is 20 years ahead of China's, which is, in turn, 30 years ahead of India's. India has 30 more years to arrive at the dividend phase, while China has just exhausted it and Japan has already been aging for years.

We can also calculate the rates of change of these support ratios. In economies with exceptionally rapid fertility transitions, such as Japan, Mexico, South Korea, Taiwan, and Thailand, the support ratio sometimes changes by more than 1% per year. Table 4-1 shows the average

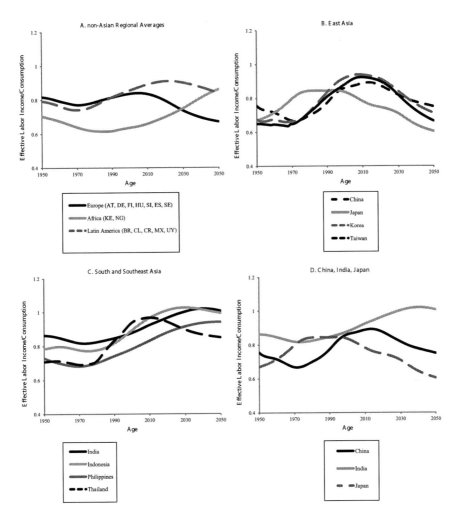

FIGURE 4-2 Support ratios for countries and regions.
NOTE: See Table 4-1 for country codes.
SOURCE: Calculated from National Transfer Accounts data and United Nations
Population Division (2009).

rate of change of the projected support ratio between 2010–2050 for
the NTA countries. We see that the majority (five out of eight) of the
Asian NTA economies have declining support ratios over this period,
indicating that population aging will reduce the rate of consumption
growth, other things being equal. In the remaining three countries, projected support ratios rise over the next four decades.

HOW DO THE ELDERLY FUND THEIR CONSUMPTION?

As discussed earlier, children's consumption is funded largely by public and private transfers, and partly by their own productive efforts, particularly in poorer countries. The elderly, however, may additionally use assets accumulated during their earlier working years through saving and/or inheritance. Where assets are an important source of funding for consumption in old age, an increase in the ratio of elderly to working age population will raise the ratio of assets to workers. This will be true whether asset accumulation takes place through funded government pension programs (as opposed to pay-as-you-go pensions), funded occupational pensions, or direct saving by individuals. If these assets are invested in domestic capital, then capital per worker will rise, raising the productivity of labor and offsetting to a greater or lesser degree the drop in support ratios (Lee, Mason, and Miller, 2003; Mason and Lee, 2007).

We first combine public and private transfers into the single measure "transfers" and consider how the funding of old age consumption is divided among transfers, labor income, and asset income. It is possible for an elderly person to own substantial assets but to save the asset income rather than use it to fund consumption. In this case, we will not count it as a funding source for consumption. On this principle, we can calculate the percentage of old age consumption that is funded by one's own labor income, by net transfers, and by assets. Net transfers can have a negative value, indicating that net transfers are made to younger people. The percentages must add to 100%.

Figure 4-3 is a triangle graph. The proportion of each of these three funding components is indicated along one side of the triangle. If a country is situated at one of the vertices of the triangle, then elder consumption is funded 100% by the source that names that vertex. If a country is situated on an edge of the triangle, then support comes entirely from a mixture of the two sources naming the vertices that the edge connects. If a country is inside the triangle, the elderly are funded by a mix of all three sources. If a country is situated to the right of the triangle, the elderly are receiving negative net transfers, meaning that they contribute to others, rather than the reverse.

In Figure 4-3, the points cluster around a line from the transfer vertex (where Austria, Hungary, Slovenia, and Sweden are funded nearly 100% by transfers) to a point on the opposite edge (between India and Indonesia). Along this line, for a given share of transfers, about one-third of the balance of the funding comes from labor income and two-thirds from assets. Most of the action in the chart reflects the tradeoff between relying on transfers and on assets, with less systematic variation in labor income as a source. Nonetheless, in economies relying more on assets,

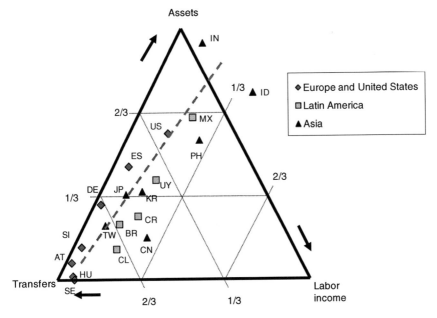

FIGURE 4-3 Shares of elder consumption funded from labor income, transfers, and asset-based reallocations in seventeen NTA countries.
NOTE: See Table 4-1 for country codes.
SOURCE: Mason et al. (2011).

people also rely more on labor income in old age. The Asian countries fall close to the line, with China, Japan, South Korea, and Taiwan closer to the transfers vertex and India, Indonesia, and the Philippines at the other end of the line. These are also the poorest NTA countries in the region, and poor countries generally have higher labor income in old age. Note also that India and Indonesia are well outside the triangle, indicating that the elderly make net transfers to others rather than receive them.

A surprising result at first glance is the extent to which the elderly are relying on assets in some relatively low-income countries like India, Mexico, and the Philippines. The imputed rent from owner-occupied housing is important for many elderly living in these countries, and if the elderly own a productive asset such as a farm used as part of a family enterprise, one-third of the income will be allocated to the asset and therefore to the elderly. Also it should be kept in mind that we are measuring the extent to which the elderly are relying on assets to fund their consumption. In many countries the elderly may save most or all asset income, rather than use it to fund their consumption.

The next step is to set labor income aside and consider how consumption net of labor income is funded. The advantage is that by looking at how elder consumption net of labor income is funded, we can distinguish public and private transfers as well as asset income. Figure 4-4 shows the result. Most countries are arrayed along the edge joining assets and public transfers, indicating that the elderly have zero net family transfers or, in most cases, they are making net familial transfers to younger people. Public transfers are a very important source of old age support for most countries. Asian countries, however, rely more prominently on the family as a source of old-age consumption. India, the Philippines, and Thailand lie on the edge joining assets and family transfers, indicating that public transfers play no role. Indonesia also lies on this edge-line, but so far above the asset vertex as to be outside the range of the chart. China, South Korea, and Taiwan are well inside the triangle, indicating that old age support is

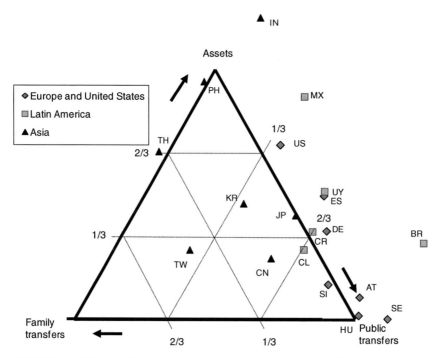

FIGURE 4-4 How is elder consumption net of labor income funded? Shares of public transfers, family transfers, and asset-based reallocations for seventeen NTA countries.
NOTE: See Table 4-1 for country codes.
SOURCE: Calculated from data in Lee and Mason (2011).

drawn from all three sources, with Taiwan drawing quite equally on the three. Japan lies on the edge connecting assets and public transfers, indicating that on net, elders neither give nor receive family transfers.

In the countries located near the public transfers vertex, the elderly have little motivation to save for retirement on average, because their consumption needs are met by public pensions and healthcare. This does not mean that there is little saving, because there are certainly many other motives to save besides provision for old age. It does mean, however, that in these countries, population aging is less likely to produce a second demographic dividend by raising asset accumulation and making the economy more capital intensive and the labor more productive.

POPULATION AGING AND HUMAN CAPITAL ACCUMULATION

The main cause of population aging is low fertility, not longer life. East Asia has had exceptionally rapid and deep fertility declines, and the average total fertility rate in the region is now 1.5 births per woman, with Taiwan lowest at 1.0. East Asia is also known for its heavy investment in education per child, and it is sometimes suggested that this is one of the explanations for its rapid economic growth over recent decades. Might the very low fertility be linked to the high investment in human capital?

A well-developed theory in economics, originally due to Becker and Lewis (1973) and Willis (1973), asserts that parents derive utility from both the quantity and the average quality of their children, as well as from their own consumption. "Quality" indicates the amount spent to rear each child on average. Quantity and quality interact in the budget constraint multiplicatively, since the total amount spent by parents on their children is the number of children times the amount spent per child, quantity times quality. In the extreme case often used for expositional purposes, the parents first decide an amount to allocate to children in total, and then decide how to allocate it between quantity and quality. In this case the quantity-quality tradeoff is particularly stark: Quality = Total Funds Pre-Allocated to Children Divided by Quantity.

When income rises over time, the demand for quality, which is posited to have a larger income elasticity than the demand for quantity, rises, and this raises the shadow price of quantity. The net result is that parents opt to have lower fertility and to invest much more in each child. Other factors can also alter the balance between quantity and quality, such as the rate of return to human capital as perceived by parents, the availability of contraceptives, or improved transportation networks that reduce the cost to parents of sending their children to school.

Although the quantity-quality theory was developed for private expenditures, it may also characterize public spending on human capital.

The rise in the support ratio may ease fiscal constraints faced by governments, allowing them to invest more in human capital. Governments might be forward-looking and invest more in human capital so as to offset the coming decline in the number of workers.

In light of these various possibilities, it is interesting to look at the cross-national relationship between investment in human capital per child and the Total Fertility Rate (TFR). (See Lee and Mason, 2010a, for a more detailed analysis of the full set of NTA countries.) First, however, we explain how we measure human capital investment. The theoretical literature (Becker et al., 1973; Willis, 1973) counts all expenditure on children as quality. We choose to focus on the explicit spending on education and health, since this is more clearly discretionary (rather than being passively tied to parental consumption such as housing and meal choices) and is more clearly linked to later life labor productivity. We sum from the NTA estimates of public and private spending per child for each single year of age. For education, these sums go from 0 to 26 to include postgraduate education, while for healthcare they go from 0 through 17. This gives a synthetic cohort estimate of human capital investment per child, with public and private spending combined. We do not attempt to take into account the opportunity cost of the children's time as a costly input. As elsewhere, we standardize the results for different countries by dividing the human capital measure by average labor income for ages 30–49. Our measure, then, can be interpreted as the number of years' worth of prime age labor income that are invested in human capital per child. For fertility we use the average TFR in the five years preceding the NTA observation year. In the stylized story, the product of quantity and quality is constant, in which case the logs of quantity and of quality should be linearly related with a slope of –1.0. We will therefore plot the logarithm of our measure of human capital investment against the logarithm of fertility.

Figure 4-5 shows the result for the eight Asian countries, for both total and private human capital expenditures. For total human capital expenditures, there is a strong negative relationship, with an elasticity of –.91, quite close to the expository model prediction of –1.0. For private expenditures alone, the elasticity is similar at –.89. However, the scatter is much tighter to the line for the total investment than for the private investment, consistent with the idea that public and private investments substitute for one another.

The log of standardized public expenditure on human capital in a country is shown by the gap between the two markers (circle and cross) for that country. Thus Japan and Taiwan invest the same amount in total, but Taiwan has low public spending and high private spending, while Japan has the opposite. China and South Korea both have low public spending, whereas Thailand has unusually high public spending.

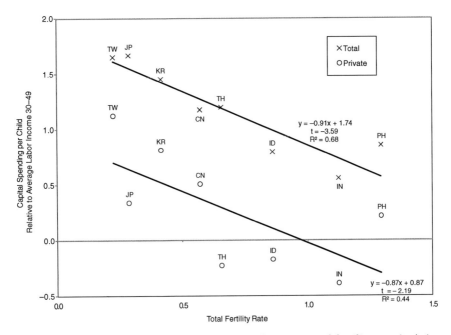

FIGURE 4-5 Investment in human capital in relation to total fertility rate in Asia.
NOTE: See Table 4-1 for country codes.
SOURCE: Calculated from data in Lee and Mason (2011).

The East Asian countries have far lower fertility than those in Southeast Asia or India, and they have correspondingly higher human capital investment per child. The per child human capital investment in Taiwan and Japan is approximately five years of prime age labor income, an amount comparable to that of Europe.

Elsewhere we have looked at the relation of changes over time in fertility and human capital in Japan, Taiwan, and the United States, and found similar results (Lee and Mason, 2010b).

We expect that as fertility falls in other Asian countries, spending per child will rise, with beneficial effects for future labor productivity and economic growth. To some degree, quality of labor will be substituted for quantity of labor, reducing the difficulties of the working ages in providing for the elderly population.

NATIONAL TRANSFER ACCOUNTS AND
HEALTH AND RETIREMENT STUDIES (HRS)

National Transfer Accounts rely on survey data as a key source of information, in addition to National Income and Product Accounts and various kinds of administrative data. The richness and quality of HRS-type data (henceforth, HRSTD) can potentially improve the quality of the NTA estimates in a number of ways, despite its restriction to respondents who are at least 45 or 50 years of age. HRSTD can provide high-quality data on interhousehold transfers to and from the elderly. While NTAs require such data for the entire age range, HRSTD can be used to check the quality of the NTA estimates where they overlap. Preliminary work along these lines for the United States has so far found good agreement between the NTA and HRS data, after appropriate adjustments are made to bring the concepts into line.

HRSTD on bequests should be particularly valuable, because data on bequests, particularly smaller bequests, are hard to come by. In some countries, data on savings and asset holdings are also not readily available. Savings rates are necessary for NTA flow accounts. Ordinarily, they are calculated in NTA as a residual, so having high quality data to check against this residual is valuable, in part because matching the residual would provide a partial confirmation of the other estimates from which it is derived. Asset holdings are necessary to construct NTA wealth accounts. The difficulties with measures of asset holdings are particularly severe in East Asia, where many elderly transfer ownership of their assets to their co-residing adult son well before the time of death. This practice makes it very difficult to trace the accumulation of assets over the life course, which is necessary for understanding how population aging affects asset accumulation. It should be possible, using longitudinal HRSTD, to trace asset transfers of this sort. With the data now used to construct NTAs, we attribute ownership of assets to the head of the household, which may obscure the behavioral processes that lead to its original accumulation.

If HRSTD can help improve NTA estimates, NTAs also broaden the picture offered by HRSTD in certain respects. Most obviously, NTAs cover the entire age range, not just the elderly. But there is much more. NTAs estimate intrahousehold transfers such as transfers to co-resident elders. Since familial transfers are a very important source of support for the elderly in Asia, as we saw in Figure 4-5, it is important to develop information about their size absolutely and relative to other sources of support available to the elderly. Familial transfers to co-resident elderly also provide for intergenerational sharing that enables the elderly to share in the benefits of very rapid economic growth long after they have left the labor force.

NTAs also provide a natural interface with macroeconomic models and analyses, including overlapping generations models and Auerbach-Kotlikoff-Gohkale style Generational Accounting (Auerbach, Gokhale, and Kotlikoff, 1991; Auerbach, Kotlikoff, and Leibfritz, 1999). Estimates derived from HRSTD can be inserted in NTAs and used for this purpose. Similarly, NTAs lend naturally to long-term projections and assessments of fiscal sustainability of public-sector programs.

Finally, the exercise of formulating NTA estimates leads to questions that can be addressed using the microanalysis of HRSTD. The question raised above about the transfer of ownership of elders' assets at the point of moving into an adult child's house is a case in point.

CONCLUSIONS

Population aging in East Asia will be early and profound, due to early fertility declines to very low levels and high and rising life expectancy. In most of Southeast Asia (Thailand is an exception) and India, aging will come later and more gradually. What can be said about the economic effects that this population aging will have? The data presented in this chapter provide some insights and raise some questions.

Japan is the richest Asian country and had the earliest fertility transition. Unlike other Asian countries, Japan has also instituted public sector transfer programs for the elderly that are quite similar to those in Europe, with generous pensions, health care, and long-term care. As a result, Japan will face similarly severe long-term fiscal problems as its population ages. As in Europe and the United States, the consequences of population aging in Japan are exacerbated by a strong upward gradient in consumption by age, a pattern that has probably emerged in recent decades as the welfare state has grown.

In the rest of Asia, the public-sector transfers to the elderly are very low, and if they remain so, then population aging will not threaten fiscal sustainability. However, it would not be surprising if they followed Japan and other rich countries in coming decades and developed similar public transfers to the elderly.

Without public transfers for the elderly, one might wonder whether the family will instead bear the costs of population aging. Indeed, in East Asia and in Thailand, net familial support of the elderly is important. In India and Southeast Asia, however, neither public transfers nor net familial transfers go to the elderly. The elderly, who continue to earn labor income, also receive substantial asset income and use it not only for their own consumption, but also to make net transfers to their children. These downward transfers, funded by assets, may reflect residence by children's families in homes owned by their elderly parents or may reflect familial work on farms owned by the elderly parents, to whom our methods impute one-third of family farm output as the asset share. In any case, in these circumstances population aging would impose smaller costs on the working age population. Furthermore, outside of Japan, consumption is flat across age from the early twenties until death, which means that population aging will be less costly for families.

Population aging may also be associated with increased physical capital and increased human capital per worker. In countries where the elderly hold substantial assets that they accumulated through their savings out of their lifetime earnings rather than through inheritance, population aging will tend to raise asset holdings per capita, and if these are invested in the domestic economy, then the rising capital labor ratio will boost productivity and wages. In addition, the low and declining fertility that is the main cause of population aging is associated with increased investments in human capital per child, raising future productivity and earnings. This has been particularly so in Asia, both through public and private spending. In this way, quality of workers may be substituted for quantity, further reducing the adverse effects of population aging in this region.

The economic consequences of population aging in Asian countries will depend on whether they follow the path of Japan or instead retain the current features of their public sectors and private economic behaviors.

REFERENCES

Auerbach, A.J., J. Gokhale, and L.J. Kotlikoff. (1991). Generational accounts: A meaningful alternative to deficit accounting. Pp. 55-110 in *Tax Policy and the Economy*, D. Bradford (Ed.). Cambridge, MA: MIT Press for the National Bureau of Economic Research.

Auerbach, A.J., L.J. Kotlikoff, and W. Leibfritz (Eds.). (1999). *Generational Accounting Around the World*. Chicago: University of Chicago Press.

Becker, G., and H.G. Lewis. (1973). On the interaction between the quantity and quality of children. *Journal of Political Economy 81*(2):S279-S288.

Costa, D.L. (1998). *The Evolution of Retirement: An American Economic History, 1880-1990*. Chicago: University of Chicago Press.

Gruber, J., and D.A. Wise. (1999). Introduction and summary. Pp. 437-474 in *Social Security and Retirement around the World*, J. Gruber and D.A. Wise (Eds.). Chicago: University of Chicago Press.

Gruber, J., and D.A. Wise. (2001). *An International Perspective on Policies for an Aging Society*. NBER Working Paper No. W8103. Cambridge, MA: National Bureau of Economic Research. Available: http://www.nber.org/papers/w8103.pdf.

Ladusingh, L., and M.R. Narayana. (2011). The role of familial transfers in supporting the lifecycle deficit in India. In *Population Aging and the Generational Economy: A Global Perspective*, R. Lee and A. Mason (Eds.). Cheltenham, UK: Edward Elgar.

Lee, R., and A. Mason. (2010a). Fertility, human capital, and economic growth over the demographic transition. *European Journal of Population 26*(2), May 2010. DOI10.1007/s10680-009-9186-x:159-182.

Lee, R., and A. Mason (2010b). Some macroeconomic aspects of global population aging. *Demography* 47(Suppl):S151-S172.

Lee, R., and A. Mason. (2011). *Population Aging and the Generational Economy: A Global Perspective.* Cheltenham, UK: Edward Elgar.

Lee, R., A. Mason, and T. Miller. (2003). From transfers to individual responsibility: Implications for savings and capital accumulation in Taiwan and the United States. *Scandinavian Journal of Economics* 105(3):339-357.

Li, L., Q. Chen, and Y. Jiang. (2011). The changing patterns of China's public services. In *Population Aging and the Generational Economy: A Global Perspective*, R. Lee and A. Mason (Eds.). Cheltenham, UK: Edward Elgar.

Mason, A., and R. Lee. (2007). Transfers, capital, and consumption over the demographic transition. Pp. 128-162 in *Population Aging, Intergenerational Transfers and the Macroeconomy*, R. Clark, A. Mason, and N. Ogawa (Eds.). Cheltenham, UK: Edward Elgar.

Mason, A., R. Lee, and S.-H. Lee. (2010). The demographic transition and economic growth in the Pacific Rim. Pp. 19-55 in *The Economic Consequences of Demographic Change in East Asia*, T. Ito and A.K. Rose (Eds.). Chicago: University of Chicago Press.

Mason, A., N. Ogawa, A. Chawla, and R. Matsukura. (2011). Asset-based flows from a generational perspective. Pp. 209-236 in *Population Aging and the Generational Economy: A Global Perspective*, R. Lee and A. Mason (Eds.). Cheltenham, UK: Edward Elgar.

United Nations Population Division. (2009). *World Population Prospects: The 2008 Revision.* New York: United Nations.

Willis, R.J. (1973). A New Approach to the economic theory of fertility behavior. *Journal of Political Economy* 81(2, Part 2):S14-S64.

5

Facilitating Longer Working Lives: The Need, the Rationale, the How[1]

David A. Wise

The theme of this paper is that social and economic choices in societies must adjust as the age structure of the population changes. In particular, some of the bounty of longer lives must be allocated to prolonging the labor force participation of older workers. The changing demographic environment over the past four or five decades represents both an achievement and a problem. Mortality rates have declined and life expectancy has increased substantially in industrialized and developing countries. This is the achievement. What is the problem? Declining birth rates and fewer young people, together with longer lives, have meant that

[1]This is a written version of a paper presented at the conference on the Challenges of Population Aging in Asia: Strengthening the Basis of Policy Development, held in Beijing, December 9–10, 2010. A very similar paper was also presented at the Collogue sur l'Emploie des Seniors, organized by DARES, and held in Paris, October 14, 2010. The paper relies heavily on the International Social Security Project that I direct with results based on analyses by research teams in 12 countries. In particular, I draw freely from the preliminary summary of the most recent phase of the project (Milligan and Wise, 2011), the summary of the prior phase of the project (Gruber and Wise, 2010), and the summary of the first phase of the project (Gruber, Milligan, and Wise, 1999). This paper also compares many of the key results with results for China, and I wish to thank Wei Huang from Peking University for providing these data. The International Social Security Project has been funded by the National Institute on Aging through grants P01 AG005842 and P30 AG012810 and by the U.S. Social Security Administration (SSA) via Inter-Agency Agreement Y3-AG-0725. The content is solely the responsibility of the authors and does not necessarily represent the official views of the National Institute on Aging, the National Institutes of Health, or the U.S. Social Security Administration. I have also benefited from the comments of two reviewers of the paper and from the comments of the volume facilitators.

the proportion of old to young is increasing. As the number of older people increases, health care costs will rise, both because of the increase in the number of older people but also because advancing technology will likely create better and perhaps more expensive health care treatments. The cost of public pension (social security) programs will also rise, but with a smaller proportion of the population in the labor force to pay for these increasing social security and health care costs. The problem has been magnified by the departure of workers from the labor force at younger ages along with substantial increases in the number of years they spend in retirement. Thus the theme above: Some of the bounty of longer lives must be allocated to prolonging the labor force participation of older workers. It will not be feasible to use all of the increase in longevity to increase years in retirement, a theme also emphasized in Wise (2010). This is the need.

Although not discussed further in this paper, the theme is based on three working assumptions. First, the increase in the labor force participation of older people will increase production and gross domestic product (GDP). Second, the increase in production will increase tax revenues. Third, the increase in tax revenues will increase the funds available to pay for increasing social security and health care costs. In addition, the increase in labor force participation at older ages would likely increase personal saving. In the United States, with the conversion from defined benefits to a personal account system based largely on 401(k) plans, this increase would happen essentially by default. Increased personal saving would be drawn down over fewer retirement years and, thus, would increase resources in each year of retirement.

Many of the conclusions reported in this paper are based on results obtained in the International Social Security Project. Researchers who have participated in this project are listed in Box 5-1.

To emphasize the theme of population aging in Asia, wherever possible I have compared labor force and mortality trends in the participating countries with trends in China. Japan, another Asian country, is a key participant of the International Social Security Project.

The paper is in three sections. The first section, which is the primary emphasis, considers the rationale for considering longer working lives in the face of the demographic trends. In particular, I emphasize healthier older populations. I note the reduction in mortality is a marker of better health, not because it is equivalent to reductions in morbidity or to other measures of health status, but because it is an indicator of health that is comparable across countries and comparable over time within the same country. I discuss the relationship between labor force participation and health and how it has changed over time. I then emphasize the relationship between mortality and self-assessed health and point to measures of the capacity to work, based on analysis by Cutler, Meara, and Richards-Shubik

BOX 5-1
International Social Security Project: List of Researchers

Belgium   Alain Jousten, Mathieu Lefèbvre, Sergio Perelman,
                   Pierre Pestieau
                   Arnaud Dellis, Raphaël Desmet, Jean-Philippe Stijns

Canada   Michael Baker, Kevin Milligan
                   Jonathan Gruber

Denmark   Paul Bingley, Nabanita Datta Gupta, Peder J. Pedersen

France   Luc Behaghel, Didier Blanchet, Thierry Debrand, Muriel Roger
                   Melika Ben Salem, Antoine Bozio, Ronan Mahieu,
                   Louis-Paul Pelé, Emmanuelle Walraet

Germany   Axel Börsch-Supan, Hendrik Juerges
                   Simone Kohnz, Giovanni Mastrobuoni, Reinhold Schnabel

Italy   Agar Brugiavini, Franco Peracchi

Japan   Takashi Oshio, Satoshi Shimizutani
                   Akiko Sato Oishi, Naohiro Yashiro

Netherlands   Adriaan Kalwij, Arie Kapteyn, Klaas de Vos

Spain   Pilar García Gómez, Sergi Jiménez-Martín, Judit Vall Castelló,
                   Michele Boldrín, Franco Peracchi

Sweden   Lisa Jönsson, Mårten Palme, Ingemar Svensson

United Kingdom   James Banks, Richard Blundell, Antonio Bozio, Carl Emmerson
                   Paul Johnson, Costas Meghir, Sarah Smith

United States   Kevin Milligan
                   Courtney Coile, Peter Diamond, Jonathan Gruber

NOTE: The participants in the current phase are listed first; others who have participated in one or more of the previous phases are listed second and shown in italics.

(2011). My concentration on the rationale is motivated by the belief that
discussion of longer working lives must be predicated by discussion of
why working longer is a plausible adjustment to the changing age structure of the population.

In the second section, I review evidence on how to facilitate working lives, drawing in large part from the International Social Security Project and discussing the false rationale for inducing older workers to leave the labor force. In many countries, the proposition that older workers must leave the labor force to provide jobs for young workers is used as a reason to induce older workers to leave the labor force. Based on results from the International Social Security Project, however, no evidence supports this "boxed economy" view of the labor market. The final section of the paper presents a summary and conclusions.

THE RATIONALE

For ease of exposition, much of this section is based on comparative data for the United States, France, the United Kingdom, and China. I begin by considering mortality trends and by documenting long-run trends in mortality. Next, I compare the change in mortality trends to labor force participation. I then discuss the relationship between mortality and self-assessed health (SAH), a common measure of health status, and discuss evidence on the capacity to work at older ages.

Declining Mortality and Equivalent Mortality Ages

There are several ways to present mortality data that highlight more clearly the implications of mortality declines for health. One way is to ask how old one would have to be today to have the same mortality as a person of a given age in an earlier year. For example, consider the mortality rate of people aged 65 in the 1960s, and then consider the age at which the same mortality rate occurred in later years. Figure 5-1 shows the ages of equivalent mortality in the United Kingdom. Men aged 74 in 2007 had about the same mortality rate as men aged 65 in the 1960s. The

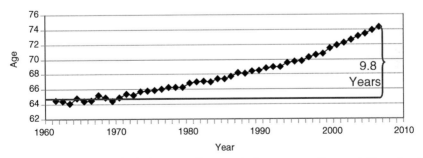

FIGURE 5-1 Age at which the mortality rate is the same as the mortality rate of a 65-year-old in the 1960s—by year, men in the United Kingdom.
SOURCE: Milligan and Wise (2011).

TABLE 5-1 Gain in Equivalent Mortality Age, Early 1980s to 2005, for Men Aged 65 in Initial Year

Country	First Year	Mortality Rate in First Year (%)	Equivalent Mortality Age in 2005	Gain in Years
Belgium	1960	3.53	72.3	7.8
Canada	1961	3.26	73.4	8.4
Denmark	1961	2.69	70.0	5.0
France	1960	3.22	73.5	8.5
Germany	1960	4.15	73.2	8.2
Italy	1960	3.06	72.8	7.8
Japan	1960	3.56	75.0	10.0
Netherlands	1960	2.35	69.7	4.7
Spain	1960	3.54	71.9	6.9
Sweden	1960	2.37	71.4	6.4
UK	1960	3.53	73.4	8.4
US	1960	3.84	74.1	9.1

SOURCE: Milligan and Wise (2011).

difference is about 9.8 years. Thus, by this measure, there has been a very large improvement in health (a reduction in the mortality rate) over the past several decades.

The same comparison has been made for each of the countries participating in the International Social Security Project. Table 5-1 shows the age in 2005 with the same mortality as men aged 65 in the early 1960s for each of the countries. Although in each country the equivalent mortality age in 2005 was substantially greater than age 65-mortality in the early 1960s, there is also substantial variation in the 2005 equivalent age—from a low of age 69.7 (an increase of 4.7 years) in the Netherlands to a high of age 75 (an increase of 10 years) in Japan, the only Asian country participating in the International Social Security Project. Below, I compare equivalent mortality ages to equivalent self-assessed health ages, which may be closer to healthy equivalent ages.

Employment by Age

I next present a series of figures to describe the change over time in the relationship between employment and mortality and the relationship between employment and age. I begin with employment by age now and then turn to employment by mortality and how it has changed over time. Figure 5-2 shows employment by age in the United States, the United Kingdom, France, and China. While the employment rate was similar for these countries through age 50, by age 63 the employment rate in France was much lower than in the other countries. The provisions of the pen-

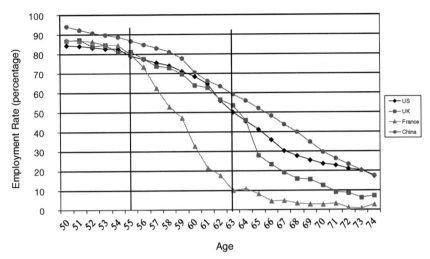

FIGURE 5-2 Employment by age, United States, United Kingdom, and France, 2007, and China, 2005.
SOURCES: Milligan and Wise (2011) and data from China Census (2005).

sion plan in France provide very substantial incentives to leave the labor force early.

Mortality by Age

I now turn to employment by mortality and begin by describing mortality by age across the countries. Figure 5-3 shows mortality by age in the same four countries. While there are differences across countries, the variation appears small relative to differences in employment by age.

Employment by Mortality

We want to understand how employment varies across countries, given health. Again, I use mortality as the measure of health, sticking with a measure that is comparable across countries. I then compare the employment rate across countries for given levels of mortality. Figure 5-4 shows employment by mortality for each of the four countries. Taking the ages at which the mortality rate in each of these countries was about 0.5 percent indicates that the employment rates are very similar, ranging from about 0.82 to 0.90. But as the mortality rate increases, the divergence across the countries increases. For example, at the age at which the mortality rate in each of the countries was 2.0%, the employment rates varied

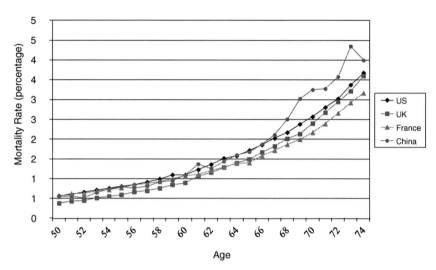

FIGURE 5-3 Mortality by age, United States, United Kingdom, and France, 2007, and China, 2005.
SOURCES: Milligan and Wise (2011) and data from National Bureau of Statistics of China (2006).

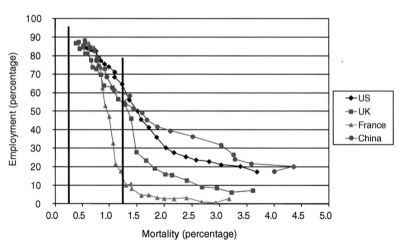

FIGURE 5-4 Employment and mortality by age, United States, United Kingdom, and France, 2007, and China, 2005.
SOURCES: Milligan and Wise (2011); data from National Bureau of Statistics of China (2006) and China Census (2005).

from about 3% in France, to 16% in the United Kingdom, to 30% in the United States, and about 40% in China. Like the increasing divergence in employment rates by age, the divergence in employment as people age and mortality increases reflects the large variation in the provisions of pathways to retirement.

To understand the cross-country comparisons in Figures 5-3 and 5-4, it helps to consider in more detail the relationship between employment and mortality. Figure 5-5a shows the relationship between age and employment in 1982 and 2005 in China. As highlighted, the employment rate at ages 62 and 63 declined by about 9% over this 23-year period. Also at these ages the mortality rates declined substantially between 1982 and 2005—about 1.3% at each age. Figure 5-5b presents a different view of the data, showing the employment rate by mortality in 1982 and 2005. Consider first the age at which 50% of men were employed. In 2005, the mortality rate when 50% of men were employed was 3.2%; 23 years later, in 2005, the mortality rate was only 1.6%, a decline of 1.6%. That is, for the employment rate to be 50% in 2005, men "had to be" much healthier (by the mortality measure) than they were in 1982. Looking at the data another way, at the age at which the mortality rate was 1.5%, in 1982 about 80% of men were employed, but in 2005, only 50% were employed.

The version of the data presented in Figure 5-5b for China is presented for the United States and for France in Figures 5-6 and 5-7, respectively.

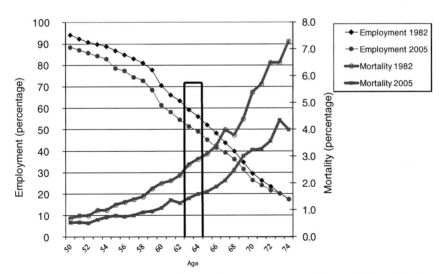

FIGURE 5-5a Employment and mortality by age, men in China, 1982 and 2005. SOURCES: Data from National Bureau of Statistics of China (2006) and China Census (1982, 2005).

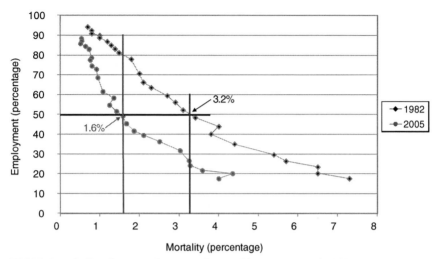

FIGURE 5-5b Employment by mortality in China, 1982 and 2005.
SOURCES: Data from National Bureau of Statistics of China (2006) and China Census (1982, 2005).

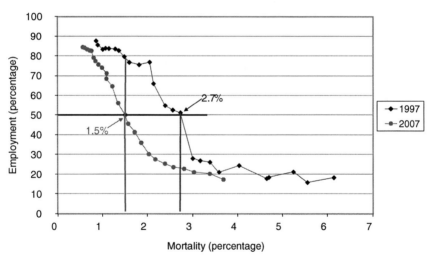

FIGURE 5-6 Employment by mortality, men in the United States, 1977 and 2007.
SOURCE: Milligan and Wise (2011).

For these countries, the data are for 1977 and 2007, instead of 1982 and 2005. For the United States, Figure 5-6 shows that in 2007, the mortality rate when 50% of men were employed was 2.7%; 30 years later in 2007, the mortality rate was only 1.5%, a decline of 1.2%. That is, for the employ-

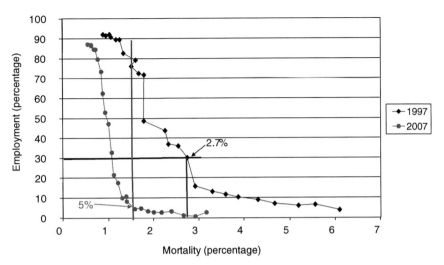

FIGURE 5-7 Employment by mortality, men in France, 1977 and 2007.
SOURCE: Milligan and Wise (2011).

ment rate to be 50% in 2007, men "had to be" much healthier (by the mortality measure) than they were in 1977. Looking at the data another way, at the age at which the mortality rate was 1.5%, in 1977 about 80% percent of men were employed, while in 2007, the rate dropped to only 50%.

In France, the employment rate at ages 62 and 63 declined by almost 30%. In addition, the mortality rate at these ages declined by about 1%, about the same as in the United States and somewhat less than in China. Figure 5-7 shows that in France, at the age at which 30% percent of men were employed, the mortality rate was 2.7% in 1977 but only 1.1% in 2007, a decline of 1.6%. That is, for the employment rate to be 30% in 2007, men "had to be" much healthier (by the mortality measure) than they were in 1977. Further, looking at the data another way, at the age at which the mortality rate was 1.5%, almost 80% of men were employed in 1977 compared to only 5% in 2007.

Mortality Versus Self-Assessed Health

The figures above highlight the changing relationship between mortality and employment. As emphasized, mortality lends itself to these comparisons because this measure is comparable across countries and across time within countries. Other potential measures of health status are not comparable across countries and may not be comparable across time within countries. Nonetheless, I explore the relationship between mortality and SAH status, perhaps the most commonly used summary measure of health status. I compare these two measures in several ways. First, I compare SAH and future mortality in the United States. Second, I compare mortality-equivalent ages over time with SAH-equivalent ages over time using data for two countries, the United States and Sweden, as illustration. Third, I consider within countries the time-trend relationship between mortality and SAH. Finally, I combine the latter comparisons to estimate the cross-country relationship between the change in mortality over time with the comparable change in SAH over the same period.

SAH and Future Mortality in the United States

Table 5-2 shows that in the U.S. Health and Retirement Study (HRS), SAH in 1992 was strongly predictive of subsequent mortality. The table shows the proportion of men and women deceased by 1996, 2002, and 2008. For example, for men in excellent health, only 11.4% were deceased by 2008, compared to 57.9% for men in poor health. More generally, although mortality is not equivalent to health status or disability, it is likely to be an important indicator of age-equivalent work potential over time. Heiss et al. (2009) used HRS data to show a striking relationship at all ages between self-reported health status and death rates and between self-reported disability status and death rates.[2]

Mortality-Equivalent Ages Versus SAH-Equivalent Ages

Figure 5-8 compares these two measures for the United States. First, the figure shows mortality by age in 1977 and 2007. The figure shows that a person aged 77 in 2007 had about the same mortality rate as a person aged 60 in 1977, a difference of about 7 years. Second, the figure shows the proportion of people who reported they were in fair or poor health, by age, in the 1970s and in the 2000s, based on the National Health Interview Survey. Comparing these two trends, men who were aged 69 in the 2000s had about the same SAH as men who were more than 9 years younger, aged 60, in the 1970s. Thus in this example, there was a greater difference

---

[2]There is substantial additional evidence of declining disability in the United States among people older than 65. Using data from the National Long-Term Care Survey, Manton, Gu, and Lamb (2006) showed that in each of three age intervals—65–74, 75–84, and 85 and older—there has been a large decline since 1982 in the percentage of older people who need help with activities of daily living. But Martin et al. (2007, 2009), examining self-assessed trends in fair/poor health, questioned whether such declines pertain to the younger old in more recent years. Weir (2007) also questioned the decline in health status among the younger old, drawing particular attention to the increase in obesity.

TABLE 5-2 Percentage of HRS Respondents, Aged 51–61 in 1992 Who Are Deceased by the Beginning of Each Wave, by Self-Assessed Health (SAH) Status in 1992, United States

Year	Self-Reported Health in 1992				
	Excellent	Very Good	Good	Fair	Poor
Men					
1996	1.0	1.5	2.1	4.3	10.8
2002	5.8	7.2	13.3	22.1	36.9
2008	11.4	15.6	25.8	36.5	57.9
% in Category	24.5	29.6	27.8	11.5	6.6
Women					
1996	0.4	0.8	0.8	2.1	4.2
2002	2.6	5.4	7.1	15.2	24.4
2008	6.4	10.3	15.2	28.8	36.8
% in Category	23.1	30.7	25.7	13.6	6.9

SOURCE: Milligan and Wise (2011).

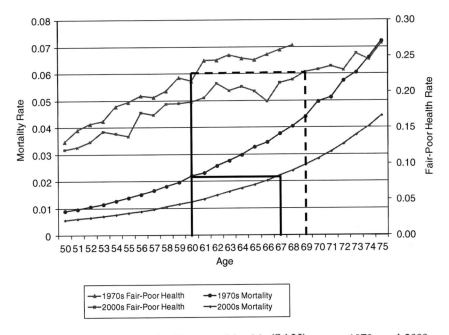

FIGURE 5-8 Mortality and self-assessed health (SAH) status, 1970s and 2000s, United States.
SOURCE: Milligan and Wise (2011).

in age-equivalent SAH than in age-equivalent mortality (about 9 versus 7 years).

Mortality-equivalent ages versus SAH-equivalent ages for Sweden are compared in Milligan and Wise (2011). Based on rough approximations, a person aged 63 in 2005 in Sweden had about the same mortality rate as a person aged 55 in 1976, a difference of about 8 years. Men who were about 64 in 2005 had about the same SAH as men who were about 9 years younger, age 55, in 1976. In this example, Sweden also shows a greater difference in age-equivalent SAH than in age-equivalent mortality (about 9 versus 8 years).

Thus, in both the United States and Sweden, there appears to be a substantial correspondence between age-equivalent mortality and age-equivalent SAH. These results must be interpreted with caution, however. Similar comparisons for the United Kingdom do not reveal the same pattern. While the difference in mortality rates between the 1970s and early 2000s are similar to the United States, differences in SAH do not follow the pattern suggested by the U.S. and Swedish data.

Cross-Country Comparison Between the Percentage Change in Mortality and the Percentage Change in SAH

Milligan and Wise (2011) find a strong relationship across countries in the percentage decline in mortality within a country and the percentage decline in SAH. For the nine countries in the International Social Security Project with data on the proportion in fair or poor health (or 1 minus the proportion in better health), there is a close relationship between the change in mortality and the change in SAH. A regression of the percentage change in fair or poor SAH on the percentage change in mortality in the nine countries yields an estimated slope coefficient of close to one (0.97). This suggests a fairly tight *within-country* relationship between improvements in mortality and improvements in self-assessed health, providing a link between the mortality analysis above and one commonly used health measure. The data also show, however, that the level of SAH varies greatly from country to country, consistent with substantial country-specific SAH response effects.

Potential for Work in the United States

An alternative approach to comparing health status and employment is to estimate the potential for work at older ages. Cutler, Meara, and Richards-Shubik (2011) followed this approach. They first estimate the relationship between labor force participation on the one hand and demographic and health characteristics on the other for people aged 62–64. Then

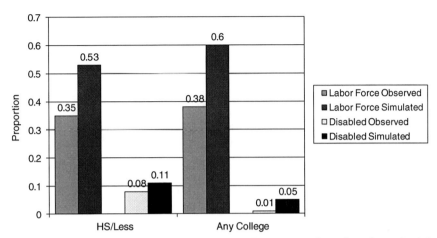

FIGURE 5-9 Labor force status in the United States, with and without Social Security and Medicare benefits, aged 65–69, men.
SOURCE: Cutler, Meara, and Richards-Shubik (2011).

they use these estimates to simulate the labor force participation for older people aged 65–69, which they call capacity for work. These simulated participation rates do not account for Medicare or Social Security provisions. Results for men with a high school degree or less and for men with any college are shown in Figure 5-9. The actual "observed" labor force participation—that is, affected by Medicare eligibility and Social Security provisions—is compared with the simulated participation that does not account for Medicare or for Social Security provisions. For both education groups, the simulated labor force participation is substantially higher than the observed rate—53 versus 35% for the high school or less group and 60 versus 38% for the any-college group. The simulated proportion on disability is also higher than the observed proportion, but the difference is very small relative to the difference in labor force participation.

THE HOW

I highlight three policy changes that can be used to facilitate longer working lives and discuss each briefly.

Social Security Provisions That Induce Early Retirement

The first policy is to eliminate Social Security provisions that induce early retirement and penalize work at older ages—implicit tax on work. Consider the compensation for working another year, say from age 60 to 61. Compensation is in two forms: the wage earnings for working another year and the increase in future retirement benefits. One might suppose that the increase in future retirement benefits would be at least large enough to offset the receipt of benefits for one fewer year. But in many countries, the present value of future social security benefits is reduced if the person works another year. That is, some of the gain in earnings from working another year is offset by the loss in future social security benefits. Following Gruber and Wise (1999), I call this the implicit tax on work or the tax force to retire.

Figure 5-10, taken from Gruber and Wise (1999), shows the strong relationship between the tax force to retire and the proportion of men aged 55–65 out of the labor force. The horizontal axis shows the sum of the tax force to retire from the early retirement age in a country to age 69. The vertical axis shows the proportion of men out of the labor force. In the countries with the lowest implicit tax rates, fewer than 40% of men in the 55–65 age range are out of the labor force, while in countries with the highest implicit tax rates, as many as 67% are out of the labor force. In making calculations like these, it is important to include disability insurance programs, special unemployment programs, and other programs that in many countries serve as early routes to retirement. These issues are discussed in detail in Gruber and Wise (1999).

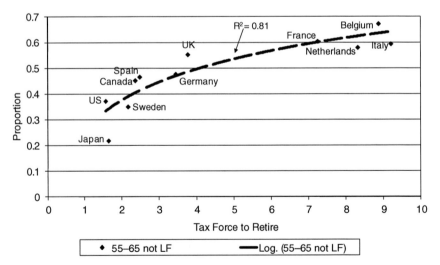

FIGURE 5-10 Proportion of men, aged 55–65, out of the labor force, by tax force to retire.
SOURCE: Gruber and Wise (1999).

The Boxed Economy View of the Labor Market

The second "policy" to facilitate longer working lives is to abandon the false assumption that economies are "boxed." This proposition holds that older people must retire to provide jobs for the young. It is often used as an excuse or as a rationale for provisions that induce older people to retire. As one example from many countries, Pierre Mauroy, then-Prime Minister of France, said this in 1981:

> And I would like to speak to the elders, to those who have spent their lifetime working in this region, and well, I would like them to show the way, that life must change; when it is time to retire, leave the labor force in order to provide jobs for your sons and daughters. That is what I ask you. The Government makes it possible for you to retire at age 55. Then retire, with one's head held high, proud of your worker's life. This is what we are going to ask you. . . . This is the *contrat de solidarité* [an early retirement scheme available to the 55+ who quit their job]. That those who are the oldest, those who have worked, leave the labor force, release jobs so that everyone can have a job (quoted in Gaullier (1982), *L'avenir à reculons*, page 230).

Gruber and Wise (2010) consider a series of methods to estimate the relationship between the employment of older people and the employment of youth, based on the analyses of the authors in the countries participating in the International Social Security Project. I show an example of the evidence, adding to Figure 5-10 above. The strong relationship between the tax force to retire and the proportion of older men out of the labor force is apparent in Figure 5-10. If the incentives that reduced the proportion of older people in the labor force (and increased the proportion out of the labor force) created more job opportunities for young people, then the tax force to retire should be related to youth employment. The greater the tax force to retire, the lower youth unemployment should be and the greater youth employment should be. Figure 5-11 is the same as Figure 5-10 but with the addition of the unemployment rate of youth aged 20 to 24. Essentially there is no relationship across countries between the tax force for older people to retire and the unemployment of youth. Indeed, the actual relationship is slightly positive—the greater the tax force to retire, the greater is youth unemployment. Similarly, the relationship between the tax force to retire and youth employment (not shown) is negative: the greater the tax force to retire, the lower the employment rate of youth.

Gruber and Wise show estimates based on several additional methods of analysis. One method is within-country "natural experiment" comparisons that help to demonstrate the relationship between within-country

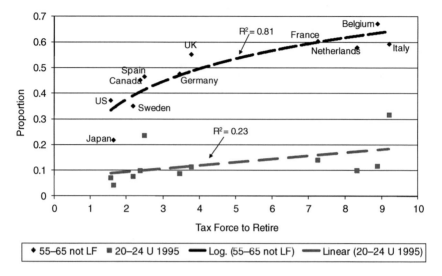

FIGURE 5-11 Men, aged 55–65, out of the labor force and youth, aged 20–24, unemployed (1995), by tax force to retire.
SOURCE: Gruber, Milligan, and Wise. (2009).

reforms and the consequent changes in the employment of the old on the one hand and changes in the employment of the young on the other hand. A second method is based on various cross-country comparisons, and a third method presents a more formal estimation based on panel regression analysis.

As it turns out, all of the various estimation methods yield very consistent results. In particular, there is no evidence that reducing the employment of older persons provides more job opportunities for younger persons, nor is there evidence that increasing the labor force participation of older persons reduces the job opportunities of younger persons.

Private Pension Provisions and Flexible Work Arrangements

The third policy to facilitate work at older ages is to remove private plan incentives to retire early and to provide flexible work arrangements for older workers. The evidence on pension plan provisions summarized above pertains to public pension systems, but these are not the only systems that contain incentives to leave the labor force early. Defined benefit systems in the private sector in the United States typically contain provisions that strongly encourage early retirement (Stock and Wise, 1990a,b). Defined benefit plans in the private sector are becoming less prevalent and are being replaced in large part by 401(k)-like plans that have none of the incentive effects of defined benefit plans. However, defined benefit plans are still common in state and local governments and in the federal government. These plans are typically very generous and typically have strong incentives to retire early. And while Social Security incentives to retire early based on non-actuarial benefit adjustments have been largely eliminated, Goda, Shoven, and Slavov (2007a,b) show that other provisions still discourage work at older ages. In addition, there are other adaptations that might encourage longer working lives. For example, institutional arrangements within firms to provide for partial retirement could well prolong work on a part-time basis.

SUMMARY AND CONCLUSIONS

I have briefly described the need for longer working lives in response to demographic trends that will greatly increase the proportion of the population that is older. The increase in the older population will increase social security and health care costs, while prolonging working lives can be an important way to pay for these rapidly increasing costs. I have emphasized that some of the bounty of longer lives must be allocated to prolonging the labor force participation of older workers.

To rationalize the plausibility of increasing working lives to adjust to demographic trends, it is important to understand the changes in health over the past four or five decades. Thus I have given primary attention to the increasing health status of older people, and I have discussed the relationship between change in health status over time and change in labor force participation. The evidence shows that the labor force participation at a given health status is much lower today than it was three or four decades ago. Much of my discussion is based on the decline in mortality rates, not because mortality is equivalent to morbidity or other measures of health, but because it is a measure comparable across countries and comparable over time within the same country. I also considered the relationship between mortality and self-reported health, also a common measure of health status, and I have considered evidence on the capacity for work at older ages.

A striking feature of the data is the correspondence between employment and mortality trends in China and the United States, as well as European countries such as the United Kingdom. Through age 65, employment of men by age is only slightly higher in China than in the United States and France, and also through age 65, mortality by age is similar in China and in European countries. But for mortality rates above 1.5%, employment for men in China is substantially greater than employment in the United States and much greater than employment in the United Kingdom and the United States, presumably due to the provisions of social security programs in the United States and in European countries.

I have also summarized how longer working lives might be facilitated. I have emphasized three policy directions: removing public social security provisions that induce older people to leave the labor force; abandoning the boxed economy view of the labor market that is often used as an excuse, or rationale, for providing incentives for older people to leave the labor force; and removing private pension plan provisions that induce early retirement and developing flexible work arrangement for older workers.

These results, based on developed countries including Japan, may have substantial implications for China. China has a very rapidly increasing older population. Yet China also has mandatory retirement ages for many workers—as young as age 50 for women and age 55 for men. Thus at a time when the cost of support for older workers is increasing, older workers are driven from the labor force (or their exit from the labor force is facilitated) by mandatory retirement ages. The data, however, suggest that many who "retire" at mandatory retirement ages remain in the labor force, perhaps in other jobs.

Finally, even in light of these trends, there are limits on work at older ages. In all countries, people with greater self-assessed disability or low health status are more likely to retire early. Policies that reduce the incentives to retire early may also limit the retirement options of people in poor health. Thus, any comprehensive analysis of the potential for longer working lives must also consider the limits on work at older ages.

REFERENCES

China Census. (1982). National Bureau of Statistics of China, Beijing, People's Republic of China.

China Census. (2005). National Bureau of Statistics of China, Beijing, People's Republic of China.

Cutler, D., E. Meara, and S. Richards-Shubik. (2011). *Healthy Life Expectancy: Estimates and Implications for Retirement Age Policy*. Available: http://www.nber.org/programs/ag/rrc/NB10-11%20Cutler,%20Meara,%20Richards%20Final,%20REVISED.pdf.

Gaullier, X. (1982). *L'avenir à Recoulons: Chomage et Retraite*. Paris: Éditions Economie et Humanisme.

Goda, G.S., J.B. Shoven, and S.N. Slavov. (2007a.) *Removing the Disincentives in Social Security for Long Careers*. NBER Working Paper No. 13110. Cambridge, MA: National Bureau of Economic Research.

Goda, G.S., J.B. Shoven, and S.N. Slavov. (2007b). *A Tax on Work for the Elderly: Medicare as a Secondary Payer*. NBER Working Paper No. 13383. Cambridge, MA: National Bureau of Economic Research.

Gruber, J., and D.A. Wise (Eds.). (1999). *Social Security and Retirement Around the World*. Chicago: University of Chicago Press.

Gruber, J., and D.A. Wise (Eds.). (2010). *Social Security Programs and Retirement Around the World: The Relationship to Youth Employment.* Chicago: University of Chicago Press.

Gruber, J., K. Milligan, and D.A. Wise. (2009). *Social Security Programs and Retirement Around the World: The Relationship to Youth Employment—Introduction and Summary.* NBER Working Paper No. 14647. Cambridge, MA: National Bureau of Economic Research.

Heiss, F., A. Börsch-Supan, M. Hurd, and D. Wise. (2009). Pathways to disability: Predicting health trajectories. Pp. 105-150 in *Health at Older Ages: The Causes and Consequences of Declining Disability Among the Elderly,* D. Cutler and D.A. Wise (Eds.). Chicago: University of Chicago Press.

Manton, K., X. Gu, and V. Lamb. (2006). Change in chronic disability from 1982 to 2004/2005 as measured by long-term changes in function and health in the U.S. elderly population. *Proceedings of the National Academy of Sciences 103(48)*:18374-18379.

Martin, L., V. Freedman, R. Schoeni, and P. Andreski. (2007). Feeling better? Trends in general health status. *Journal of Gerontology: Series B 62*:S11-S21.

Martin, L., V. Freedman, R. Schoeni, and P. Andreski. (2009). Health and functioning among baby boomers approaching 60. *Journal of Gerontology: Series B 64*:369-377.

Milligan, K., and D.A. Wise. (2011). *Social Security Programs and Retirement Around the World: Historical Trends in Mortality and Health, Employment, Disability Insurance Participation and Reforms-Introduction and Summary.* NBER Working Paper No. 16719. Cambridge, MA: National Bureau of Economic Research.

National Bureau of Statistics of China. (1987). *China Statistical Yearbook 1987.* Beijing: China Statistics Press. Available: http://tongji.cnki.net/overseas/engnavi/HomePage.aspx?id=N2010100096&name=YINFN&floor=1.

National Bureau of Statistics of China. (2006). *China Statistical Yearbook 2006.* Beijing: China Statistics Press. Available: http://tongji.cnki.net/overseas/engnavi/HomePage.aspx?id=N2010100096&name=YINFN&floor=1.

Shoven, J.B. (Forthcoming). New age thinking: Alternative ways of measuring age, their relationship to labor force participation, government policies and GDP. Pp. 17-36 in *Research Findings in the Economics of Aging,* D.A. Wise (Ed.). Chicago: University of Chicago Press.

Stock, J.H., and D.A. Wise. (1990a). Pensions, the option value of work, and retirement. *Econometrica 58*:1,151-1,180.

Stock, J.H., and D.A. Wise. (1990b). The pension inducement to retire: An option value analysis. Pp. 205-230 in *Issues in the Economics of Aging,* D.A. Wise (Ed.). Chicago: University of Chicago Press.

Weir, D. (2007). Are baby boomers living well longer? Pp. 95-112 in *Redefining Retirement: How Will Boomers Fare?,* B. Madrian, O.S. Mitchell, and B.J. Soldo (Eds.). Oxford: Oxford University Press.

Wise, D. (2010). Facilitating longer working lives: International evidence on why and how. *Demography 47*:S131-S149.

6

The Labor Supply and Retirement Behavior of China's Older Workers and Elderly in Comparative Perspective[1]

John Giles, Dewen Wang, and *Wei Cai*

There is keen awareness across developed and middle-income countries of the developing world that increased longevity and aging populations will place significant and growing burdens on working age adults in the relatively near future. In the United States and other economies with pay-as-you-go social security systems, these burdens will be transmitted through fiscal systems. Even where public transfer mechanisms are not as important, working-age adults may nonetheless face increasing burdens associated with supporting the elderly through both financial and in-kind transfers.[2] Increasing the retirement age is frequently viewed as one feasible means of easing burdens on working-

[1]This chapter has benefited from conversations with Fang Cai, Xiaoyan Lei, Philip O'Keefe, Albert Park, James Smith, John Strauss, Firman Witoelar, Kyeongwon Yoo, Xiaoqing Yu, and Yaohui Zhao, and also from comments of David Wise, Yaohui Zhao, and other participants in the Conference on Aging in Asia, sponsored by the U.S. National Academy of Sciences and Chinese Academy of Social Sciences (Beijing, December 9–10, 2010). We are grateful for financial support for this work from two sources at the World Bank: the Gender Action Program of the PREM Network and the Knowledge for Change Trust Fund managed by the Development Economics Vice Presidency (DEC) of the Bank. The findings, interpretations, and conclusions expressed in this paper are entirely those of the authors. They do not necessarily represent the views of the International Bank for Reconstruction and Development/ World Bank and its affiliated organizations, or those of the executive directors of the World Bank or the governments they represent.

[2]Lee and Mason (2011) highlight the implications of population aging for sustainability of public and private transfer systems across Africa, Asia, Europe, Latin America, and the United States.

age populations, and yet it is likely that exits from productive activity are shaped by household wealth and individual preferences, as well as by institutions and policy. Alternatively, continued participation in the workforce may reflect the ability of workers to learn new skills and to remain productive into older age. With an eye toward providing insight into the retirement decision in East Asia, this chapter presents descriptive evidence on retirement and labor supply patterns in China, Indonesia, and Korea.

While China's rapid demographic transition is frequently highlighted in news accounts because of the sheer size of its aging population, Korea and Indonesia are also confronting rapidly aging populations.[3] In contrast to most developed countries, however, rural and urban populations face significantly different retirement systems. Differences across rural and urban areas in both retirement patterns and access to financial support are most extreme in China, where most long-term residents in urban areas have had formal wage employment, retire at a relatively young age, and receive substantial support from pensions. Rural residents, by contrast, have lacked pension support and may expect to work in farming or other agriculture-related activities until relatively late in their lives.[4] In this sense, urban residents of China with formal sector employment face retirement decisions that are more similar to those of residents in developed countries. Residents of China's rural areas, by contrast, share more in common with residents of other developing countries, and make labor supply decisions in the absence of both pension availability and the constraint imposed by a mandatory age of retirement from the formal sector.

This chapter brings together information from several data sources to highlight differences in labor supply of older workers across urban and rural China, Indonesia, and Korea, and to review patterns and trends in the context of institutional differences across these three countries and between urban and rural areas. For perspective on retirement patterns in East Asian economies, we then place the retirement decision in China, Indonesia, and Korea in the context of employment patterns of older

---

[3]Recent research by demographers at the U.S. Census Bureau suggests that the old age dependency rates in 2020 will reach 22, 19, and 13%, for Korea, China, and Indonesia, respectively, and by 2040 these rates will rise to 53, 40, and 25% (Kinsella and He, 2009). A preliminary release from China's 2010 census informs us that 13.3% of China's population is now over 60 as opposed to 10.3% in 2000, while the size of the future workforce has dwindled, with individuals under 14 accounting for 16.6% of the population, down from 23% in 2000 (National Bureau of Statistics, 2011).

[4]New initiatives are currently under way in rural China. A government-subsidized contributory rural pension piloted in 2009 will be rolled out to cover all rural counties over the next three years. In cities, a new pension scheme, modeled on the rural pension program, was first introduced in July 2011 with the aim of providing financial protection in old age to nonworking urban residents and informal sector workers.

workers in the United States and the United Kingdom. In common with findings from the retirement literature focusing on developed economies, the descriptive evidence presented in this chapter is suggestive of the role that ability to collect a pension (or social security benefit) plays in the retirement decision.[5]

Mandatory retirement provisions in each of these East Asian economies, however, condition decisions of when and how to exit from productive activity. While significant numbers of retirees return to work in self-employed activities or informal work after reaching mandatory retirement age, the types of work that "retirees" are able to find may be unattractive for some older workers. Differences in the mandatory retirement age for men and women in China likely contributes to differences across genders in participation in work later in life, with important consequences for relative pension wealth and relative financial security of older men and women.

After reviewing descriptive trends, we lay out an empirical model to examine correlates of labor supply with own and spouse eligibility to receive a pension, own and spouse health status, and proxies for household wealth. We next review data sources and correlates of employment separately for China, Indonesia, and Korea. The chapter presents comparative descriptive evidence from East Asia and highlights important questions on retirement behavior in developing countries that may be addressed from new panel data initiatives currently under way.

EMPLOYMENT PATTERNS AND THE RETIREMENT OF OLDER WORKERS

In China, long-term urban residents with formal sector employment can expect to receive a pension upon retirement, but face mandatory retirement at a relatively young age.[6] Where urban employed men confront mandatory retirement at age 60, women in blue collar occupations are frequently required to retire at age 50, those in white collar occupations at

---

[5]Blau (1994) suggests that social security eligibility contributes to relatively high exit from the labor force at age 65; Krueger and Pischke (1992) exploit design features of the U.S. social security system to demonstrate the effects of benefits on labor force participation. Gruber and Wise (1999, 2004) present evidence from Organisation for Economic Co-operation and Development economies of the effects of social security and public pension systems on labor supply decisions of older workers.

[6]We define a long-term urban resident as an urban dweller with an urban (nonagricultural) residential registration (*hukou*) status. While considerable efforts have been made recently to extend social insurance benefits to migrants living in the city, migrants are much less likely to have employment contracts and to have employers who are making mandated contributions to pension, health, and disability insurance programs (Giles, Wang, and Park, 2012).

age 55, with women in some categories (e.g., university professors) able to work until age 60. Among current retirement-age residents of urban areas, a large share is receiving relatively generous pension support. By contrast, rural elderly, who had lower incomes during their working lives and less accumulated wealth than their urban counterparts (Kanbur and Zhang, 1999; Ravallion and Chen, 2007), do not typically have pension income. According to the 2005 1% population sample, 45.4% of urban residents over age 60 report pension income as their most important source of financial support, but only 4.6% of rural residents note an important role for pension income. Instead, 38% of rural respondents over age 60 report that income from their own labor is their most important source of support.[7]

The stark difference in employment rates of rural and urban residents reflects differences in both pension wealth and mandatory retirement provisions across urban and rural areas.[8] As evident in Panel A of Figure 6-1, which presents locally weighted regression (LOWESS) estimates of employment rates by age, China's rural residents are far more likely to be employed well after the mandatory retirement ages faced by urban residents. From the China Health and Retirement Longitudinal Study (CHARLS) pilot conducted in 2008, we note 45% of urban men aged 60–64 were still employed at least one hour per week (Panel A), but in rural areas nearly 86% of men in this age range were still working. The difference in employment of urban and rural women aged 60–64 was even wider, with only 16% working in urban areas and nearly 57% still employed in rural areas.

If anything, the CHARLS pilot, with relatively small sample sizes in urban Zhejiang and Gansu and representative of only two provinces, may overstate the employment rates of older men and women. Also presented in Panel A of Figure 6-1 are the 1991 and 2009 estimates from the China Health Nutrition Survey (CHNS), which show a substantially lower employment rate of 31% for urban men in the 60–64 age range. When comparing employment rates across the age distribution over time using the CHNS, one observes declines for both men and women in urban

---

[7]Additional descriptive statistics on sources of support from the 2005 1% population subsample are reported in Cai et al. (2012) and Giles, Wang, and Zhao (2010).

[8]In defining "employment" in this chapter, we include wage employment in the informal sector, casual work, self-employed activities, and unpaid work in family-run enterprises, all of which may be important for older workers in these economies. We focus on employment as opposed to labor force participation, per se, for two reasons. Job search is often not well documented, and where it is (e.g., the CHARLS data for China), there are a vanishingly small number of respondents (five in CHARLS) aged 45 and older who are not employed but report active searches for work. We have no doubt that a search process exists for older workers who wish to work, but it is difficult to capture, and this is particularly true when large shares of older workers are self-employed.

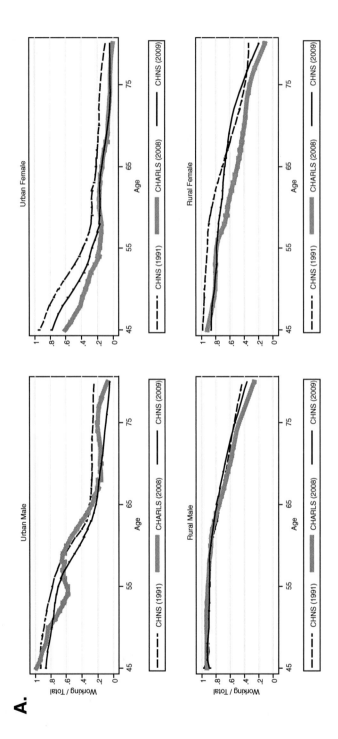

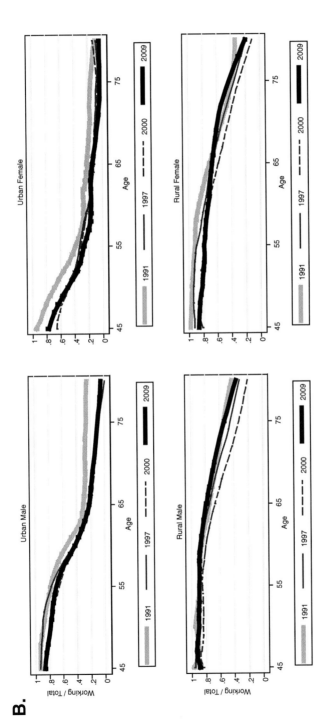

FIGURE 6-1 Employment rates by age cohort of older workers and elderly in urban and rural China.
NOTE: Employment rates by age cohort are calculated using nonparametric locally weighted regression (LOWESS) with a band-width of 0.3.
SOURCES: Panel A and B use data from the common provinces surveyed across waves of the China Health and Nutrition Survey (CHNS) conducted from 1991 to 2009. Panel A also includes data from the 2008 China Health and Retirement Longitudinal Study (CHARLS) pilot.

areas, but less pronounced declines in employment rates in rural areas.[9] Rural women between age 45 and 65 were somewhat less likely to be working in 2009 than in 1991, but this does not appear to be true for older women or for rural men.

One of the sharper changes from 1991 to 2009, as viewed from the CHNS, lies in the decline in employment rates of women over age 45 in urban China.[10] The decline in older women's labor force participation raises an important question for labor research in China: Does the decline in women's employment reflect a resurgence of gender discrimination in post-reform China or the effects of increases in household wealth and the ability of women to exit the labor force at a younger age? Differences across genders in mandatory retirement ages likely create an institutional bias against women's employment. Even in the absence of discrimination, the employment decision of older women in urban China reflects a constrained choice. Women may return to work as consultants or in self-employed activities after reaching mandatory retirement age, but retired women are frequently receiving pensions, which raises reservation wages for new employment. Those urban women uninterested in working in typical self-employed activities held by blue collar workers (e.g., nannies or housekeepers) may choose to stay out of work if their pension incomes are sufficient.

Earlier research on labor force participation in China has noted the drop in employment rates of urban residents, and urban women in particular (Cai, Park, and Zhao, 2008; Maurer-Fazio et al., 2011) and attributed the drop to the effects of state sector restructuring after 1997. After losing work during state sector restructuring, men, the young, and the well educated generally faced shorter durations out of work (Appleton et al., 2002; Giles, Park, and Cai, 2006a; Maurer-Fazio, 2007). Moreover, some researchers found that a woman's decision to reenter the workforce was affected not only by permanent and relatively generous pensions, but also by family circumstances (Giles, Park, and Cai, 2006b).

Given support available through pensions to relatively young workers

---

[9]We review evidence from the CHNS as it is the publicly available data source that researchers used (pre-CHARLS) to study labor supply, health status, and retirement of older workers in China (e.g., Benjamin, Brandt, and Fan, 2003; Dong, 2010). As it is based on a panel of households that does not enumerate complete information on family members who have split off of households, one should be concerned that later waves of the CHNS over-represent those who remain in the households. As we are interested in the over-45 population, this is less of a problem than if we were considering the employment decisions of individuals who were children in 1991 and likely to have moved out of households.

[10]Additional corroborating evidence on the decline in women's labor force participation from the census and the China Urban Labor Survey (CULS) can be found in the expanded working paper version of this paper (Giles, Wang, and Cai, 2011).

during economic restructuring and potential biases against hiring dis-placed workers relatively close to retirement age, one would expect to see sharp drops in employment of urban women from 1991 to 1997 and 2000, as is shown in Panel B of Figure 6-1. If reduced employment rates of urban women over 45 were simply the effect of restructuring in the late 1990s, however, we would expect that employment of women in the 45–55 age range would return to higher pre-1997 levels by 2009. The fact that older working-age women, who have not yet reached mandatory retirement age, continue to have lower employment rates, even after labor markets tight-ened during the 2000s, raises the possibility that exits from the labor force may be a choice facilitated by higher wealth or by increasing demands on time for nonmarket activities, such as caring for children, elderly, or other ill family members.

Exits from employment among older workers as they approach pen-sion eligibility are not unusual in more developed economies such as the United Kingdom and the United States, but exit rates in the years before retirement age are not typically as high as one observes in China. Figure 6-2 highlights differences in employment rates across five countries and shows that 68 and 70% of women aged 50 to 54 are still employed in the United States and United Kingdom, respectively. Employment rates of women in this age range are somewhat lower in urban Indonesia at 63%, but above the 38 and 30% employment rates witnessed in urban Korea and China, respectively.[11] Relative employment patterns of men in the 55 to 59 age range follow a similar pattern: 68 and 67% of urban men in this age range in China and Korea, respectively, are employed, while 82% of urban Indonesia men of this age are still working.

Mandatory Retirement Provisions and Retirement Patterns

Incentives created by gender differences in the mandatory retirement age may encourage early exits from the labor force by women, particu-larly for women who face the prospect of a job search in their 40s. Career changes and job changes later in working life can be difficult in devel-oped and developing economies alike. As beginning a new job requires learning processes, technology, and culture of the new workplace, a new employee will not reach peak productivity in a position immediately upon being hired. An employer may be less likely to consider hiring a worker who is close to mandatory retirement age simply because there is not sufficient time to earn a return on initial training and start-up costs relative to a younger worker. In the United States, where many workers

---

[11]Note that this is the urban employment rate for women using the CHARLS sample; in the CHNS sample, the rate is higher at 42%.

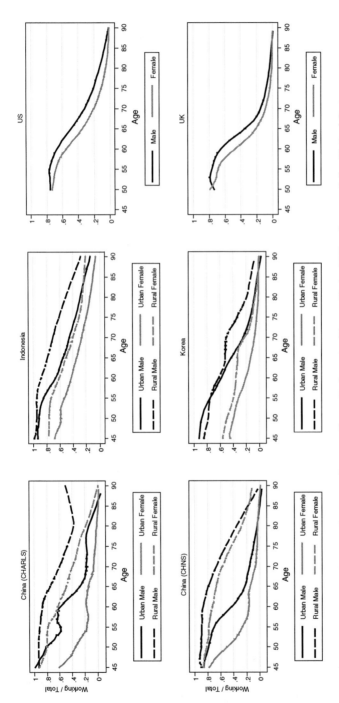

FIGURE 6-2 Employment rates by age cohort in China, Indonesia, Korea, United Kingdom, and the United States.

NOTE: Employment rates by age cohort are calculated using non-parametric locally weighted regression (LOWESS) with a bandwidth of 0.3.

SOURCES: Data from China: 2009 CHNS and the 2008 CHARLS pilot; Indonesia: 2007 Indonesia Family Life Survey (IFLS); Korea: 2006 Korean Longitudinal Study of Aging (KLoSA); United States: 2008 Health and Retirement Study (HRS); United Kingdom: 2008/9 English Longitudinal Study of Ageing (ELSA).

start to leave the workforce upon eligibility for Social Security benefits, difficulties finding new employment among older displaced workers are well documented. Research using the U.S. Health and Retirement Study (HRS), for example, has demonstrated that of workers who lose jobs after age 55, only 60% of men and 55% of women are employed again within two years, while 80% of nondisplaced workers are employed (Chan and Stevens, 2001).

In China, and to some extent Indonesia and Korea, a mandatory retirement age for some occupations and types of employers is even more binding than Social Security eligibility in the United States. Differences in mandatory retirement ages of men and women in China may have a significant impact on how employers view the relative returns to hiring male and female employees who are in their 40s and older.[12]

In Korea and Indonesia, retirement ages are not mandated by the law, but employment laws allow for firms to set mandatory ages, and government employees and civil servants face mandatory retirement. After the East Asian financial crisis in 1997/1998, firms that had not implemented mandatory retirement started to do so as a way of slowing wage increases associated with seniority-based wage systems (Cho and Kim, 2005).

The higher employment rates of older urban men and women in Indonesia and Korea (Figure 6-2) suggest that mandatory retirement from some occupations and types of employers does not mechanically lead to permanent exit from productive employment. Existing research on older workers in both countries suggests that an impending retirement creates incentives for forward-looking workers to leave employers preemptively, either to start their own businesses or to start second careers working for smaller private-sector employers.[13]

One significant difference across workers in urban and rural areas of China, Indonesia, and Korea lies in the share of the retirement-age workforce with access to pensions. In China, evidence from the CHARLS pilot suggests that, of urban residents aged 60 and older, 79% of men and 54% of women have access to pension support. In urban areas of Indo-

---

[12]Of course, employers may already perceive older workers to be less productive (Chan and Stevens, 2001; Dalen, Henkens, and Joop, 2010), but this is a problem faced by both older men and women when looking for work.

[13]McKee (2006) finds that in Indonesia, half of government workers move into either the private sector or into self-employment, and 61% of workers who leave their private-sector jobs move into self-employment. In Korea, self-employment was one response to lay-offs from larger employers in the wake of the 1997/1998 financial crisis (Sohn, 2007) and continues to be an important source of employment for older males (Lee, 2009). Lee and Lee (2011) note differences in the retirement ages of self-employed and wage-salary earners, but do not discuss the incentive to move into self-employment ahead of mandatory retirement among wage and salary earners who wish to continue working.

nesia and Korea, by contrast, fewer than 35% of men and 15% of women have access to pensions.[14] Another unique feature of pension eligibility in Korea lies with an imperfect correspondence between mandatory retirement age and age at which pension-eligible retirees may start receiving pension benefits. The National Pension scheme, the largest of the three main sources of pensions in Korea, does not begin paying benefits until age 60, yet a significant share of employees face mandatory retirement at age 55 (Cho and Kim, 2005). This imperfect correspondence likely increases incentives for those employees facing mandatory retirement to look for new career opportunities, including in the self-employed sector.

Across rural areas of China, Indonesia, and Korea, both men and women remain actively employed until much later in their lives than urban residents. In rural areas of all three economies, agricultural production on the family farm continues to be a significant source of employment for older workers, and this is necessitated by the fact that rural residents tend to accumulate less wealth over their working lifetimes. In addition, older workers in rural China and Indonesia are far less likely to have access to pensions than their urban counterparts. Both the CHARLS and the 2005 Population Census suggest that, of rural residents over 60, roughly 5% of men and less than 1% of women have pension support. Similarly, in rural Indonesia, the Indonesia Family Life Survey (IFLS) shows that only 8% of men and 3% of women aged 60 and older have access to pensions.

Rural Korea is a somewhat different matter. Efforts to bring rural residents into the National Pension scheme established in 1988 have led to pension coverage rates in rural areas that do not differ significantly from urban areas; indeed, 34% of older rural men in the 2006 Korean Longitudinal Study of Aging (KLoSA) wave report receiving pensions. Nonetheless, the continued labor supply of rural men is viewed as an important factor contributing to high rates of economic activity among older Koreans (Lee, 2009). In spite of availability of pensions, levels of support are not sufficient to permit retirement of the rural elderly. Lee (2009) suggests that the out-migration of the young has left elderly who remain behind with both a lack of young labor and insufficient wealth to cease productive activity. Given that the history of rapid urbanization in Korea mirrors the process of rural-to-urban migration taking place in China, one might be concerned that incidence of delayed retirement of China's rural farmers, who are less affluent and have lacked pension support, may follow a similar pattern to Korea.

---

[14]More specifically, in Korea, 34% of urban men and 15% of urban women have access to pensions; and in Indonesia, 27% of urban men and 10% of urban women have access to pensions. Figures on pension coverage are drawn from the 2006 wave of KLoSA and the 2007 wave of IFLS.

RETIREMENT IN CHINA, INDONESIA, AND KOREA

The descriptive patterns shown above make use of data from early stages of longitudinal studies from China and Korea that are modeled on the Health and Retirement Study (HRS) from the United States and the English Longitudinal Study on Ageing (ELSA) in the United Kingdom. New survey efforts, like CHARLS in China, promise to facilitate the study of retirement and labor supply behavior in regions where pension and social security systems are not well established and population aging is occurring at a rapid pace. In the analytical models that we estimate, we make use of the cross-sections from China, Indonesia, and Korea used for basic descriptive statistics presented above.[15] Below, we provide some additional discussion of the analysis sample used for each country.

China

The China Health and Retirement Longitudinal Study (CHARLS), directed by Yaohui Zhao at the National School of Development at Peking University, was developed and implemented by an accomplished team of collaborators from China and abroad. The sample used in this analysis is from the pilot survey conducted in 2008 in Gansu and Zhejiang provinces and is representative of adults over 45 years of age in these provinces. Gansu, in the northwest, is a relatively poor province, and Zhejiang, on the coast south of Shanghai, is relatively affluent. CHARLS follows the model of the HRS, ELSA, and KLoSA in the United States, United Kingdom, and Korea, and enumerates information on respondent and spouse socioeconomic status, health conditions, work and employment, and incomes and pensions, and it also includes household and community-level information. In the pilot sample used in the analysis below, there are 1,570 households and 2,685 eligible respondents.[16]

Indonesia

The Indonesia Family Life Survey (IFLS) is an ongoing project conducted by the RAND Corporation and universities in both Indonesia and the United States. To date, four waves have been conducted in 1993, 1997/1998, 2000, and 2007/2008. The survey covers individuals, households, communities, and the community-level health and educational

---

[15]Additional summary statistics for important variables used in the analysis are shown in Table 1 of the longer working paper version of this paper (Giles, Wang, and Cai, 2011).

[16]The CHARLS project has funding for nationally representative surveys in 2011 and 2013, and fieldwork on the first national wave began in July 2011. Public-use data should be available for the research community by June 2012.

facilities that respondent households access in their daily life. While it is not a formal member of the "HRS family" of aging surveys, the data are comprehensive and include information on respondent health status, employment and labor allocation, pension participation, and household and family characteristics, all of which are crucial for study of retirement and labor supply decisions of the elderly. The original survey was representative of 83% of the Indonesian population and 13 of 27 provinces. As it tracks the movers and split-offs from the original sample, IFLS was a pioneer among household surveys in the developing world. Tracking is important when working with the 2007/2008 round of IFLS, because it allows us to avoid using a selected sample of individuals who have not moved.[17] The most recent round has 50,583 observations and 13,507 households. The analytical work below uses detailed information collected from 7,283 direct respondents aged 45 and over for whom information on pension eligibility was enumerated.

Korea

The Korean Longitudinal Study of Ageing (KLoSA) is a nationally representative survey conducted by the Korea Labor Institute to investigate the overall conditions of people aged 45 and older in South Korea (excluding Jeju island). KLoSA belongs to the same family of aging surveys as CHARLS, HRS, and ELSA. The first baseline survey was conducted in 2006, and it was followed by a job history survey in 2007. While KLoSA is a longitudinal survey, only the baseline survey is publically available. In common with CHARLS and ELSA, but differing from the HRS, the first baseline survey does not cover the institutionalized elderly. Overall, 6,171 households and 10,254 individuals participated in the baseline survey, and there are 10,030 observations with complete information.

A MODEL OF THE EMPLOYMENT OF OLDER ADULTS

Below, we examine determinants of the labor supply (employment) of older workers, recognizing that important correlates, such as access to pensions, may be systematically related to both the ability to retire and unobservable characteristics (e.g., ability). While these models should be viewed as providing descriptive evidence, we choose measures of health status and proxies for wealth and family characteristics with the aim of minimizing endogeneity biases.

---

[17]Even though older residents of both this survey, as well as the CHNS in China, do not move or split off with the same frequency as household members who were under 25 during the initial wave, one might nonetheless be concerned about this potential source of bias.

The three data sources used to examine employment outcomes in China (CHARLS 2008), Indonesia (IFLS, 2007), and Korea (KLoSA, 2006) provide roughly comparable information on labor supply, health status, and education of both the respondent and spouse, and information on parents and children regardless of current residence in the household.[18] We estimate the reduced form labor supply model in each country:

$$L_i^S = \beta_1 E_i + \beta_2 E_i^2 + \beta_3 Pen_i + \beta_4 Pen_{-i} + $$
$$ADL_i'' \beta_5 + \beta_6 \overline{E}_{-i} + X_i' \gamma + V_j + u_i \qquad (1)$$

where labor supply, L_i^S, is a binary indicator of whether individual i worked for one hour or more during the previous week. We expect that higher values of educational attainment of elderly, E_i, will be associated with higher wealth and savings and, as leisure is a normal good, may be negatively related to elderly labor supply.[19] Similarly, we expect that access to own pension income, Pen_i, and pension income of a spouse, Pen_{-i}, will be negatively related to employment.

The health of older workers and the elderly are measured using two z-scores calculated from responses to a set of activities of daily living questions, ADL.[20] For each of the three data sources, we make use of questions related to activities of daily living to construct two indices: one is based on the number of activities that the respondent may perform with difficulty (Difficulty), and the second is based on the number of activities that a respondent cannot perform (Unable). Because each survey has some differences in activities and asks a different number of activities, we use these responses to construct within country z-scores

---

[18]An important benefit of knowing the numbers of grandchildren and living parents independent of whether they are members of the household is that we are able to control for potential demand for a family care-provider without introducing biases related to endogenous household composition, as would occur if relying on information about household members alone.

[19]Of course, an individual with more education may also be able to earn significantly higher returns, and so the coefficient on education will reflect the net effect of returns and accumulated wealth on employment.

[20]Bound (1991) cautions that general health status questions are likely to be correlated with unobservable individual characteristics and, further, that they may suffer from justification bias. Several studies (e.g., Bound, 1999; Dwyer and Mitchell, 1999) have suggested that proxies constructed from ADLs do not suffer from such serious bias. Bound, Stinebrickner, and Waidmann (2010) cautions that financial wealth may affect ADL outcomes, and that even proxies developed from ADLs may lead to underestimating the negative effects of poor health on labor supply. As we do not yet have appropriate panel data for the three countries in this study, we are not able to control for dynamic relationships between health and wealth.

(respondent count – average count)/(standard deviation of count).[21] Increases in each of these two z-scores reflect declining physical ability and worsening general health status. A particular value of the Unable-ADL z-score will be associated with more severe limitations than the same value of the Difficulty-ADL z-score.

We expect that declining health will have a negative impact on work activity, particularly for those workers in occupations in which physical strength and mobility are important (Bound, 1999). As the education of a spouse or adult children will be related to additional sources of income (from spouse income or transfers from children), we include average education of these family members, $\overline{E}_{-i}$. Finally, we control for a vector of individual and household characteristics, X_i, which include age and age-squared and are associated with own productivity, numbers of grandchildren, and living parents of the head and spouse, which are associated with preferences for employment, and the ln (1 + per capita value of the household dwelling), as a proxy for household wealth.

Within the retirement literature in the United States, recent research has focused on the important roles of spouse employment and spouse health status in labor supply and retirement decisions. First, the retirement decisions of husbands and wives may be interdependent. Structural models (Blau, 1994; Gustman and Steinmeier, 2004) suggest that labor supply decisions of older couples reflect preferences for shared retirement. Second, work decisions may be affected by the health status of a spouse. One may plausibly observe an added worker effect, in which a spouse's health shock leads to increased labor supply so as to ensure income against the earnings-loss associated with the health shock (e.g., Coile, 2004a), or alternatively find that spouse care requirements will require exit from the labor force (e.g., McGeary, 2009). To gauge the potential importance of these factors in China, Indonesia, and Korea, we next estimate model (2) below:

$$L_i^S = \beta_1 E_i + \beta_2 E_i^2 + \beta_3 Pen_i + \beta_4 Pen_{-i} + ADL_i'' \beta_5 + \beta_6 \overline{E}_{-i} + ADL_{-i}' \beta_7 + \beta_8 L_{-i}^S + X_i' \gamma + V_j + u_i \qquad (2)$$

where L_{-i}^S is an indicator of whether or not a spouse is employed, and ADL_{-i} are measures of spouse health status. As the labor supply decisions of husbands and wives are likely to be determined jointly and have a

---

[21]CHARLS asks 19, IFLS asks 18, and KLoSa asks 17. Each of the surveys asks questions related to functional abilities such as the ability to walk for a kilometer, go up and down stairs, lift 10 or 20 lbs., draw water from a well, and perform household chores, bathe oneself, or take medication.

dynamic relationship with health and shocks to health and employment, we view these models as purely descriptive but informative of the extent to which joint labor supply decisions may affect the timing of retirement. As the HRS-type surveys mature into full panel studies, it will be feasible to control for unobservables and to unlock directions of causality among these variables.[22]

DETERMINANTS OF "RETIREMENT" IN CHINA, INDONESIA, AND KOREA

Employment and Pension Availability

Descriptive patterns of employment in productive activity across urban and rural areas of China, Indonesia, and Korea (see Figure 6-3) are suggestive of the role that eligibility for a pension may play in retirement of older workers and elderly. In these figures, the line shows the share of population in two-year age cohorts that is employed in some productive activity (salaried work, informal sector wage labor, casual work, self-employed activities, or unpaid employment in family-run enterprises) and the bars represent the pension-eligible share. In urban China, the employed share decreases sharply with increases in the pension-eligible share. In rural areas of China, one does not observe a similar decline in employment, and shares of workers with access to pensions are quite low. In Indonesia and Korea, where pension coverage rates at young ages are lower than for urban China, one observes a much more gradual decline in the employment of men in urban areas, and a far less pronounced decline in rural areas of both countries.

In Table 6-1, we show results from estimating the labor supply model presented in model (2) above.[23] The results are suggestive of the role that pension income plays in decisions to exit from employment and the labor

---

[22]In estimating models (2) and (3), it should be noted that for each country, there are subsamples of the population for which there is no spouse or for which spouse information is not available, and this may lead to concerns about biases introduced by selection into marriage. In the models presented in this paper, we have handled this problem by including indicator variables for marital status and for absence of spouse information, and then set spouse information to zero for those observations for which no data on a spouse are available (for ADL z-scores, of course, this corresponds to the mean). We have also estimated these models on the subset of the data for which we have information on both spouses. We take comfort in the fact that there is no appreciable difference in the coefficients of interest across models using the full sample and the one estimated on married couples with spouse information.

[23]We present linear probability models by gender and residence location (urban and rural). While magnitudes differ somewhat, marginal effects using probit models do not lead to significant qualitative differences in results.

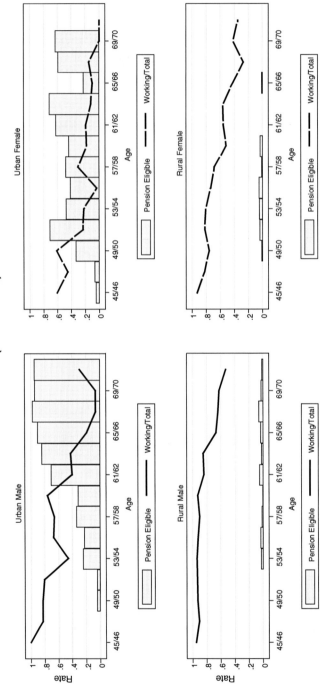

FIGURE 6-3 Employment patterns and access to pensions across rural and urban areas of China, Indonesia, and Korea.
SOURCES: Calculated using the 2008 CHARLS pilot (China), 2007 IFLS (Indonesia), and the 2006 KLoSA (Korea).

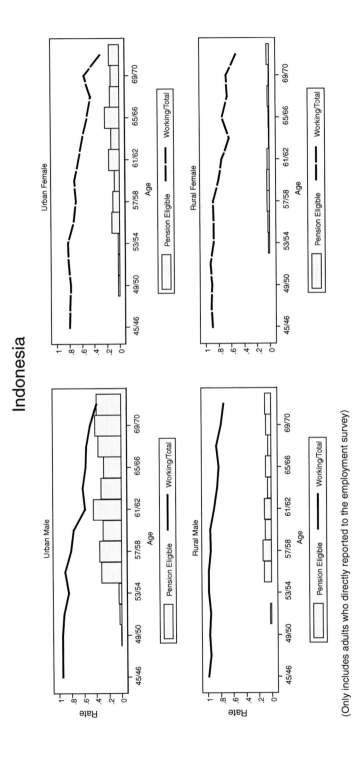

Indonesia

(Only includes adults who directly reported to the employment survey)

FIGURE 6-3 Continued

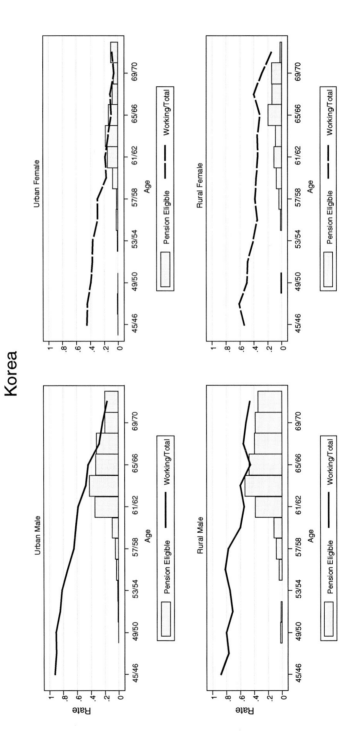

FIGURE 6-3 Continued

force. After controlling for age, education, health status of respondent and spouse, proxies for wealth, and family demographic characteristics, men and women in urban China are 15.2% and 18.3% less likely to be working if eligible for a pension. Among the rural population, we observe a marginally significant negative relationship between pension eligibility and employment for men, but no effect on employment of women. In Indonesia, where coverage by pensions is most common among retired civil servants, access to pensions is also negatively associated with work activity for both genders in rural and urban areas. In Korea, by contrast, access to a pension only affects the employment status of men in urban areas. This may not be surprising if pension coverage or income is particularly low in Korea, or is earned by wealthier households whose labor force participation is affected by other factors. Lee (2009) has noted that although coverage expansion to rural areas was an objective of the National Pension Scheme after 1988, wealth distribution in rural areas remains skewed and that the majority of rural households lacked sufficient pension income or wealth to retire.

Ability to retire, of course, not only depends on pension access, but also on whether a household has sufficient accumulated wealth to allow for retirement. A respondent's years of schooling will be associated both with lifetime wealth, and with potential current returns available in the labor market. In the models reported in Table 6-1, we observe a nonlinear relationship between years of education for urban and rural women and their probability of working. For urban Chinese women, probability of working declines with each additional year of schooling through completion of middle school, and then starts to increase with higher levels of education. We also observe that increases in housing wealth per capita in urban China are associated with reduced probability of employment. In rural China, the probability of male and female employment declines with education through 11 years of schooling. As educational attainment is not very high in rural China, increasing education (and lifetime accumulated wealth) is associated with reduced likelihood of employment for all but those individuals who have completed high school. The more highly educated rural women are likely to be working in village administration, run small enterprises, or be involved in other activities that have higher returns and do not require the same physical demands as work in agriculture. Turning to Indonesia and Korea, we only observe a similarly strong negative relationship between years of schooling and participation in work among women in urban Indonesia.

The pension income of a spouse, as well as other incentives affecting spouse retirement decisions, may also influence the retirement decision (Coile, 2004b). In the results shown in Table 6-1, we find that spouse pension eligibility has a significant impact on the employment status of rural

TABLE 6-1 Pension Eligibility and Health Status in the Labor Supply of Adults Aged 45 and Older

	Linear Probability Models, Dependent Variable: Worked at Least One Hour per Week			
	China (CHARLS)			
	Urban		Rural	
	Male	Female	Male	Female
Age	−0.067	−0.088***	0.016	0.005
	(0.04)	(0.03)	(0.01)	(0.01)
Age-Squared	0.000	0.001***	−0.000*	−0.000*
	(0.00)	(0.00)	(0.00)	(0.00)
Years of Education	0.003	−0.032*	−0.009	−0.040**
	(0.02)	(0.02)	(0.01)	(0.02)
Years of Education-Squared	0.000	0.003***	0.001	0.004**
	(0.00)	(0.00)	(0.00)	(0.00)
Pension Eligible	−0.152*	−0.183***	−0.123*	0.003
	(0.08)	(0.06)	(0.07)	(0.12)
Spouse Pension Eligible	0.048	0.029	0.060	−0.182***
	(0.07)	(0.08)	(0.10)	(0.06)
Average Education of Spouse and Adult Children	−0.006	0.003	−0.008	0.007
	(0.01)	(0.01)	(0.01)	(0.01)
Ln(Housing Wealth P.C.+1)	−0.061**	−0.013	−0.010	−0.028*
	(0.03)	(0.02)	(0.02)	(0.02)
Number of Living Parents	0.011	0.065**	0.018	−0.003
	(0.03)	(0.03)	(0.01)	(0.02)
Number of Grandchildren	0.005	−0.009	−0.009**	−0.006
	(0.02)	(0.02)	(0.00)	(0.00)
ADL Z-Score (w/difficulty)	−0.049	−0.027	−0.075***	−0.072***
	(0.04)	(0.03)	(0.01)	(0.01)
ADL Z-Score (unable)	−0.003	−0.010	−0.080***	−0.050***
	(0.04)	(0.03)	(0.01)	(0.01)
Observations	256	236	1,000	1,103
R-squared	0.464	0.458	0.308	0.325

NOTES: These regression models contain an indicator for married, spouse information not present, and dummy for no-existence of adult children. Control variables not presented in the table are (Dummy = 1 if spouse is not present), (Dummy == 1 if the individual does not have non-schooling adult children), and location dummies (China: county; Indonesia: Kabupaten; Korea: metropolitan city and province). Standard errors in parentheses. * denotes $p < 0.1$; ** $p < 0.05$; *** $p < 0.01$.
SOURCES: Calculated using the 2008 CHARLS pilot (China), 2007 IFLS (Indonesia), and the 2006 KLoSA (Korea).

	Indonesia (IFLS)				Korea (KLoSA)			
	Urban		Rural		Urban		Rural	
	Male	Female	Male	Female	Male	Female	Male	Female
	0.021**	0.075***	0.023***	0.032***	−0.058***	−0.051***	−0.015	−0.023*
	(0.01)	(0.01)	(0.01)	(0.01)	(0.01)	(0.01)	(0.02)	(0.01)
	−0.000***	−0.001***	−0.000***	−0.000***	0.000***	0.000***	−0.000	0.000
	(0.00)	(0.00)	(0.00)	(0.00)	(0.00)	(0.00)	(0.00)	(0.00)
	−0.009	−0.015**	−0.002	−0.004	0.011	0.008	0.031**	0.018*
	(0.01)	(0.01)	(0.00)	(0.01)	(0.01)	(0.01)	(0.01)	(0.01)
	0.000	0.002***	0.000	0.000	−0.000	−0.000	−0.002**	−0.001*
	(0.00)	(0.00)	(0.00)	(0.00)	(0.00)	(0.00)	(0.00)	(0.00)
	−0.238***	−0.246***	−0.132***	−0.126*	−0.107***	−0.021	−0.039	0.014
	(0.03)	(0.05)	(0.03)	(0.07)	(0.02)	(0.03)	(0.04)	(0.05)
	−0.119**	−0.040	0.103	−0.055	−0.051	−0.040*	0.043	−0.070*
	(0.05)	(0.04)	(0.08)	(0.05)	(0.05)	(0.02)	(0.10)	(0.04)
	−0.004	−0.010***	−0.000	−0.003	0.007***	−0.009***	−0.001	−0.000
	(0.00)	(0.00)	(0.00)	(0.00)	(0.00)	(0.00)	(0.01)	(0.01)
	0.002	−0.001	0.002	0.003	0.017**	−0.016***	0.008	−0.024
	(0.01)	(0.01)	(0.01)	(0.01)	(0.01)	(0.01)	(0.02)	(0.02)
	0.011	0.029**	−0.003	0.005	0.008	−0.011	0.031	−0.017
	(0.01)	(0.01)	(0.01)	(0.01)	(0.01)	(0.01)	(0.02)	(0.02)
					−0.006**	−0.003	0.009*	0.007**
					(0.00)	(0.00)	(0.00)	(0.00)
	−0.100***	−0.068***	−0.066***	−0.072***	−0.035***	−0.013**	−0.066***	−0.008
	(0.01)	(0.01)	(0.01)	(0.01)	(0.01)	(0.01)	(0.02)	(0.01)
	−0.110***	−0.070***	−0.135***	−0.093***	−0.033***	−0.007	−0.036***	−0.026*
	(0.02)	(0.02)	(0.01)	(0.01)	(0.01)	(0.01)	(0.01)	(0.01)
	1,505	2,004	1,613	2,161	3,413	4,356	1,005	1,262
	0.328	0.133	0.316	0.154	0.384	0.169	0.247	0.192

women. A rural woman married to someone with a pension is likely to be in a much wealthier household. Pension recipients in rural areas tend to be retired cadres with much greater lifetime savings. Lack of an effect of spouse pension eligibility on employment of women in urban China likely reflects the fact that urban women, who are 5 to 10 years younger than their spouses, are frequently pension-eligible and already out of the labor force. A husband's pension eligibility does not have an independent effect on labor supply.

Work and Health Status

For those workers in developing countries involved in manual tasks, such as work in agriculture, we would expect to observe a strong relationship between health status and labor force participation. From the results shown in Table 6-2, health status has a far more pronounced effect on work activities of China's rural residents than urban residents. A one standard deviation increase in the Difficulty-ADL z-score is associated with 7.5% and 7.2% declines in probabilities of working for rural men and women, respectively, and a one standard deviation increase in the ADL-Unable z-score is associated with an 8.0% reduction for men and 5.0% reduction for women. In contrast to China, decline in physical functioning has a negative effect on work status of men and women in both urban and rural areas of Indonesia. Given that urban residents of Indonesia tend to work until much later in their lives, frequently in self-employed activities, the difference in importance of health status between urban residents of China and Indonesia makes sense. China's urban residents retire before marked declines in physical functioning. Finally, in Korea, poor health status has a statistically significant negative effect on employment of men in both urban and rural areas, but the effect is more pronounced in rural areas where work is likely to be more strenuous.

Family Care Provision and Employment?

One frequently raised hypothesis concerning the exit of older women from the labor force lies with growing demands for provision of elder care and care of grandchildren. In order to reduce potential bias, the models estimated in Table 6-2 use numbers of living parents and grandchildren, respectively, rather than presence of parents or grandchildren as *household* members as covariates. This distinction is important as a significant negative correlation when an elder is present in the household may lead to misleading causal interpretations if arrangements for care-provision and older worker labor supply are jointly determined.[24] The lack of a systematic negative relationship between employment of China's older urban workers and the number of family members for whom they might provide care, suggests that the explanation for decline in women's labor force participation lies elsewhere. In Indonesia and Korea as well, the composition of the extended family does not seem to be strongly and systematically associated with labor supply and retirement decisions.

Interdependence of Spouse Retirement Decisions

In Table 6-2, we present results from estimates of model (2), which provide insight into the joint retirement decisions of spouses and the role of spouse health status in retirement. Across rural and urban areas of China, Indonesia, and Korea, men are more likely to work if their spouses are working as well. In urban China, where the effect of a spouse working is associated with a 19.6% and 20.2% higher probability of employment for men and women, respectively, one policy implication of joint retirement decisions is that efforts to encourage retirement at older ages for both men and women will likely have a positive impact on employment of spouses (Falkinger, Winter-Ebmer, and Zweimuller, 1996). Moreover, in rural China and both urban and rural areas of Indonesia, we find that a woman's employment is more strongly correlated with spouse work status than men's. In part, this reflects the youth of wives relative to their husbands and the likelihood that women will choose to retire at roughly the same time as their older husbands when there are (effectively) no gender differences in mandatory retirement and pension eligibility ages. In Korea, we observe a positive correlation between employment of men and the work status of wives in urban areas, but a strong and roughly equal positive association between the employment of husbands and wives in rural Korea, which likely reflects joint decisions to retire from farming among older rural Koreans.

Employment and Spouse Health Status

Inclusion of Spouse Difficulty-ADL and Spouse Unable-ADL z-scores among covariates in model (2), and presented in Table 6-2, allow us to shed light on the relationship between spouse health status and respon-

---

[24]Research using census data, which is unable to control for endogeneity of household composition, provides weak evidence that eldercare and childcare may explain a small share of women's exits from the labor force (Maurer-Fazio et al., 2011). Giles et al. (2006b) find that urban women are more likely to work if they have a college-age adult child, which may reflect a labor supply response to the sharp increase in postsecondary tuitions after 1996.

TABLE 6-2 Spouse Health and Work Status in Labor Supply
Decisions of Adults Aged 45 and Older

	Linear Probability Models, Dependent Variable: Worked at Least One Hour per Week			
	China (CHARLS)			
	Urban		Rural	
	Male	Female	Male	Female
Pension Eligible	−0.134*	−0.194***	−0.127*	−0.031
	(0.08)	(0.06)	(0.07)	(0.12)
Spouse Pension Eligible	0.106	0.087	0.084	−0.136**
	(0.07)	(0.08)	(0.10)	(0.06)
Spouse Working	0.196***	0.202***	0.121***	0.193***
	(0.07)	(0.07)	(0.03)	(0.04)
Ln(Housing Wealth P.C.+1)	−0.062**	−0.001	−0.007	−0.026
	(0.03)	(0.02)	(0.02)	(0.02)
ADL Z-Score (w/difficulty)	−0.061	−0.027	−0.083***	−0.083***
	(0.04)	(0.03)	(0.01)	(0.01)
ADL Z-Score (unable)	0.005	−0.005	−0.079***	−0.048***
	(0.04)	(0.03)	(0.01)	(0.01)
Spouse ADL Z-Score (w/difficulty)	0.068	0.031	0.031**	0.052***
	(0.04)	(0.04)	(0.01)	(0.02)
Spouse ADL Z-Score (unable)	−0.016	−0.014	0.003	0.003
	(0.05)	(0.04)	(0.01)	(0.02)
Observations	256	236	1,000	1,103
R-squared	0.489	0.482	0.320	0.343

NOTES: These regression models include age, age-squared, years of education, years of education-squared, average education of spouse and adult children, number of living grandparents, number of grandchildren, indicator variables for married, for spouse information not present and for no adult children, and city dummies (China: county; Indonesia: Kabupaten; Korea: metropolitan city and province). Standard errors in parentheses. * denotes $p < 0.1$; ** $p < 0.05$; *** $p < 0.01$.
SOURCES: Calculated using the 2008 CHARLS pilot (China), 2007 IFLS (Indonesia), and the 2006 KLoSA (Korea).

| Indonesia (IFLS) | | | | Korea (KLoSA) | | | |
| Urban | | Rural | | Urban | | Rural | |
Male	Female	Male	Female	Male	Female	Male	Female
−0.235***	−0.240***	−0.129***	−0.136*	−0.104***	−0.020	−0.008	0.024
(0.03)	(0.05)	(0.03)	(0.07)	(0.02)	(0.03)	(0.03)	(0.05)
−0.104**	−0.015	0.110	−0.028	−0.050	−0.037*	0.047	−0.061*
(0.05)	(0.04)	(0.08)	(0.05)	(0.05)	(0.02)	(0.09)	(0.03)
0.047**	0.091**	0.088***	0.231***	0.054***	0.025	0.354***	0.339***
(0.02)	(0.04)	(0.02)	(0.05)	(0.02)	(0.02)	(0.03)	(0.03)
0.002	−0.001	0.002	0.003	0.018**	−0.016***	0.015	−0.023
(0.01)	(0.01)	(0.01)	(0.01)	(0.01)	(0.01)	(0.02)	(0.02)
−0.101***	−0.069***	−0.063***	−0.071***	−0.034***	−0.012*	−0.062***	−0.007
(0.01)	(0.01)	(0.01)	(0.01)	(0.01)	(0.01)	(0.01)	(0.01)
−0.107***	−0.070***	−0.133***	−0.093***	−0.032***	−0.007	−0.038***	−0.019
(0.02)	(0.02)	(0.01)	(0.01)	(0.01)	(0.01)	(0.01)	(0.01)
0.016	0.005	−0.020**	0.031**	−0.016	0.003	0.005	0.008
(0.01)	(0.02)	(0.01)	(0.01)	(0.01)	(0.01)	(0.02)	(0.01)
0.030	−0.052	0.008	0.016	−0.011	−0.008	−0.038	0.016
(0.02)	(0.03)	(0.01)	(0.02)	(0.01)	(0.01)	(0.03)	(0.01)
1,505	2,004	1,613	2,161	3,413	4,356	1,005	1,262
0.332	0.138	0.330	0.164	0.386	0.169	0.329	0.265

dent work decisions. Similar to the relationship with own health status, we find no correlation between spouse health status and employment in urban China. In rural China, by contrast, increases in the number of functions that a spouse has difficulty performing (Spouse Difficulty-ADL z-score) are positively associated with labor supply, suggesting an added worker effect dominates. A one standard deviation increase in the Spouse Difficulty-ADL z-score is associated with 3.1% and 5.2% increases that men and women, respectively, will be employed. The gender difference in the added worker effect, evident in rural areas of China and Indonesia, stands in contrast to the results using data from the U.S. Health and Retirement Study, which suggest that shocks to health of a spouse have a small positive effect on labor force participation of men and no effect on women (Coile, 2004a). While results for the United States can be interpreted as suggesting that there is little opportunity to smooth income loss associated with health shocks through the labor market (as Coile concludes), the employment response for both genders in rural China and men in rural Indonesia likely reflects both a stronger need to smooth income and fewer constraints to returning to work on the family farm than when looking for formal wage work.

CONCLUSIONS

As in other regions of the developing and developed world, population aging in China raises the prospect that both formal and informal mechanisms for supporting the elderly will come under strain over the next 20 years. In common with Indonesia and other developing countries, however, China is experiencing population aging at lower income levels and prior to the extension of pensions to rural residents and to urban residents in the informal sector. In a sense, China has two retirement systems: a *formal* system, under which urban employees receive generous pensions and face mandatory retirement by 60, and an *informal* system, under which rural residents and individuals in the urban informal sector rely on family support in old age and have much longer working lives. The retirement patterns presented in this chapter illuminate the employment context for the decisions that China's policymakers are currently facing as they work to extend new pension programs in rural areas and to the urban informal sector. Several issues warrant consideration when thinking about employment-related policy for an aging population.

First, as researchers have found in the United States, the United Kingdom, and Organisation for Economic Co-operation and Development (OECD) economies, we observe a strong association between pension eligibility and exit from productive employment in China, Indonesia, and Korea. Moreover, in rural areas of China and Indonesia, where work is physically demanding, we observe a strong correlation between employment status and physical functioning abilities. In China, this raises concerns that the "ceaseless toil" characterization of rural elderly lives (Davis-Friedman, 1991) may remain accurate for a significant share of the rural elderly population. China's government has taken steps recently to improve pension support for the elderly. In 2009, a Rural Pension Pilot scheme was rolled out, and current plans are to extend it to all counties before the end of the 12th Five-Year Plan in 2012. The New Rural Pension Plan is a contributory plan with matched public contributions. Participants are eligible to receive the pension at age 60 with 15 years of contributions (or an equivalent buy-in).[25] Receiving pensions from these sources would not contain a mandate that the recipient stopped working, but also the income would facilitate reduced work, whether complete or gradual.

Second, the gender disparity in mandatory retirement and pension eligibility ages for formal sector workers creates strong incentives for women to exit productive work at younger ages. While labor force participation rates of women are similar to those of men at younger ages, they fall precipitously after age 40. The evidence presented and reviewed in this chapter suggests that the probability an urban woman is employed is strongly related to pension eligibility, which also corresponds to working for an employer enforcing mandatory retirement. Changing the age of pension eligibility rapidly may cause hardship for those women who are close to the current retirement age and want to retire, but allowing women to retire at the same age as their male counterparts would remove an obstacle that women face relative to men when looking for work later in life. In Indonesia and Korea, where there is no difference in mandatory retirement ages for men and women in the civil service or formal sector, women's labor force participation also declines after 45, but these declines are not nearly as steep as those observed for urban Chinese women.

Apart from the disparity between mandatory retirement age for men and women from government and formal sector employers, retirement ages are quite low for those with formal sector employment in urban China. Given the rate of population aging, the argument that mandatory retirement is important for providing opportunities for younger workers makes less sense.[26] Indeed both macroeconomic and fiscal considerations warrant encouraging workers to remain employed until older ages. As noted above, eliminating (or raising) mandatory retirement ages will be

---

[25]To cover the urban informal sector (the self-employed and workers whose employers are not participating in employer-based programs), a New Urban Residents Pension Scheme was announced in June 2011, with roll-out of pilots beginning in July 2011.

[26]Gruber and Wise (2010) raise questions as to whether older and younger workers are substitutes, and the extent to which raising retirement ages could limit opportunities for new entrants into the workforce.

less problematic than increases in the age of pension eligibility, but both are likely to be unpopular because they force changes in expectations and long-term planning. One politically palatable approach may be to gradually raise the retirement age in three-month increments. Were such a reform started during the 12th Five Year Plan period, the retirement age for men would reach 65 by 2030, though it would take longer at this pace for full equalization for women. Research conducted in the United States and Europe, however, suggest that one might provide incentives within the pension system to encourage retirement later in life.[27] Moreover, correlations in retirement of spouses, reflecting coordination of retirement planning, raises the prospect that eliminating disincentives for women to remain in the labor force after 50 may encourage delayed retirement of their husbands as well.[28]

Among older residents who work, the paper has shown that reductions in work hours are quite gradual. A key area of employment experimentation in OECD countries is through introduction of flexible work arrangements, accompanied by removal of mandatory retirement ages and promotion of "job-sharing," which has received positive reviews as a component of labor market reforms in Germany. China could benefit from assessment of international lessons and expansion of pilots domestically in these areas.[29]

While this study has focused primarily on the relationship between pension eligibility, mandatory retirement, and work activity, the positive relationship in urban China between educational attainment and continued employment at the high end of the education distribution (for those with more than high school education) reflects the possibility that workers with more skills, or with the ability to learn new skills, may find it easier to work at older ages. In a review of policies followed in Europe, the OECD has recognized this phenomenon and noted that support for skills-upgrading at mid-career can be attractive for employers and employees alike, and may help to enhance the skills and employability of workers later in their careers.

---

[27]Coile and Gruber (2007) find that changes in expected Social Security benefits in the United States have an impact on retirement planning well ahead of retirement. Gustman and Steinmeier (2009) and Vere (2011) find that changes in social security rules or benefits help to increase the labor force participation of older workers, and may even lead to increases in hours worked "after retirement" in one's 70s. Robalino et al. (2009) suggest that changes to social insurance policies in Brazil could have an important impact on the labor supply and retirement decisions of older workers.

[28]Falkinger, Winter-Ebmer, and Zweimuller (1996) find that increasing the retirement age of women through social security reforms may lead to longer working lives for men as well.

[29]OECD (2006) provides a useful review of policies and approaches to reducing barriers and disincentives to continue working.

REFERENCES

Appleton, S., J. Knight, L. Song, and Q. Xia. (2002). Labor retrenchment in China: Determinants and consequences. *China Economic Review 13*:252-275.

Benjamin, D., L. Brandt, and J. Fan. (2003). Health and labor supply of the elderly in rural China. Unpublished manuscript, Department of Economics, University of Toronto.

Blau, D.M. (1994). Labor force dynamics of older men. *Econometrica 62(1)*:117-156.

Bound, J. (1991). Self-reported versus objective measures of health in retirement models. *Journal of Human Resources 26(1)*:106-138.

Bound, J. (1999). The dynamic effect of health on labor force transition of older workers. *Labor Economics 6*:179-202.

Bound, J., T. Stinebrickner, and T. Waidmann. (2010). Health, economic resources and the work decisions of older men. *Journal of Econometrics 156(1)*:106-129.

Cai, F., J. Giles, P. O'Keefe, and D. Wang. (2012). *Old-Age Support in Rural China: Challenges and Prospects*. Directions in Development Monograph. Washington, DC: World Bank.

Cai, F., A. Park, and Y. Zhao. (2008). The Chinese labor market in the reform era in China's great economic transformation. Pp. 167-214 in *The Chinese Labor Market in the Reform Era*, L. Brandt and T. Rawski (Eds.). Cambridge: Cambridge University Press.

Chan, S., and A.H. Stevens. (2001). Job loss and employment patterns of older workers. *Journal of Labor Economics 19*:484-521.

China Health and Retirement Longitudinal Survey. (2008). China Center for Economic Research, Peking University. Available: http://charls.ccer.edu.cn/charls/data.asp.

China Health and Nutrition Survey. (1991, 2009). Available: http://www.cpc.unc.edu/projects/china.

Cho, J.M., and S.W. Kim. (2005). On using mandatory retirement to reduce workforce in Korea. *International Economic Journal 19*:283-303.

Coile, C.C. (2004a). *Health Shocks and Couples' Labor Supply Decisions*. NBER Working Paper 10810. Cambridge, MA: National Bureau of Economic Research.

Coile, C.C. (2004b). Retirement incentives and couples' retirement decisions. *Topics in Economic Analysis and Policy 4(1)*:1-28.

Coile, C.C., and J. Gruber. (2007). Future social security entitlements and the retirement decision. *The Review of Economics and Statistics 89(2)*:234-246.

Dalen, H.P.V., K. Henkens, and S. Joop. (2010). Productivity of older workers: Perceptions of employers and employees. *Population and Development Review 36*:309-330.

Davis-Friedman, D. (1991). *Long Lives: Chinese Elderly and the Communist Revolution, Expanded edition*. Stanford, CA: Stanford University Press.

Dong, X. (2010). Parental care and married women's labor supply in urban China. *Feminist Economics 16(3)*:169-192.

Dwyer, D.S., and O.S. Mitchell. (1999). Health problems as determinants of retirement. *Journal of Health Economics 18*:173-193.

English Longitudinal Study of Ageing. (2008/2009). Available: http://www.esds.ac.uk/longitudinal/access/elsa/l5050.asp.

Falkinger, J., R. Winter-Ebmer, and J. Zweimuller. (1996). Retirement of spouses and social security reform. *European Economic Review 40*:449-472.

Giles, J., A. Park, and F. Cai. (2006a). How has economic restructuring affected China's urban workers? *China Quarterly 185* (March 2006):61-95.

Giles, J., A. Park, and F. Cai. (2006b). Reemployment of dislocated workers in urban China: The roles of information and incentives. *Journal of Comparative Economics 34(3)* (September 2006):582-607.

Giles, J., A. Park, and D. Wang. (2011). Expanding social insurance coverage in urban China: The evololution of policy and participation. Mimeo, World Bank.

Giles, J., D. Wang, and W. Cai. (2011). *The Labor Supply and Retirement Behavior of China's Older Workers and Elderly in Comparative Perspective.* Policy Research Working Paper 5853. Washington, DC: World Bank.

Giles, J., D. Wang, and A. Park. (2012). *Expanding Social Insurance Coverage in Urban China.* Policy Research Working Paper. Washington, DC: World Bank.

Giles, J., D. Wang, and C. Zhao. (2010). Can China's rural elderly count on support from adult children? Implications of rural to urban migration. *Journal of Population Ageing* 3(3):183-204.

Gruber, J., and D. Wise. (1999). *Social Security and Retirement around the World.* Chicago: University of Chicago Press.

Gruber, J., and D. Wise. (2004). *Social Security Programs and Retirement around the World: Micro-estimation.* Chicago: University of Chicago Press.

Gruber, J., and D. Wise. (2010). *Social Security Programs and Retirement around the World: The Relation to Youth Employment.* Chicago: University of Chicago Press.

Gustman, A.L., and T.L. Steinmeier. (2004). Social security, pensions and retirement behavior within the family. *Journal of Applied Econometrics* 19:723-737.

Gustman, A.L., and T.L. Steinmeier. (2009). How do changes in social security affect retirement trends? *Research on Aging* 31:261-290.

Health and Retirement Study. (2008). Available: http://hrsonline.isr.umich.edu/.

Indonesia Family Life Survey, Wave 4. (2008). Available: http://www.rand.org/labor/FLS/IFLS/ifls4.html.

Kanbur, R., and X. Zhang. (1999). Which regional inequality? The evolution of rural-urban and inland-coastal inequality in China from 1983 to 1995. *Journal of Comparative Economics* 27(4):686-701.

Kinsella, K., and W. He. (2009). *An Aging World: 2008.* U.S. Census Bureau, International Population Reports, PS95/09-1. Washington, DC: U.S. Government Printing Office.

Korean Longitudinal Study of Ageing. (2006). Available: http://www.kli.re.kr/klosa/en/about/introduce.jsp.

Krueger, A.B., and J. Pischke. (1992). The effect of social security on labor supply: A cohort analysis of the notch generation. *Journal of Labor Economics* 10:412-437.

Lee, C. (2009). *Labor Force Participation of Older Males in Korea: 1955-2005.* NBER Working Paper Series 14800. Cambridge, MA: National Bureau of Economics Research.

Lee, C., and J. Lee. (2011). *Employment Status, Quality of Matching and Retirement in Korea: Evidence from the Korean Longitudinal Study of Aging.* RAND Working Paper Series WR-834. Santa Monica, CA: RAND.

Lee, R., and A. Mason. (2011). *Population Aging and the Generational Economy: A Global Perspective.* Abingdon, Oxon, UK: Edward Elgar .

Maurer-Fazio, M. (2007). The role of education in determining labor market outcomes in urban China. Pp. 260-275 in *Education and Reform in China,* E. Hannum and A. Park (Eds.). London and New York: Routledge.

Maurer-Fazio, M., R. Connelly, L. Chen, and L. Tang. (2011). Childcare, eldercare, and labor force participation of married women in urban China, 1982-2000. *Journal of Human Resources* 46(2):261-294.

McGeary, K. (2009). How do health shocks influence retirement decisions? *Review of Economics of the Household* 7:307-321.

McKee, D. (2006). *Forward Thinking and Family Support: Explaining Retirement and Old Age Labor Supply in Indonesia.* CCPR Working Paper No. 005-06. Los Angeles: California Center for Population Research, University of California.

National Bureau of Statistics. (2011). *Communiqué of the National Bureau of Statistics of People's Republic of China on Major Figures of the 2010 Population Census* (No. 1). National Bureau of Statistics of China, Beijing. Available: http://www.stats.gov.cn/english/newsandcomingevents/t20110428_402722244.htm.

Organisation for Economic Co-operation and Development. (2006). *Live Longer, Work Longer.* Paris: OECD Publishing.

Ravallion, M., and S. Chen. (2007). China's (uneven) progress against poverty. *Journal of Development Economics 82(1)* (January 2007):1-42.

Robalino, D.A., E. Zylberstajn, H. Zylberstajn, and L.E. Afonso. (2009). *Ex Ante Methods to Assess the Impact of Social Insurance Policies on Labor Supply with an Application to Brazil.* World Bank Social Protection Discussion Paper No 0929. Washington, DC: World Bank.

Sohn, M.J. (2007). The characteristics of the recent trend of self-employment. *SERI Economic Focus 146*:39-55.

Vere, J.P. (2011). Social security and elderly labor supply: Evidence from the Health and Retirement Study. *Labor Economics 18*(5):676-686.

7

Relying on Whom?
Poverty and Consumption
Financing of China's Elderly[1]

Albert Park, Yan Shen, John Strauss, and *Yaohui Zhao*

Because of increases in longevity and strict family planning policies for three decades, China is facing rapid population aging at a relatively early stage of development. It is projected that the proportion of those aged 60 and older will increase from 10% of the population in 2000 to about 30% in 2050 (United Nations, 2002). China's elderly support ratio, defined as the number of prime-aged adults 25–64 divided by the number aged 64 and older, is projected to fall from nearly 13 in 2000 to just 2.1 by 2050. China is not alone in facing this challenge. According to United Nations projections, there are 42 countries with income per capita less than $10,000 in 2005 for which the share of those aged 65 and older will be greater than 15% by 2050 (Lee, Mason, and Cotlear, 2010).

China faces significant challenges in its effort to provide adequate financial support to its elderly population in the years to come. Because of strict family planning policies, tomorrow's elderly will have many fewer children than today's elderly, and large-scale migration as well as modernizing values also could undermine traditional family support systems. Public pension programs remain immature, and most elderly lack

[1]This research was supported by the National Institute on Aging (Grant Number R21AG031372), Natural Science Foundation of China (Grant Numbers 70773002 and 70910107022), the World Bank (Contract 7145915), and the Fogarty International Center (Grant Number R03TW008358). The content is solely the responsibility of the authors and does not necessarily represent the official views of any of the funders.

pension coverage, especially in rural areas.[2] Privatization and increasing informalization of the labor market have made it difficult for local governments to effectively extend social insurance coverage (including pensions) to the entire population.

With these future challenges in mind, this chapter analyzes how China's current elderly finance their consumption expenditures. We focus on household expenditure per capita as the preferred measure of living standards, since it best captures consumption, which directly enters individuals' utility functions, and because annual consumption reflects permanent income better than annual income, which is subject to greater year-to-year fluctuations, especially for rural households.

We utilize a unique data set with highly detailed information on income, consumption, and public and private transfers of China's elderly—the China Health and Retirement Longitudinal Study (CHARLS) pilot survey conducted in Gansu and Zhejiang provinces in 2008. We calculate elderly consumption poverty rates and analyze the extent to which the elderly rely upon their own income (including from pensions), income from other household members, public transfers, private transfers, and savings to finance their consumption. Using regression analysis, we further examine how poverty status and the use of different financing sources are related to different characteristics of the elderly, such as the number of children, living arrangements, and availability of pensions.

Throughout the analysis, we make a point of distinguishing between urban versus rural residents because of the significant differences in economic and social institutions affecting the two populations. We define urban versus rural status based on whether an individual's official family residential registration (*hukou*) is nonagricultural (urban) or agricultural (rural). There is a long history in China of preferential policies toward nonagricultural residents. Urban residents for many years enjoyed an "iron rice bowl" of guaranteed employment, housing, health insurance, pension support, and other subsidies that were unavailable to rural residents even if they migrated to cities (Chan and Zhang, 1999; Solinger, 1999). Even after three decades of reform, urban residents continue to enjoy more generous subsidies to support minimum standards of living, and better health insurance and access to housing. Under housing reforms in the late 1990s, state-supplied housing was sold to nonagricultural residents at highly subsidized prices. Family planning policies were stricter for urban residents. As a result of all of these differences, the sources of consumption financing are likely to be very different for urban versus rural residents. One limitation we face in our analysis is that only 18.5%

---

[2] A new rural pension program initiated after the CHARLS pilot in 2008 had reached 23% of rural counties by year-end 2010 and will eventually be scaled up nationally.

of our sample has nonagricultural residential registration.[3] Nonetheless, we report all of the main results separately for urban and rural residents.

In this study, relationships that we quantify statistically are best interpreted as partial correlations rather than causal relationships. This is because individuals and households alter their labor supply, living arrangements, and private transfer decisions in complex ways in response to individual circumstances, including access to pensions as well as public and private transfers. These decisions, as well as education and fertility choices, also reflect unobserved individual attributes that are likely be correlated with the determinants of poverty status and use of different financing sources.

The chapter is divided into five sections. The next section describes the CHARLS data and the measurements used in the analysis. Section 3 estimates income and consumption poverty rates and describes how different financing sources help to reduce consumption poverty, and analyzes which characteristics of the elderly are most closely associated with poverty status. Section 4 describes financing sources in greater detail, analyzes the determinants of reliance on different financing sources, and assesses the extent to which saving behavior contributes to poverty. The final section concludes with a discussion of implications for how China can successfully provide adequate support to the elderly in the future.

CHARLS DATA AND MEASUREMENTS

CHARLS is modeled after the Health and Retirement Study (HRS) in the United States and other similar aging studies worldwide. A distinguishing feature of HRS-type surveys is that they are longitudinal and collect detailed data on both socioeconomic status and physical and mental health. This study uses data from the CHARLS pilot survey conducted in 2008 in two provinces: Zhejiang, China's richest province in 2008 in terms of income per capita (both urban and rural) located on the coast, and Gansu, China's poorest province in terms of income per capita located in China's northwest. The two provinces capture much of China's great diversity but are not fully representative of China as a whole. The simple average of urban income per capita in the two provinces in 2008 is 7% greater than the national average, and the share of urban household

---

[3]This is much lower than the urban share of the populations in the two provinces according to China's Statistical Yearbook. This is partly because of a lower response rate among urban residents, which is corrected by using appropriate sampling weights when reporting means for the full sample. A more important reason is that the definition of urban in the statistical yearbooks is based on population density criteria and so includes a large number of people with agricultural residential registration living in administrative villages in suburban or peri-urban areas, especially in Zhejiang.

income from wages, self-employment, property income, and transfers in the two provinces is almost identical to the national average. Mean rural income per capita for the two provinces is 26% greater than the national average in 2008, due mainly to high rural incomes in Zhejiang, and the share of rural income in the two provinces that comes from self-employment (wages) is 6% greater (lower) than the national average; shares of property and transfer income are nearly the same as the national average.

The pilot survey sampled individuals aged 45 and older plus their spouses, and it included interviews of 2,685 individuals in 1,562 households.[4] The response rate was 85%. Sampling was conducted in three stages. First, 16 county-level units were selected in each province, based on probability proportionate to size (PPS) sampling after county units were first stratified by whether they were urban districts or rural counties and by subregions of each province. Three communities (administrative villages or urban neighborhoods) were then randomly sampled within each county unit, again using PPS sampling. Sampling frames for county and village sampling were based on population data provided by China's National Bureau of Statistics. Finally, households within each community were randomly sampled based on a full map-based enumeration of all dwellings in each neighborhood. One main respondent was randomly selected in each household with eligible members (those aged 45 and older), and the spouse of each main respondent was also interviewed.[5] The resulting sample of main respondents thus is representative of the populations of Gansu and Zhejiang provinces. The sample's demographic structure is similar to that found in the 2005 population mini-census in the two provinces.[6]

In this study, we focus attention on the subsample of main respondents aged 60 and older, which we refer to as the elderly sample. Occasionally, we also examine the younger sample of those aged 45 to 59. For all descriptive tables, in order to maximize representativeness, we

---

[4]The sample size is 1,531 households in this study, after dropping 31 households with missing data.

[5]See Zhao et al. (2009) for full details of the sampling procedure and construction of sampling weights. Tibetan counties in Gansu were excluded; they accounted for 3.8% of the provincial population in 2007.

[6]The population structure by age group of those aged 45 and older in China's 2005 population census (2008 CHARLS pilot survey) in Gansu and Zhejiang is as follows: 17.5 (17.9)% aged 45–49, 22.7 (18.5)% aged 50–54, 17.8 (14.3)% aged 55–59, 13.0 (16.4)% aged 60–64, 11.0 (14.7)% aged 65–69, 8.8 (8.6)% aged 70–74, 5.2 (5.2)% aged 75–79, 4.0 (4.5)% aged 80+ (all numbers based on authors' calculations). Thus, relative to the 2005 mini-census, CHARLS slightly undersamples those aged 50–59 and oversamples those aged 60–69; however, these differences are relatively small and could be due to the surveys being conducted three years apart.

restrict attention to the sample of main respondents, excluding spouses. Regressions are unweighted and also include spouses aged 60 and older to increase power.

Understanding how the elderly support their consumption requires detailed information on income, including that of the elderly themselves and that of other household members, as well as on transfers and consumption. Such complete data are typically not collected in household surveys, but CHARLS made great efforts to collect all of the necessary information in order to better understand the financial situation of the elderly. Income was measured at both the individual and household levels. Main respondents and their spouses were asked about all sources of income and public transfers that went to them individually, and a financial respondent—the person most familiar with the household's finances—answered questions about the individual income of other household members, income from household activities such as agriculture, household expenditures, and household-level transfers, including private transfers from nonhousehold members.

These data were then aggregated to calculate several different income-per-capita measures that exclude different types of transfers. Respondents and their spouses (RS) own income per capita includes wage income, self-employment income, agricultural income, pension income, and net asset income received by the respondent and spouse. Their share of income from activities undertaken with other family members, such as family farming, is calculated based on an equal division of income among all household members who were reported to have engaged in the activity.[7] Household pre-transfer income per capita is calculated by adding up the income of all household members (for respondents and spouses living alone, this is the same as RS own income) and dividing by the total number of household members.[8] Household income per capita can be greater or less than RS own income per capita, depending on whether the respondent and spouse are net givers or receivers of resources when they pool their income with other household members. Our third income measure is post-transfer

---

[7]Unfortunately, no information is available on the time spent on different activities by other household members.

[8]Although we can clearly distinguish each source of individual income for main respondents and their spouses, who were asked about each separately, for other household members, we can only distinguish two types of individual income: earnings from work and all unearned income (including pensions, public transfers, asset income, and other sources of income). Given our strong prior belief that public transfers are likely to account for the bulk of such income (because other members tend to be too young to have pension income and asset income is relatively rare), we have chosen to categorize all unearned individual income of other household members as public transfer income when calculating household income from different sources.

income per capita, which is calculated by adding private and public transfers to pre-transfer income. To discern whether private or public transfers are playing a more important role, we also calculate post-transfer income separately for private transfers and public transfers.

Household consumption expenditure items are measured by recall questions covering the past week, month, or year depending on the expected frequency of different types of expenditures. The survey asks about food expenditure during the past week, including expenditures on dining out, food bought from the market, and the value of home-produced food.[9] Monthly expenditures include fees for utilities, communications, nannies, and other costs. Yearly expenditures occur occasionally throughout the year, for example, for travel, purchases of durable goods, or education and training fees. Household expenditure per capita is calculated by aggregating consumption expenditure at the household level over a full year and dividing by the total number of household members.[10]

We categorize the difference between post-transfer income per capita and expenditure per capita as savings (or dissavings if the values are negative). Thus, our measure of savings is likely to also include measurement error in income, transfers, or expenditures.

Before examining in detail differences in income and expenditure per capita, it is informative to describe the components of income, transfers, and expenditures.[11] The importance of pensions is very different in urban and rural areas. In urban China, pension income accounts for 53% of the income of respondents and spouses and 57% of total household (pre-transfer) income per capita. About two-thirds of urban residents receive pensions or have a spouse who receives pensions. In contrast, in rural areas, only 17% of the income of respondents and spouses and 13% of total household (pre-transfer) income per capita are from pensions; only 12% of the rural elderly receive pensions or have spouses who receive pensions.

Wage income is the second most important source of income for respondents and spouses (24 and 38% for urban and rural residents, respectively) and the most important source of income for households (30 and 50% for urban and rural residents, respectively). The third most important is self-employed income, which accounts for 13 (27)% of the income of respondents and spouses who are urban (rural) residents, and

---

[9]Food expenditures spent on guest meals are subtracted from expenditures to better reflect household food expenditure per capita in a normal week.

[10]For food expenditures, the number of household members is the number of persons who ate regularly in the household in the past week. For other expenditures, household members are those who lived in the household for at least 6 months in the past year.

[11]Mean shares described in this paragraph are calculated as the mean of each category divided by the mean of the total, not the mean of household-specific shares.

7 (29)% of household pre-transfer income per capita. Of note is the relative unimportance of agricultural income to the elderly, accounting for just 7% of rural household income per capita, as well as asset income. Only 47% of the rural elderly live in households with any agricultural income.

The composition of consumption expenditures of elderly households can be divided into 16 categories. The largest spending category is food (49 and 53% in urban and rural households, respectively) followed by medical expenditures (16 and 19%, respectively). All other categories account for 6% or less. Public transfers include 19 categories, which include both transfers to individuals as well as to households.[12] The largest category is other individual public transfers (42 and 28% for urban and rural households, respectively), which includes all individual public transfers received by household members other than the respondent and spouse. This is due to the fact that although we have a detailed breakdown by type for the main respondent and spouse, for other household members all categories are aggregated together in one question and so categorized as "other" (see also footnote 4). We do not provide a breakdown of private transfers, but note that these transfers are asked only at the household level and include both cash and in-kind transfers, most of which come from children of the main respondent and spouse. To prompt respondents, separate questions are asked about private transfers received at different major holidays (e.g., spring festival) and about transfers that are received regularly (e.g., every month) or irregularly.

Table 7-1 presents the mean and median of household per capita income and expenditure measures for the two subsamples of those less than aged 60 and those aged 60 and older. For the elderly, we also report urban and rural outcomes separately. At the time of the survey in July 2008, the RMB/US$ exchange rate was 6.82. The means show large differences between average income levels and average consumption levels, likely because of the influence of richer households in the sample. We get a somewhat different picture looking at medians. Comparing age groups, it appears that the role of transfers is quite different for the two groups. For those older than 60, the mean post-transfer income per capita is 44% greater than respondent and spouse income per capita. Medians portray an even more drastic picture, with median post-transfer income per capita (3,712 yuan) being almost five times the median respondent and spouse income per capita. Median expenditure per capita is 4,418 yuan, which, in

---

[12]Public transfers include medical expenditure subsidies, workers' compensation, rural and urban minimum living standards subsidies, subsidies for those unable to work (*wubaohu*), compensation for land seizure, agricultural subsidies, family planning subsidies, elderly pension subsidies, reforestation subsidy, unemployment benefits, rural poverty subsidies, disaster relief subsidies, and social donations.

TABLE 7-1 Household per Capita Income and Expenditure by Age and by Urban Versus Rural (in RMB)

	HH	R/S Income		Pre-Transfer Income		Post-Transfer Income		Expenditure	
	Number	Mean	Median	Mean	Median	Mean	Median	Mean	Median
Age 45–59	794	17,649	8,400	15,886	7,200	15,958	7,624	8,401	6,416
Age ≥ 60	737	5,114	650	5,897	1,600	7,365	3,712	6,192	4,418
Urban	136	14,502	12,000	12,843	11,400	14,654	10,633	9,876	8,000
Rural	601	2,955	400	4,299	1,000	5,689	2,783	5,345	3,920
Urban/rural		4.91	30.00	2.99	11.40	2.58	3.82	1.85	2.04

SOURCE: Authors' calculations using sample of main respondents in CHARLS pilot data.

contrast to the mean, is higher than that of median post-transfer income per capita, suggesting that most elderly are net dissavers. Overall, it is evident that China's elderly rely heavily on sources other than their own income to finance their consumption. Those below age 60 earn much higher incomes (respondent and spouse mean income per capita of 17,649 yuan), and are net givers of resources to other household members since household income per capita is lower than respondent and spouse income per capita.

Table 7-1 reveals interesting differences between urban and rural elderly. First, across all income and consumption measures, urban standards of living are much higher than rural standards of living. The most extreme gap is in the differences in respondent and spouse own income per capita, for which the urban/rural ratio based on means (medians) is 4.91 (30.0). But as one moves to pre-transfer income, post-transfer income, and finally expenditures, the urban/rural ratio declines steadily from 2.99 (11.40) to 2.58 (3.82) to 1.85 (2.04) using means (medians). Interestingly, for urban residents, median values decline monitonically in this progression while rural residents' median values increase monitonically, suggesting that the rural elderly are made increasingly better off by living with others, receiving transfers, and dissaving while urban residents are made increasingly worse off because they subsidize the consumption of people they live with, give money to relatives, and save funds rather than spend them. The picture is less clear when looking at means, which reveal that urban residents on average receive transfers and that rural residents also save.

Table 7-2 provides descriptive statistics for CHARLS main respondents, again broken down by age group (those 45 to 60 and those 60 and above) and for the older group by urban versus rural. Compared with the younger group, the elderly have more children, with two-thirds of the elderly having three or more children, compared to just one-quarter of those aged 45–60. However, in terms of living arrangements, the elderly are more likely to live with children (49%, compared to 30% for those aged 45–60) and more likely to live alone (24% versus 8% for the younger group). They are less educated (53% illiterate), poorer in health, and rely much more on public and private transfers. These facts suggest that China's elderly are vulnerable in their socioeconomic status and more dependent on others, making it important to assess the extent to which they are able to finance adequate standards of living. Elderly living in urban areas differ from those in rural areas mostly in access to pensions (67% for urban, just 12% for rural), propensity to live with children (34% for urban, 53% for rural), health status (urban are healthier), and education (share with educational attainment of junior high or above is 38% for urban and 5% for rural).

TABLE 7-2 Descriptive Statistics for Main Respondents

Variables	Age 45–59	Age ≥ 60	Age ≥ 60 Urban	Rural
Age	51.65	70.63	71.11	70.58
Male	0.50	0.48	0.49	0.48
Pension (1 = yes)	0.12	0.22	0.67	0.12
Children = 0	0.04	0.03	0.00	0.04
Children = 1	0.27	0.08	0.12	0.08
Children = 2	0.44	0.21	0.24	0.20
Children > 2	0.25	0.67	0.64	0.68
Live Alone	0.08	0.24	0.27	0.24
Live w/Spouse Only	0.26	0.19	0.29	0.16
Live w/Adult Children	0.30	0.49	0.34	0.53
Live w/Others	0.36	0.08	0.11	0.07
Poor	0.19	0.29	0.19	0.32
Health-Fair	0.40	0.39	0.51	0.36
Health-Good or Above	0.41	0.32	0.30	0.33
Illiterate	0.31	0.53	0.31	0.58
Informal Education	0.19	0.22	0.18	0.23
Primary School	0.16	0.13	0.14	0.13
Junior High or Above	0.34	0.12	0.38	0.05

SOURCE: Authors' calculations using CHARLS pilot data.

ELDERLY POVERTY

The most direct way to study the adequacy of consumption financing is to calculate poverty rates for the elderly. In this section, we use our detailed measurements of income and consumption expenditure to calculate the extent of poverty among the elderly, and the contributions made by different sources of finance in altering the extent of poverty among China's elderly. These measurements are of obvious policy concern because older individuals may have lower productivity because of poorer health, lower education, and outdated skills, and have fewer work opportunities, making them more reliant on public assistance to maintain living standards.

The starting point for poverty calculations is to identify a poverty line. In this study, we use the most recent World Bank international poverty line of $1.25/day converted to Chinese RMB using the Purchasing Power Parity (PPP) exchange rate estimated for China in 2005. This gives us a poverty line in 2005 domestic currency, which we then adjust to 2008 using national urban and rural consumer price indices as well as an urban/ rural price deflator.[13] In 2008 RMB, the World Bank international poverty line translates to 2,089 yuan per capita for urban areas and 1,552 yuan per capita for rural areas. We use these poverty lines to calculate the poverty headcount ratio, poverty gap, and poverty gap squared for the elderly, which are presented in Table 7-3. These poverty indices are calculated using the familiar formula of Foster, Green, and Thorbecke (1984):

$$FGT_\alpha(y,z) = \sum \frac{w_i}{N} I(y_i - z)[1 - (y_i - z)]^\alpha, \alpha = 0,1,2,$$

where y_i is income or expenditure per capita of individual i, z is the poverty line, w_i is a sampling weight with mean of one, and α is a "poverty aversion" parameter (larger α gives greater weight to larger poverty gaps, i.e., poorer people).

The first column of Table 7-3 presents the poverty headcount ratio ($\alpha = 0$) using different income per capita measures as well as expenditure per capita. The results show clearly the important role played by transfers in keeping the elderly out of poverty. If we only consider the income of respondents and spouses, 60% of the elderly are poor; when income from other household members is also factored in, the poverty rate falls by 9%, reflecting the implicit financial support of the elderly that occurs through co-residence. When we then add private transfers but not public transfers to household income, the poverty rate falls from 51 to 41%; when we add public transfers but not private transfers, the poverty rate falls to 44%, and when we add both public and private transfers, the poverty rate falls to 34%. Thus, co-residence and transfers reduce the headcount poverty ratio by 26 percentage points. The poverty headcount ratio for expenditure per capita is much lower still—16%, suggesting that dissaving (or unmeasured income or transfers) accounts for a significant share of consumption for the income poor. This consumption poverty rate is not far from the 12.9% poverty headcount ratio estimated for the elderly in all of China in 2003 using National Bureau of Statistics national household survey data and a lower poverty line (World Bank, 2009).[14] That World Bank report

---

[13]The 2005 PPP exchange rate for household consumption is 4.09 yuan/$ and reflects urban costs of living (Chen and Ravallion, 2008). Following Chen and Ravallion (2008), we assume that urban costs of living are 37% higher than rural cost of living in 2005, based on analysis of the cost of actual consumption bundles of the poor in urban and rural China that they estimated in collaboration with China's National Bureau of Statistics. We then use China's rural and urban consumer price indexes to calculate poverty lines for 2008.

[14]The 2003 estimate uses the previous World Bank poverty line of $1.08 per day using a PPP exchange rate from 1993 of only 1.419. The World Bank report (2009) assumed that this exchange rate reflected rural costs of living at the time and that the urban cost of living was 27.2% higher than the rural cost of living in 2002 using the Brandt-Holz price deflator.

TABLE 7-3 Poverty Status of Elderly Aged 60 and Older*

Income Measures	Total	Urban	Rural
Headcount			
RS own income	0.60	0.28	0.68
Pre-transfer income	0.51	0.26	0.57
plus public transfers only	0.44	0.19	0.49
plus private transfers only	0.41	0.15	0.47
Post-transfer income	0.34	0.09	0.40
Expenditure	0.16	0.08	0.17
Poverty Gap			
RS own income	0.51	0.27	0.57
Pre-transfer income	0.40	0.23	0.44
plus public transfers only	0.31	0.16	0.34
plus private transfers only	0.27	0.11	0.31
Post-transfer income	0.21	0.07	0.24
Expenditure	0.07	0.04	0.08
Poverty Gap^2			
RS own income	0.47	0.27	0.52
Pre-transfer income	0.35	0.22	0.38
plus public transfers only	0.25	0.15	0.28
plus private transfers only	0.22	0.09	0.25
Post-transfer income	0.16	0.06	0.18
Expenditure	0.05	0.03	0.05

NOTE: *Negative incomes are set to zero in calculating the poverty measures.
SOURCE: Authors' calculations using main respondent sample in CHARLS pilot data.

found that the poverty rate of the elderly was only slightly higher than that of the working population (12.1%) but much lower than the poverty headcount rate of the young aged less than 16 years (16.8%).

Again, there are important differences between urban and rural residents. Expenditure-based poverty rates are much lower for urban residents (8%) than rural residents (17%). Transfers play a key role in reducing poverty in both urban and rural areas, by 17 percentage points in both cases when we compare poverty rates based on pre-transfer and post-transfer income. In both cases, private transfers are more important than public transfers. However, in rural areas, co-residence and dissaving also play key roles, accounting for decreases in poverty rates of 11 and 23 percentage points, respectively, while for urban residents these sources of finance are relatively unimportant.

To examine not just the frequency but also the depth of poverty, we calculate the normalized poverty gap ($\alpha = 1$) and normalized squared poverty gap ($\alpha = 2$) for different income and expenditure per capita measures. As α increases, the FGT measure puts increasing emphasis on the degree of poverty. The results presented in Table 7-3 reveal that for rural residents, co-residence and transfers play an even more important role in reducing the degree of poverty than they do in reducing poverty head-count rates, while dissaving matters less. This is not surprising given that more severely deprived individuals are less likely to have savings to draw upon in bad times. Overall, external support via co-residence and trans-fers reduce a greater share of rural poverty the greater the weight given to the severity of poverty. When using post-transfer income per capita instead of the income per capita of respondents and spouses, the rural normalized poverty gap falls from 0.57 to 0.24, or by nearly 50%, while the rural poverty gap squared falls from 0.52 to 0.18, or by 65%. These declines are both greater than the 41% fall in the poverty headcount ratio. Interestingly, the same does not appear to be true for urban residents, for whom co-residence matters slightly more when poverty severity is given greater weight and transfers matter slightly less. This suggests that sup-port mechanisms for urban residents are less well targeted to the poorest of the poor than for rural residents.

To illustrate more clearly the importance of distinguishing between income poverty and consumption poverty, we note the relatively low correlation between income poverty and consumption poverty in the data. Using the sample of 743 main respondents aged 60 and older, we find that among the 52% of the elderly who are poor as measured by pre-transfer income per capita, 75% are not poor when poverty is measured using expenditure per capita. Of the 48% of the elderly who are not poor using pre-transfer income, 8% are poor using expenditure per capita.

Economic well-being can vary considerably with differences in loca-tion, living arrangements, health status, etc. A poverty profile of the elderly presented in Table 7-4 shows sharp differences in poverty for different population subgroups. For example, headcount poverty ratios based on pre-transfer income are very high for those living alone (73.8% for women and 61.7% for men), those living in rural Gansu (74.6%), those in poor health (65.4%), those without pensions (62.6%, compared to just 7.6% of those with pensions), and the illiterate (60.6%). However, mea-sured by expenditures per capita (after accounting for transfers and dis-saving), for all of these population groups the poverty rates are less than 25% (with the exception of poverty rates of 29.7% in rural Gansu). Like income poverty, consumption poverty is associated with living in rural Gansu, poor health, living alone, less education, and lacking pensions. For both income and consumption, poverty is slightly higher for women than men (51.2 and 16.7%, compared to 49.0 and 14.4%).

Next, we analyze the determinants of poverty separately for urban and rural households using different income and consumption measures in a multivariate setting by estimating probit models of poverty status and calculating the marginal probabilities of different individual char-acteristics. Results are reported in Table 7-5. We find that for both urban

TABLE 7-4 Income and Consumption Poverty Headcount Ratios for the Elderly

		Poverty Headcount Ratio		
		Pre-transfer Income	Post-transfer Income	Expenditure
Gender				
	Women	0.512	0.328	0.167
	Men	0.490	0.333	0.144
Rural or Urban				
	Urban	0.236	0.058	0.078
	Rural	0.562	0.393	0.174
Pension Status				
	Without pension	0.626	0.418	0.190
	With pension	0.076	0.033	0.040
Number of Children				
	Children = 0	0.890	0.201	0.139
	Children = 1	0.543	0.481	0.236
	Children = 2	0.360	0.234	0.100
	Children > 2	0.521	0.348	0.165
Education Background				
	Illiterate	0.606	0.404	0.192
	Informally educated	0.428	0.237	0.152
	Primary	0.452	0.331	0.111
	Junior or above	0.217	0.170	0.049
Living Arrangements				
	Men living alone	0.617	0.233	0.187
	Women living alone	0.738	0.358	0.228
	Live w/spouse only	0.353	0.242	0.109
	Live w/adult children	0.445	0.352	0.154
	Live w/others	0.647	0.493	0.121
Health Status				
	Poor health	0.654	0.489	0.234
	Fair health	0.432	0.260	0.103
	Good health or above	0.408	0.266	0.134
Residence				
	Urban Zhejiang	0.225	0.062	0.076
	Rural Zhejiang	0.476	0.260	0.117
	Urban Gansu	0.252	0.053	0.081
	Rural Gansu	0.746	0.675	0.297
With or Without Agricultural Income				
	Without agri income	0.728	0.705	0.343
	With agri income	0.495	0.320	0.151
Total		0.501	0.330	0.156

SOURCE: Authors' calculations using main respondents sample of CHARLS pilot data.

TABLE 7-5 Determinants of Income and Consumption Poverty (marginal probabilities from probit estimation)

	RS Own Income Poor (1 = yes)	
	Urban	Rural
Age	0.0004	0.0260**
	(0.0023)	(0.0031)
Male	−0.0080	−0.0937*
	(0.0332)	(0.0377)
Pension (1 = yes)	−0.5681**	−0.6946**
	(0.0909)	(0.0399)
Children = 0		0.2565**
		(0.0451)
Children = 1	0.0279	−0.0156
	(0.0927)	(0.0759)
Children > 2	−0.0790	−0.0190
	(0.0589)	(0.0429)
Live Alone	0.0819	−0.0145
	(0.0938)	(0.0666)
Live w/Spouse Only	−0.0158	−0.0509
	(0.0335)	(0.0413)
Live w/Others	0.0505	0.0484
	(0.0811)	(0.0562)
Health-Fair	0.0338	−0.1139**
	(0.0341)	(0.0431)
Health-Good or Above	−0.0140	−0.1175*
	(0.0342)	(0.0459)
Informal Education	−0.0092	−0.0026
	(0.0295)	(0.0460)
Primary School	−0.0402	0.0556
	(0.0260)	(0.0499)
Junior High or Above	−0.1043**	−0.0847
	(0.0403)	(0.0726)
Zhejiang	−0.0096	−0.2905**
	(0.0266)	(0.0339)
Observations	222	932

NOTE: Standard errors in parentheses. * denotes $p < 0.05$; ** $p < 0.01$.
SOURCE: Authors' estimates using elderly sample of CHARLS pilot data.

Pre-Transfer Income Poor (1 = yes)		Post-Transfer Income Poor (1 = yes)		Expenditure Poor (1 = yes)	
Urban	Rural	Urban	Rural	Urban	Rural
−0.0009	0.0114**	0.0000	0.0093**	−0.0006	0.0061**
(0.0032)	(0.0029)	(0.0015)	(0.0028)	(0.0011)	(0.0019)
0.0400	−0.0059	0.0437	−0.0296	0.0338	−0.0113
(0.0434)	(0.0402)	(0.0253)	(0.0395)	(0.0206)	(0.0275)
−0.4554**	−0.5537**	−0.0769	−0.4256**	−0.0676	−0.1354**
(0.0884)	(0.0369)	(0.0495)	(0.0307)	(0.0469)	(0.0287)
	0.2166		−0.0436		−0.0081
	(0.1305)		(0.1334)		(0.0962)
0.0828	0.0383	0.3019	0.1929*		0.0742
(0.1445)	(0.0810)	(0.2144)	(0.0816)		(0.0667)
−0.0056	0.0249	0.0188	0.0533	0.0001	0.0354
(0.0504)	(0.0471)	(0.0223)	(0.0465)	(0.0148)	(0.0318)
0.1543	0.3055**	−0.0256	0.1341	0.0143	0.1446*
(0.1244)	(0.0487)	(0.0165)	(0.0690)	(0.0344)	(0.0620)
−0.0568	0.1906**	−0.0010	0.0866*	−0.0330	0.0318
(0.0424)	(0.0407)	(0.0207)	(0.0442)	(0.0195)	(0.0325)
0.0611	0.2604**	0.0203	0.2922**	−0.0128	−0.0170
(0.0945)	(0.0503)	(0.0444)	(0.0600)	(0.0109)	(0.0404)
−0.0065	−0.1232**	−0.0072	−0.0925*	−0.0313	−0.0193
(0.0421)	(0.0429)	(0.0198)	(0.0405)	(0.0199)	(0.0284)
−0.0058	−0.1273**	−0.0202	−0.1024*	−0.0223	0.0030
(0.0509)	(0.0457)	(0.0181)	(0.0428)	(0.0154)	(0.0315)
0.0161	−0.0341	−0.0370	0.0074	0.0125	0.0441
(0.0526)	(0.0503)	(0.0189)	(0.0503)	(0.0236)	(0.0390)
−0.0758*	−0.0111	−0.0343	0.0640	0.0256	0.0109
(0.0343)	(0.0587)	(0.0177)	(0.0588)	(0.0300)	(0.0421)
−0.1434**	−0.0921	−0.0708*	−0.0906		−0.0205
(0.0441)	(0.0756)	(0.0286)	(0.0698)		(0.0480)
−0.0277	−0.3058**	−0.0093	−0.3887**	−0.0026	−0.2251**
(0.0384)	(0.0366)	(0.0194)	(0.0349)	(0.0131)	(0.0291)
222	932	222	932	222	932

and rural households, pensions have a large and significant effect on poverty status measured by respondent and spouse own income, but that the magnitude of this effect weakens as we move to pre-transfer income, post-transfer income, and finally expenditures. For urban households, the pension variable is not statistically significant for post-transfer income or expenditure, suggesting that transfers play a key role in alleviating poverty among the urban poor who lack pensions. For rural households, having pensions reduces consumption poverty by 13.5 percentage points (still much less than the 69.5% reduction in poverty based on respondent and spouse own income).

Not living with children increases poverty rates substantially for rural households when measured by pre-transfer income, but all of the living arrangement variables are much smaller in magnitude and statistically insignificant in the corresponding urban regression. For rural households, compared to those living with children, income poverty based on pre-transfer income is 31% higher for those living alone, 19% higher for those living with their spouse only, and 26% higher for those living with others. These differences are much less pronounced for those living alone or with spouse using post-transfer incomes, but grow larger for those living with others. However, using expenditure per capita, only living alone affects the poverty rate significantly, increasing the probability of being poor by 15%.

Another factor that only affects the poverty of rural respondents is poor health, which increases poverty probability by about 9 to 12% using different income measures. However, health does not significantly affect rural poverty based on expenditures. These results suggest surprisingly that co-residence and transfers do not significantly alleviate poverty for those in poor health, but that the unhealthy do manage to dissave more relative to the healthy to maintain consumption levels. We also find that in rural areas, poverty increases with age, but that this effect is smaller (but still significant) as one moves from respondent's own income (2.6% higher poverty for each extra year) to expenditures (0.6% higher). Education is also negatively associated with poverty. Having a junior high school education or greater reduces the probability of the urban elderly being income-poor by 7 to 14% compared to those with no education, and none of the urban elderly with a junior high school education are consumption poor.[15] The results show a negative effect of junior high education on income poverty of similar magnitude for rural elderly, but the results are not statistically significant and education does not predict consumption poverty for the rural elderly. Finally, being in Zhejiang instead of Gansu

---

[15]This is why colinearity causes the junior high school dummy variable to drop out of the urban consumption poverty regression.

has a very large impact on reducing poverty rates for all measures of income or expenditure (23 to 39% difference).

Overall, these results suggest that co-residence, transfers, and dis-saving together effectively compensate for much of the income shortfall associated with vulnerable characteristics to alleviate poverty.[16] Many factors that predict poverty based on the income of the respondent and spouse are no longer strong predictors of poverty when measured by expenditure per capita.

SOURCES OF EXPENDITURE FINANCE

The differences in income poverty and consumption poverty point to the fact that a significant portion of the elderly are consuming more than their income. While life cycle theory implies that the elderly may support themselves by depleting savings that they have accumulated during their prime working years, it is unclear how important dissaving is for Chinese elderly.

The descriptive statistics presented in Table 7-6 show that dissaving is actually negative for the elderly on average, equal to 47% of urban expenditures and 8% of rural expenditures. This is consistent with high household savings rates in China, especially by the urban elderly as found also by Chamon and Prasad (2010), and with mean expenditures of the elderly being less than mean incomes (see Table 7-1). Private and public transfers account for 14 (19) and 6 (9)% of expenditures for urban (rural) elderly households, while the income of respondents and spouses account for 140 (56)% of expenditures and pooling income with other household members accounts for –13.4 (23.7)%. These last findings suggest that the urban elderly are net providers of support to other household members while the rural elderly are net receivers.

The mean financing shares just described mask a great deal of diversity and reflect the behavior of the rich more than that of the poor because they are weighted by expenditures per capita. To better understand the diversity of financing arrangements for those with different income levels, in Table 7-6 we divide the urban and rural elderly each into quintiles based on pre-transfer income per capita, where quintile 1 is the poorest group and quintile 5 is the richest group. The next five columns then record the amount of financing from each source as a share of expenditure per capita. We can see that the poorest two quintiles in both urban

---

[16]We also found that the severity of inequality using different measures falls as one takes into account the incomes of other household members as well as public and private transfers. In addition, as one moves from post-transfer income per capita to expenditure per capita, the Gini coefficient falls from 0.61 to 0.45.

TABLE 7-6 Expenditure Financing Shares (%) for Elderly Aged 60 and Older

Pre-Transfer Income Quintile	RS Income	Other Family	Private Transfers	Public Transfers	Dissaving
Urban	140.3	−13.4	14.3	5.8	−47.1
Lowest	0.2	0.0	70.9	21.6	7.4
2nd	12.4	23.5	20.0	13.4	30.7
3rd	147.9	−32.5	51.4	11.5	−78.3
4th	132.8	−19.1	−4.9	2.0	−10.8
Highest	191.8	−9.6	2.8	2.3	−87.4
Rural	56.1	23.7	19.0	9.3	−8.2
Lowest	1.5	0.3	24.5	20.8	52.9
2nd	27.6	3.1	26.5	9.8	33.1
3rd	65.6	24.3	11.7	2.0	−3.7
4th	114.8	61.5	20.7	2.5	−99.5
Highest	193.1	105.8	0.8	2.1	−201.9

SOURCE: Authors' calculations using main respondents sample of CHARLS pilot data.

and rural areas are net dissavers. Among rural households in the bottom two quintiles, dissaving accounts for 53 and 33% of expenditures, respectively. For the poorest rural quintile, transfers are also important, with private and public transfers accounting for 25 and 21% of expenditures, respectively. Their own income only supports 2% of their expenditure, and 0.3% of their expenditure comes from pooling income with other family members. For urban households, the dominant source of financing for the poorest quintile is private transfers (71%) followed by public transfers (22%) and dissaving (7%), suggesting that poor urban residents have much greater ability to obtain private assistance than rural residents. Public transfers have similar importance for those in the poorest quintile among urban and rural residents and seem relatively well-targeted overall. But they seem even better targeted to the poor in rural areas, as seen in the sharper drop off in public transfers for those in the second and third rural quintiles compared to those in the second and third urban quintiles.

We noted earlier that 8% of those who are not poor based on post-transfer income per capita are poor based on expenditure per capita. Because the nonpoor represent a large base, this suggests that a large share of the consumption poor may be saving. In fact, separate calculations find that 57% of the consumption poor are net savers. Note that this is not to say that the income poor are saving a lot. In fact, among those who are poor based on post-transfer income per capita, only 9% are savers. This contrasts with 61% of the nonpoor who save. In fact, as one would expect, the share of savers increases steadily with income; the share of savers is 21%, 32%, 57%, 80%, and 95% going from lowest to highest post-transfer income per capita quintiles. Still, saving by some of the income poor, as well as by the nonincome poor in sufficient amounts to make them poor, may seem concerning.

One possible explanation for this finding is measurement error, that is, the poor savers are households who have under-reported income. Another is that some of the elderly and their families choose low consumption levels out of habit, for precautionary motives, or out of altruism to preserve resources for their children or grandchildren. To get a sense of how much savings by the poor contribute to measured consumption poverty, we can run a simulation in which we do not allow anyone who is consumption-poor to save; in other words we add the amount of savings to their consumption level, and calculate what the poverty rate would have been had they consumed rather than saved. We find that consumption poverty falls from 14.9 to 8.7%.

In Table 7-7, we study the determinants of expenditure financing shares for the elderly. Emphasizing relationships that are statistically significant, we find that for urban residents, pensions increase reliance on own income and significantly reduce reliance on other household members and public transfers. Urban residents living alone or in poor health rely significantly more on private transfers; interestingly, these relationships are not statistically significant for rural households, although the estimated magnitude of private transfer response to poor health is similar. Having three or more children increases reliance on private transfers and reduces reliance on public transfers.

For rural households, greater age reduces reliance on own income while access to pensions increases reliance on own income. In contrast to urban residents, living arrangements have a statistically powerful relationship to sources of finance. Those not living with children rely much less on pooling income with other family members (urban households do not benefit much from co-residence), those living alone or with their spouse rely more on public transfers, those living with their spouse rely more on private transfers, and those living with others rely more on dissaving. Having one child or especially no children significantly increases reliance on public transfers, consistent with the goals of targeted programs for rural residents (e.g., family planning subsidies, subsidies for those with no children, or other income support). Having a junior high school education increases reliance on own income, and living in Zhejiang increases the financing shares from own income, gains from pooling income with other household members, private transfers, and substantially reduces reliance on dissaving.

TABLE 7-7 Determinants of Expenditure Financing Shares for Elderly Aged 60 and Older

Variables	RS Own Share		Other Family Share	
	Urban	Rural	Urban	Rural
Age	−0.05	−2.82**	−1.22	−0.16
	(2.50)	(0.60)	(1.54)	(0.78)
Male	−5.33	11.67	−1.47	−2.83
	(32.45)	(8.48)	(19.90)	(11.13)
Pension	139.59**	87.04**	−101.38**	−27.81
(1 = yes)	(37.72)	(13.47)	(23.14)	(17.70)
Live Alone	−66.13	−14.43	−46.79	−80.06**
	(56.43)	(14.73)	(34.61)	(19.35)
Live w/Spouse Only	−20.83	7.05	3.12	−65.60**
	(33.00)	(9.11)	(20.24)	(11.96)
Live w/Others	38.58	−8.13	−52.00	−65.11**
	(51.30)	(13.08)	(31.47)	(17.18)
Children = 0	0.00	−23.92	0.00	30.99
	(0.00)	(30.75)	(0.00)	(40.39)
Children = 1	−54.55	−12.16	−56.39	46.59*
	(60.38)	(16.81)	(37.03)	(22.08)
Children > 2	−29.47	−15.57	−7.35	20.46
	(36.96)	(9.77)	(22.67)	(12.83)
Health-Fair	−30.70	23.62**	30.97	11.66
	(34.49)	(9.05)	(21.16)	(11.89)
Health-Good or Above	−13.23	12.65	−5.68	11.45
	(41.44)	(9.70)	(25.42)	(12.74)
Informal Education	−18.07	4.81	−16.80	−10.84
	(46.26)	(10.61)	(28.37)	(13.94)
Primary School	125.16**	1.46	14.09	−18.14
	(47.39)	(12.12)	(29.07)	(15.92)
Junior High or Above	51.79	55.69**	−22.45	3.76
	(45.73)	(15.64)	(28.05)	(20.54)
Zhejiang	20.54	18.69*	24.52	49.28**
	(30.17)	(8.38)	(18.51)	(11.00)
Constant	88.08	226.77**	159.38	29.64
	(175.29)	(41.62)	(107.52)	(54.66)
Observations	221	924	221	924
R-squared	0.18	0.14	0.16	0.06

NOTE: Standard errors in parentheses. * denotes $p < 0.05$; ** $p < 0.01$.
SOURCE: Authors' estimates using elderly sample of CHARLS pilot data.

	Private Transfer Share		Public Transfer Share		Dissaving Share	
	Urban	Rural	Urban	Rural	Urban	Rural
	−0.55	2.10	0.29	0.13	1.53	0.75
	(0.68)	(1.27)	(0.76)	(0.46)	(2.69)	(1.64)
	−5.12	−0.41	8.25	1.03	3.66	−9.45
	(8.76)	(18.05)	(9.90)	(6.48)	(34.90)	(23.22)
	−7.80	−0.23	−55.27**	−1.30	24.87	−57.70
	(10.18)	(28.68)	(11.51)	(10.31)	(40.57)	(36.90)
	58.73**	12.61	29.11	37.85**	25.07	44.03
	(15.23)	(31.36)	(17.22)	(11.27)	(60.70)	(40.35)
	2.47	54.37**	3.18	14.59*	12.07	−10.41
	(8.91)	(19.39)	(10.07)	(6.97)	(35.50)	(24.94)
	0.68	−1.98	−8.79	0.87	21.53	74.35*
	(13.85)	(27.85)	(15.66)	(10.01)	(55.18)	(35.83)
	0.00	−37.09	0.00	115.71**	0.00	−85.69
	(0.00)	(65.46)	(0.00)	(23.52)	(0.00)	(84.23)
	−15.79	−31.03	−20.12	25.35*	146.86*	−28.75
	(16.30)	(35.79)	(18.43)	(12.86)	(64.95)	(46.05)
	19.90*	19.44	−33.43**	7.04	50.36	−31.36
	(9.98)	(20.80)	(11.28)	(7.47)	(39.76)	(26.76)
	−29.44**	−25.88	0.39	10.39	28.78	−19.78
	(9.31)	(19.27)	(10.53)	(6.92)	(37.10)	(24.79)
	−23.70*	−21.89	−15.76	7.53	58.36	−9.73
	(11.19)	(20.65)	(12.65)	(7.42)	(44.58)	(26.58)
	2.95	−14.59	18.99	6.37	12.93	14.25
	(12.49)	(22.59)	(14.12)	(8.12)	(49.76)	(29.07)
	6.88	−3.80	2.58	−7.17	−148.72**	27.66
	(12.80)	(25.81)	(14.46)	(9.27)	(50.98)	(33.20)
	−3.66	−7.29	1.73	−8.28	−27.40	−43.87
	(12.35)	(33.29)	(13.96)	(11.96)	(49.19)	(42.84)
	20.74*	37.55*	−3.09	6.76	−62.71	−112.28**
	(8.15)	(17.83)	(9.21)	(6.41)	(32.46)	(22.95)
	54.58	−144.14	53.05	−16.50	−255.09	4.23
	(47.33)	(88.59)	(53.50)	(31.83)	(188.55)	(113.98)
	221	924	221	924	221	924
	0.21	0.03	0.19	0.07	0.12	0.05

DISCUSSION

Analysis of the CHARLS pilot data collected in 2008 finds that poverty rates of the elderly calculated based on consumption expenditures are much lower than those calculated based on pre-transfer income. For the income poor, co-residence, transfers, and dissaving play key roles in financing consumption expenditures and in keeping the elderly out of poverty. Results of regression analysis suggest that such mechanisms are relatively effective in protecting those with vulnerable characteristics such as lack of children, low education, and poor health. However, 15% of the elderly consume at levels below the World Bank's $1.25/day international poverty line. Also, mean expenditures per capita are significantly lower for the elderly than for those aged 45–60, suggesting that China's elderly are vulnerable relative to other demographic groups, unlike in some other countries (Lee and Mason, 2009). Those living alone appear to be particularly at risk, a result consistent with the findings of Saunders and Sun (2006) who analyze data on Chinese urban households.

Looking forward, one advantageous factor for dealing with the needs of the future elderly is that they will be much better educated than today's elderly and so will have higher incomes and wealth, which will improve their ability to be self-reliant in financing their consumption.

However, the future will also bring significant challenges to providing adequate consumption levels for the elderly. Life expectancy will continue to rise, increasing the years of life requiring support unless work-leisure choices change. As seen in the comparisons between those aged 45 to 60 and those aged 60 and older, tomorrow's elderly will have much fewer children and are much more likely to live separately from their children—an ongoing trend in China (Giles, Wang, and Zhao, 2010). Although to date there is no strong evidence that migration by children is associated with lower living standards on average, there is evidence that it is associated with greater variance in living standards, suggesting that some elderly are neglected by their migrant children (Giles, Wang, and Zhao, 2010). Anthropologists point out that modernization may be undermining filial values (e.g., Yan, 2003), which may be part of longer-term trends dating to the early 20th century (Benjamin, Brandt, and Rozelle, 2000). The sustainability of private support systems for the elderly is a common issue facing many developing countries (Lee and Mason, 2009; Lee, Mason, and Cotlear, 2010).

To meet these challenges, China is aggressively increasing public support for the elderly in the form of expanded pension coverage, as well as social assistance programs, such as subsidies to maintain minimum living standards and family planning subsidies for those elderly who followed family planning guidelines throughout their lives and so have fewer children to support them (World Bank, 2009). Significantly, these programs are being scaled up in rural areas, which is where most of China's poor continue to reside. Our analysis finds that pension payments can significantly reduce the likelihood of the elderly being poor, providing some optimism that current policy initiatives will have a significant impact on elderly poverty. The shift from private to public transfer systems to support the elderly is a path that has been followed by many Latin American countries (Calvo and Williamson, 2008).

Such programs may make it possible for the rural elderly to afford retirement in their older years rather than being forced to work until they drop, an unfortunate condition of rural life in China and other developing countries (Giles, Wang, and Cai, 2011; Goldstein and Ku, 1993; Pang, de Brauw, and Rozelle, 2004). Although as noted earlier agricultural income of the elderly accounts for a relatively small share of income, we find that simulating the loss of such income would increase the rural poverty rate based on post-transfer income per capita by 5%.

One important issue in scaling up public support for the elderly in the form of pensions or public transfers is that such support may crowd out private sources of support (Cai, Giles, and Meng, 2006) or reduce elderly labor supply, reinforcing dependence on public programs. Although this could increase the burden placed on China's public finances, in addition to the direct benefits for the elderly, other factors could mitigate these costs from a public policy perspective. Retirement by the rural elderly could enable them to transfer their land to others who could use the land more productively, and a steady reliable source of income from public programs could reduce the perceived need for precautionary savings and so increase consumption spending.

One limitation of this study is that it examines the situation of the elderly in two provinces that are diverse but not fully representative of China. Studies of other regions or using data from the first nationally representative wave of CHARLS will be of great value. Another limitation of this study is that it takes the different sources of consumption financing as exogenous, and so does not consider how changes in the availability of one type of resource will lead to responses that increase reliance on other sources of finance. Individuals with no children may anticipate future financing needs and work more hours to increase savings in advance of old age. As noted, public transfers may reduce elderly labor supply and private support for the elderly. Studies that address behavioral responses to public policies and impact evaluations of current policies may help shed important light on how different policies will ultimately affect the welfare of China's elderly.

REFERENCES

Benjamin, D., L. Brandt, and S.D. Rozelle. (2000). Aging, wellbeing, and social security in rural northern China. *Population and Development Review 26*:89-116.

Cai, F., J. Giles, and X. Meng. (2006). How well do children insure parents against low retirement income? An analysis using survey data from urban China. *Journal of Public Economics 90(12)*:2,229-2,255.

Calvo, E., and J.B. Williamson. (2008). Old-age pension reform and modernization pathways: Lessons for China from Latin America. *Journal of Aging Studies 22*:74-87.

Chamon, M.D., and E.S. Prasad. (2010). Why are saving rates of urban households in China rising? *American Economic Journal: Macroeconomics 2(1)*:93-130.

Chan, K.W., and L. Zhang. (1999). The *Hukou* system and rural–urban migration in China: Processes and changes. *The China Quarterly 160*:818-855.

Chen, S., and M. Ravallion. (2008). *China Is Poorer Than We Thought, but No Less Successful in the Fight against Poverty.* World Bank Policy Research Working Paper #1421. Washington, DC: World Bank.

China Health and Retirement Longitudinal Survey. (2008). China Center for Economic Research, Peking University. Available: http://charls.ccer.edu.cn/charls/data.asp

Foster, J., J. Greer, and E. Thorbecke. (1984). A class of decomposable poverty measures. *Econometrica 52(3)*:761-766.

Giles, J., D. Wang, and W. Cai. (2011). *The Labor Supply and Retirement Behavior of China's Older Workers and Elderly in Comparative Perspective.* Policy Research Working Paper #5853. Available: http://elibrary.worldbank.org/docserver/download/5853.pdf?expires=133 3378587&id=id&accname=guest&checksum=334AF620736554D339D707C93C0FCF4E.

Giles, J., D. Wang, and C. Zhao. (2010). Can China's rural elderly count on support from adult children? Implications of rural-to-urban migration. *Journal of Population Ageing 3(3-4)*:183-204.

Goldstein, M.C., and Y. Ku. (1993). Income and family support among rural elderly in Zhejiang Province, China. *Journal of Cross-Cultural Gerontology 8(3)*:197-223.

Lee, R., and A. Mason, A. (2009). *New Perspectives from National Transfer Accounts for National Fiscal Policy, Social Programs, and Family Transfers.* Paper prepared for the Expert Group Meeting on Population Ageing, Intergenerational Transfers and Social Protection, Santiago, Chile.

Lee, R., A. Mason, and D. Cotlear, D. (2010). *Some Economic Consequences of Global Aging.* World Bank Health Nutrition and Population (HPN) Discussion Paper. Washington, DC: World Bank.

Pang, L., A. de Brauw, and S.D. Rozelle. (2004). Working until you drop: The elderly of rural China. *The China Journal 52*:73-94.

Saunders, P., and L. Sun. (2006). Poverty and hardship among the aged in urban China. *Social Policy and Administration 42(2)*:138-157.

Solinger, D. (1999). *Contesting Citizenship in Urban China: Peasant Migrants, the State, and the Logic of the Market.* Berkeley: University of California Press.

United Nations (2002). *World Population Aging: 1950-2050.* New York: United Nations.

World Bank. (2009). *From Poor Areas to Poor People: China's Evolving Poverty Reduction Agenda.* Washington, DC: World Bank.

Yan, Y. (2003). *Private Life Under Socialism: Love, Intimacy, and Family Change in a Chinese Village 1949-1999.* Stanford, CA: Stanford University Press.

Zhao, Y., J. Strauss, A. Park, Y. Shen, and Y. Sun. (2009). *China Health and Retirement Longitudinal Study, Pilot, User's Guide.* National School of Development, Peking University.

8

Retirement Process in Japan: New Evidence from the Japanese Study on Aging and Retirement[1] (JSTAR)

Hidehiko Ichimura and *Satoshi Shimizutani*

One of the most distinct characteristics of the Japanese labor market of the elderly is "late retirement," compared to the other countries of the Organisation for Economic Co-operation and Development (OECD). The data on effective retirement age, which is most frequently quoted for an international comparison, show that the average effective retirement age for Japanese males is 69.5 years and for females is 66.5 years. These are the oldest ages among developed countries (Organisation for Economic Co-operation and Development, 2008).

Clearly, this measure alone is insufficient to capture decisions about retirement. At least three limitations are pointed out in the literature. First, the definition of retirement depends on subjective perceptions that may differ across individuals (Lazear, 1986; Lumsdaine and Mitchell, 1999). For example, several studies have revealed that the timing of retirement does not coincide with the decision to leave the labor force or to receive pension benefits (e.g., Banks and Smith, 2006, for the United Kingdom, and Shimizutani, 2011, for Japan). Second, individuals may not retire at once

[1]This study was prepared for the Conference on Policy Research and Data Need to Meet the Challenges and Opportunities of Population Aging in Asia, New Delhi, on March 14–15, 2011. We are grateful to the Indian National Science Academy, the host of the conference, and other sponsoring organizations. We also thank Asako Jufuku, Hirokazu Matsuyama, and Yuta Kikuchi for excellent research assistance. In addition, we thank the referees and Daigo Nakata, as well as participants at the conference for their constructive comments. Ichimura thanks the Japan Society for the Promotion of Science for its support through the Basic Research Grant.

but gradually, and the process of retirement may take some time. In addition, retirement may not be an absorbing state (Banks and Smith, 2006). Third, the retirement decision may be jointly made by a married couple (Gustman and Steinmeier, 2009). If this is the case, retirement behavior needs to be considered as an outcome of intrahousehold decision-making, in addition to a variety of factors including socioeconomic, health, and other circumstances.

In this chapter, we will describe Japanese workers' retirement processes using the Japanese Study on Aging and Retirement (JSTAR). JSTAR, for the first time, provides publicly available panel data on individuals who were between the ages of 50–75 in 2007. To our knowledge, this study is the first to explore the retirement process in Japan using panel data. Thus, the contribution of this study is to provide new evidence on the process uncovered by JSTAR.

While research on retirement in Japan has been accumulated, the studies are limited in two ways.[2] First, the studies use cross-sectional data, which makes it impossible to uncover a retirement "process." Second, the studies use data sets with a very limited variety of variables. In particular do they contain family demographics, such as spouses' work status or if they have elderly or other dependents?[3]

JSTAR, a sister survey of the Health and Retirement Study (HRS), English Longitudinal Survey on Ageing (ELSA), and Survey on Health, Ageing and Retirement in Europe (SHARE), overcomes those two obsta-

---

[2]Research carried out in Japanese workers' retirement behavior is largely limited to two areas: the labor supply effect of social security earnings test and the effect of mandatory retirement on the transition from a primary job to a secondary job.

[3]Some existing surveys are often used in analysis of aging in Japan. The National Survey of Family Income and Expenditure collects data every five years on a wide variety of economic variables and family demographics but less information on health. The Comprehensive Survey of People's Living Conditions is implemented every three years with small-scale surveys in between years to collect rich information on health, family, and some economic variables. The Survey on Employment of the Elderly focused on working conditions and experience of the elderly between 55 and 69 but ended in 2004. Those surveys are large but cross-sectional. On the other hand, there are three panel data sets on elderly people. The National Long-run Panel Survey on the Life and Health of the Elderly started in 1987 and collects data every three years, which is a Japanese version of AHEAD. Together with the Nihon University Japanese Longitudinal Study of Aging, these surveys provide detailed information on the health status of the elderly aged 60 (or 65) and older and less information on economic status. Thus, the retirement process is not captured well. Lastly, the Ministry of Health, Labour, and Welfare started a panel survey of the senior population (Chukonen Jyudan Chosa), tracking individuals in their 50s in 2007 every two years. The sample size is larger than that of JSTAR with nationwide regions, but the information is insufficient to capture precise amounts of pension income or medical/long-term care expenses. It also lacks data on previous working experiences or future expectations. In most cases, microdata are not accessible or only limitedly accessible.

cles. JSTAR contains a variety of variables comparable to those in HRS/ ELSA/SHARE and intends to address a variety of socioeconomic issues related to the aging population, with an emphasis on both interdisciplinarity and international comparability (see Ichimura, Hashimoto, and Shimizutani, 2009).

MEASUREMENT OF RETIREMENT

Retirement depends on definition. The definitions include an affirmative answer to a question regarding retirement status: "Are you currently retired?" as well as a state in which the individual is out of the labor force with the intention of remaining out permanently, and a state in which the individual receives some of his or her income as pension benefits (Lazear, 1986).[4] We explore retirement behavior using the three measures by examining the first wave (baseline) of JSTAR in this section. The sample in the baseline are those who are aged 50–75 and randomly chosen from household registration after regional stratification in each of the five municipalities in 2007.[5] The sample size is more than 4,000, excluding those who did not provide information on work status from the total sample size of about 4,200.

Figures 8-1a and 8-1b illustrate nonworking status and its decomposition for males and females separately.[6] For males, the proportion of the nonworking very gradually increases from less than 5% at age 50 to about 8% at age 59, but the share jumps at age 60 to about 17% and increases along with age in the 60s. However, the nonworking proportion is still only slightly above 60% at around age 70. Most nonworkers are accounted for by retirement, but only slightly above 50% classify themselves as retired at age 70. The results differ from those by Banks and Smith (2006),

---

[4]Lazear (1986) includes further definitions such as (1) a state the individual has reduced his/her hours substantially from some lifetime average and intends to maintain hours at or below the current level, (2) a state that the individual appears on some company's retirement roll, and (3) a state that the individual receives a primary social security payment. We will refer to (1) below.

[5]Note that JSTAR does not employ a probabilistic national sampling but has an emphasis on securing a larger number of samples in the same socioeconomic environment.

[6]JSTAR asked respondents and spouses, if any, to choose one among the following choices when asked about their current working status: (1) currently working, (2) leave of absence, (3) not currently working, (4) don't know, and (5) refuse to answer. Respondents who choose (1) or (2) are "working" and those who choose other choices are further asked whether they are searching for a job currently or plan to search in the future. If the answer is affirmative, they are categorized as "unemployed." The respondents who are neither explicitly working nor unemployed are further divided into retired, homemakers, or medically treated. As explained above, these questions are also asked for the spouses, but we only use the data on the respondents in this chapter.

A. Male

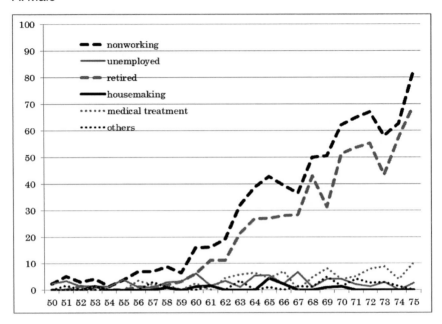

B. Female

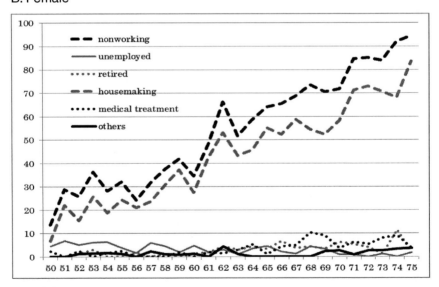

FIGURE 8-1 The proportion of males and females who are nonworking.
SOURCE: Data from JSTAR (2007).

which reveal that nonworking status and retirement is identical for people aged 65 and older in the United Kingdom. For females, the proportion of those nonworking is higher than that for males and increases with age after 50, compared to 60 for males. At a closer look, the proportion starts at about 12% at age 50 and increases to about 40% at age 60. It continues to increase in the 60s, reaching 70% at age 70. In contrast to males, a larger fraction of women's nonworking status is accounted for by homemaking, not by retirement. We should note that this must be women who are now no longer working and describe themselves as "homemakers" rather than "retired," although they are retired in the sense of having left the labor force as they reach traditional retirement ages. Those patterns do not differ much across different educational attainment either for males or females (results are omitted to save space).[7]

Figures 8-2a-d present the distribution of actual and expected retirement age in the first wave. We use the term "actual retirement age" for those who have already retired to differentiate from "expected retirement age" referring to those who have yet not retired.[8] For males, the left panel of the figure shows twin peaks in the histogram of actual retirement age, and the mode (25%) is found at age 60, followed by age 65 (15%). In contrast, the right panel shows that the age to retire in the future is concentrated at age 65, followed by age 70 and age 60. While omitted to save space, the distribution of actual retirement age is homogeneous across different levels of educational attainment, while that of expected retirement age is later for lower educational attainment. The largest fraction is observed at age 70 among those who completed junior high school only.

For females, the largest fraction in distribution of actual retirement age (left panel) is observed at age 60, which is also the case for males but the distribution is flatter, implying the distribution has a single peak at age 60. In contrast, the largest fraction in expected retirement age (right panel) is found at age 65, identical with the case for males, but the second peak is found at age 60 in contrast to age 70 for males. When decomposing by educational attainment, females' expected retirement age is later at age 70 for lower educational attainment.

In sum, the most frequently observed retirement age for those who have already retired is age 60 for both sexes, followed by age 65 for males. The most popular retirement age for those who are expecting to retire

---

[7]The proportions of nonworking persons from the Labor Force Survey are 6.9% (39.2%) for those aged 55–59, 25.6% (57.8%) for those aged 60–64, and 51.5% (74.2%) for those aged 65–75 for males (females).

[8]A very small portion of the respondents had retired before reaching age 50, and they are omitted from the figures. The sample size is 438 (797) for males and 57 (450) for females for actual (expected) retirement age. Seven respondents answered in a range (i.e., I expect to retire between age A and age B) and are excluded.

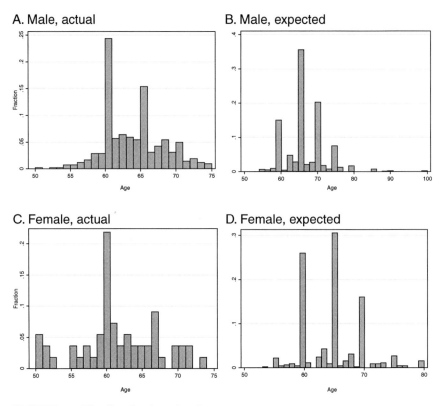

FIGURE 8-2 The distribution of retirement age.
SOURCE: Data from JSTAR (2007).

is age 65 for both sexes, followed by age 70 for males and by age 60 for females.[9] The distribution of actual retirement age does not differ much across educational attainment for both sexes, but the expected retirement age tends to be later for those with lower education.

Of course, these patterns may be a reflection of employment institutions, such as the start year to receive pension benefits. Thus, we turn to an examination of the distribution of the age to receive a pension.

The public pension program in Japan consists of three programs: the Employees' Pension Insurance (EPI, Kosei Nenkin) whose pensioners

---

[9]Rust (1989) found "twin peaks" in the retirement ages for older Americans who file for Social Security benefits using the Retirement History Survey (RHS) in the 1970s. The two peaks are observed at age 62 when the individual is eligible to receive a reduced benefit and at age 65 when the individual is eligible to full benefits. Lumsdaine and Mitchell (1999) argue that the two marked peaks remain after controlling for pension income available at those ages.

are private-sector employees; the Mutual Aid Insurance (MAI; Kyosai Nenkin) covering employees in the public sector and private schools; and the National Pension Insurance (NPI; Kokumin Nenkin) whose pensioners are not covered by EPI or MAI.[10] NPI has a flat-rate benefit only, and the normal eligibility age is 65 for both sexes. The minimum years of contribution is 25 years, and the monthly benefit for the fully insured (with 40 years of contribution) is about 66,000 yen per month (about US $800). The NPI program allows a 10-year window in claiming benefits. Individuals who claim benefits between ages 60 and 64 undergo benefit reduction, and individuals who claim benefits between ages 66 and 70 enjoy benefit rewards.[11]

The EPI program consists of flat-rate and wage-proportional components. The flat-rate component has the same contribution-benefit structure as NPI and the wage-proportional component depends on age, months of contributions, and a benefit multiplier that differs across gender and birthday. The normal eligibility ages for both components of EPI are set at age 65, but EPI beneficiaries are also entitled to receive a "special benefit" before age 65 that is close to formal benefits in most cases. The normal eligibility ages for special benefits differs between males and females and between flat-rate and wage-proportional components. As of 2011, the eligibility age for the wage-proportional component is 60 for both sexes, not allowing earlier or later claiming. Meanwhile, the eligibility age for the flat-rate component has gradually risen since 2001, and it was 63 for males and 61 for females in 2007. EPI beneficiaries were able to enjoy earlier claiming of the flat-rate component of a special benefit for males aged 60–62 and females aged 60 in 2007. One can delay either the flat-rate or wage-proportional component. (See the detail formula in Shimizutani and Oshio, 2011.) In contrast with some European countries that have high take-up rates, the disability program participation is still low and the effect on labor force participation is very limited in Japan. The main reason is the strict eligibility rules, although major revisions to the disability program have slightly expanded the eligibility for these programs (Oshio and Shimizutani, 2011).

Together with the social security program, the employment policies for the elderly have been reformed, focusing on extension of mandatory retirement age. In 2004, the Employment Measures Law was revised to include an obligatory clause that requires firms to raise the mandatory

---

[10]In terms of the number of pensioners, EPI and NPI contributed to the total by slightly less than one-half respectively, and MAI occupies the remaining small portion.

[11]For those who were born after April 2, 1941, the actuarial reduction rate before age 65 is 0.5% per month and the actuarial credit rate after age 65 is 0.7% per month (Shimizutani and Oshio, 2011).

retirement age to 65 or above by 2013 or to completely abolish it. The proportion of firms with mandatory retirement steadily increased to above 90% in the mid-1990s, and the most dominant retirement age is now 60. Some firms have indeed started extending it further to age 65 (Oshio, Oishi, and Shimizutani, 2011).

Figures 8-3a and 8-3b depict the distribution of age to start receiving any type of public pension benefits. The sample is confined to those who have received any benefits. For both sexes, close to one-half of the respondents started to receive pension benefits at age 60. The second largest fraction is found at age 65: one-quarter for males and more than 30% for females. This observation reflects the eligible ages to receive public pension benefits.

That the proportion of those who started to receive pension benefits at age 65 is larger for females reflects the fact that a larger fraction than males are NPI pensioners. By educational attainment, females who are junior high school graduates represent the largest proportion at age 65, followed by age 60, which also is a reflection that a larger proportion of NPI pensioners are females rather than males. The distribution of males is not changed across educational level.

The observation in this section is that age 60 is a specific age in Japan to retire, probably because it is the age at which people become eligible to receive pension benefits. Because the eligible age for EPI pension benefits is now in transition from 60 to 65, it is natural that the expected retirement age is changing to age 65 for the yet-to-be-retired group. However, we should keep in mind that the proportion of people working exceeds more than 30% at age 70 and some portion of the elderly keep working in their later age. In other words, the institutional reason is an important factor to account for retirement behavior but cannot completely explain labor supply behavior of the elderly.[12] This is what we examine in the next section.

TRANSITION IN WORKING STATUS BETWEEN
JSTAR FIRST AND SECOND WAVES

This section focuses on the transition of work status, using both the first and second waves in JSTAR. By doing so, we capture retirement "process," which has been unexplored in Japan. The sample is confined to the respondents who were interviewed in both waves in the five municipalities.

First, we preview retirement process transition between two years in terms of the change of work status and hours worked before retirement.

---

[12]Banks and Smith (2006) provide evidence that the proportion of nonworking and retirement jumps to 100% at age 65 in the United Kingdom because of an institutional reason: pension benefits depend on the last salary.

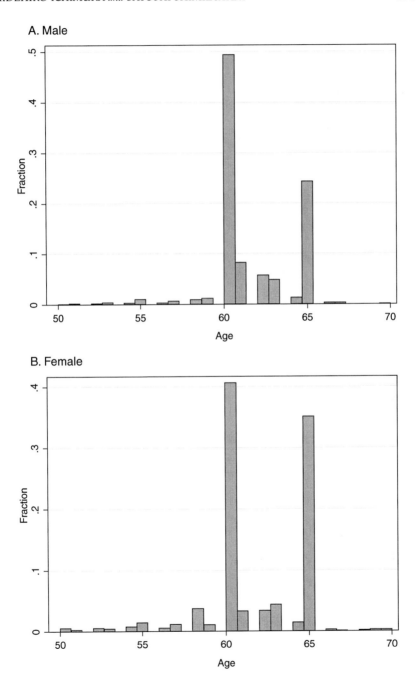

FIGURE 8-3 The distribution of starting age to receive benefits.
SOURCE: Data from JSTAR (2007).

The work status and hours worked are measured at the time of interview. Table 8-1 shows the change in work status between the first and the second wave in three definitions (working/nonworking, employed/self-employed, and full-time/part-time status) in three age ranges (60–64, 65–69, and 70 and older as of the first wave). In what follows, we call those who are wage earners and not self-employed "employed" and those who are working on a regular basis "full-time" workers. For males, the upper panel of the table shows that the transition probability into "not working" from "working" increases after age 65 from about 20 to 25%. The transition probability into "working" from "not working" drops sharply after age 65 from 17 to 5% and remains the same for the age group 70–75. For females, the transition probability into "not working" from "working" increases after age 70 from less than 20 to 27% while the transition probability into "working" from "not working" gradually drops from about 8 to 3% from age 60–75. The middle panel shows that there is very little transition between self-employment and employment status from age 60–75 for both sexes.

TABLE 8-1 Transition of Work Status Between Two Years

Male				Female			
		2009				2009	
Age 60–64		Working	Not Working	Age 60–64		Working	Not Working
2007	Working	80.3%	19.7%	2007	Working	83.0%	17.0%
	Not Working	17.1%	82.9%		Not Working	8.2%	91.8%
		2009				2009	
Age 65–69		Working	Not Working	Age 65–69		Working	Not Working
2007	Working	75.0%	25.0%	2007	Working	85.1%	14.9%
	Not Working	5.4%	94.6%		Not Working	5.6%	94.4%
		2009				2009	
Age 70–75		Working	Not Working	Age 70–75		Working	Not Working
2007	Working	77.5%	22.5%	2007	Working	73.0%	27.0%
	Not Working	5.0%	95.0%		Not Working	2.6%	97.4%

continued

TABLE 8-1 Continued

Male				Female			
	2009				2009		
Age 60–64		Employed	Self-Employed	Age 60–64		Employed	Self-Employed
2007	Employed	98.0%	2.0%	2007	Employed	98.5%	1.5%
	Self-Employed	0.0%	100.0%		Self-Employed	1.8%	98.2%
	2009				2009		
Age 65–69		Employed	Self-Employed	Age 65–69		Employed	Self-Employed
2007	Employed	100.0%	0.0%	2007	Employed	97.1%	2.9%
	Self-Employed	4.1%	95.9%		Self-Employed	3.8%	96.2%
	2009				2009		
Age 70–75		Employed	Self-Employed	Age 70–75		Employed	Self-Employed
2007	Employed	100.0%	0.0%	2007	Employed	100.0%	0.0%
	Self-Employed	0.0%	100.0%		Self-Employed	0.0%	100.0%
Male				Female			
	2009				2009		
Age 60–64		Full time	Part time	Age 60–64		Full time	Part time
2007	Full time	28.6%	71.4%	2007	Full time	42.1%	57.9%
	Part time	5.4%	94.6%		Part time	2.0%	98.0%
	2009				2009		
Age 65–69		Full time	Part time	Age 65–69		Full time	Part time
2007	Full time	40.0%	60.0%	2007	Full time	37.5%	62.5%
	Part time	2.0%	98.0%		Part time	0.9%	99.1%
	2009				2009		
Age 70–75		Full time	Part time	Age 70–75		Full time	Part time
2007	Full time	16.7%	83.3%	2007	Full time	50.0%	50.0%
	Part time	0.2%	99.8%		Part time	0.1%	99.9%

SOURCE: Data from JSTAR (2007).

The lower panel shows the transition probability between full-time and part-time work. The information on full-time/part-time status is available only for the respondents who were employed or were high-ranked managers, so the sample size is reduced. As stated, full-time status is defined as whether one worked on a regular basis or not. For males, the transition probability into "part time" from "full time" is more than 70% and 60% in their 60s, and it increases to more than 83% after age 70. The transition probability into "full time" from "part time" is low, at 5% for the first half of the 60s and lower for the older group. For females, the transition into part time from full time remains at around 50 to 60% throughout the age range. The transition probability into "full time" from "part time" for female is low at 2% for the first half of the 60s and lower for the older group.

Second, we examine changes in working hours before retirement. Figures 8-4a and 8-4b present evidence on working hours in the first wave (2007) for those who had retired by the second wave (2009). The working hours are converted into an annual basis using hours worked per week and weeks worked, i.e., 52 weeks minus nonworking weeks. Figure 8-4a reports the mean of annual working hours in three age groups (60–64, 65–69, and 70 and older) in the first wave for males and females, respectively. For males, the average annual working hours are 1,890 hours for ages 60–64, decline to 1,390 for ages 65–69, and remain at the same level for age 70 and older (1,380 hours). Males who retire at ages 60–64 seem to retire from close to full-time work, but this tendency is weakened in the older age group. For females, the average working hours is 1,620 hours for ages 60–64 and decreases to 940 hours for ages 65–69. Surprisingly, the average working hours jumps up to 1,870 hours, which corresponds to working hours for full-time workers, probably because only full-time workers keep working after 70 and older.

Figure 8-4b verifies this result further by examining 25th percentile, 50th percentile, and 75th percentile of hours worked per year for those who retired in the age categories we examined. For males, individuals below 65 seem to retire directly from full-time work. In older age categories, however, the majority of males seem to retire after reducing some work hours. For females, although the majority seem to retire from full-time work below age 65, more than 25% retire via reduced working hours. Most individuals who retire in the 65–69 category seem to retire via reduced work hours while individuals who retire above 70 seem to retire directly from full time.

A. Annual average of hours worked (mean)

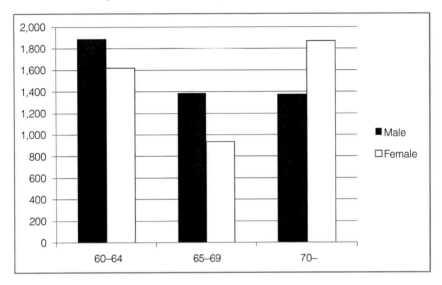

B. Annual average of hours worked (25 percentile, median, 75 percentile)

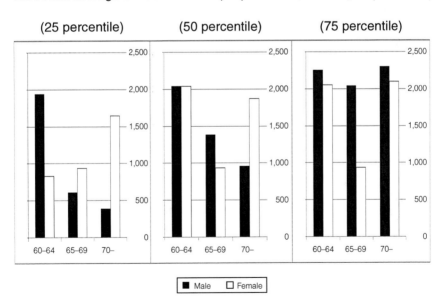

FIGURE 8-4 Hours worked before retirement.
SOURCE: Data from JSTAR (2007).

EMPIRICAL FRAMEWORK

We empirically examine the retirement process above using a regression framework. Our emphasis is on fact-finding, taking advantage of the first opportunity to explore the retirement process with JSTAR. Thus, we employ a reduced-form specification to examine how specific pre-determined variables are associated with endogenous variables.

We first examine the retirement decision in 2009, R_{2009}, given the work status (working or not working) in 2007, W_{2007}, and other variables. We employ the linear probability model for the ease of interpretation of the coefficients where we conduct the empirical analysis separately for males and females with different working status in 2007. For those who were working in 2007, we introduce dummy variables indicating different hours of work status: less than 30 hours per week, between 30–40 hours per week, and above 40 hours a week. These dummy variables are denoted by d_{HW}.

We also include age (in 2007) dummy variables: 50–59, 60–64, 65–69, and 70 and older. These dummy variables are denoted by d_A. Age and hours-worked dummy variables are interacted completely. By fully interacting the dummy variables, we intend to capture the effects of age and working hours on the outcome variables flexibly. The interaction terms are denoted by $d_A \cdot d_{HW}$.

We wish to control for a host of other variables. We gather these variables in three categories: health-related variables (denoted x_H), socioeconomic-related variables (denoted x_{SE}), and family-related variables (denoted x_F).

Health-related variables include word recall measuring the memory, grip strength, Activities of Daily Living (ADL) limitation , and a measure of depression in 2007. The socioeconomic variables include net assets over lifetime in 2007, educational attainment, and employment status (employed or self-employed) if working. Family-related variables include marital status, as well as its change between 2007 and 2009, the youngest child's age, and the number of parents for whom the individual provides care.

In order to conserve the number of parameters, we assume that these variables affect an outcome only via three linear indices ($x'_H \theta_H$, $x'_{SE} \theta_{SE}$, and $x'_F \theta_F$) representing each of the three categories using the variables discussed above. We then interact each of these three indices completely with the age and hours-worked dummy variables and also with the interaction terms of age and hours-worked dummy variables to allow for flexible ways these variables affect the outcome. We keep the index structure to conserve the number of parameters.

The estimated model is

$$R_{2009} = \beta_0 + d'_A \beta_A + d'_{HW} \beta_{HW} + (d_A \cdot d_{HW})' \beta_{A \cdot HW}$$
$$+ \beta_H (x'_H \theta_H) + \beta_{SE}(x'_{SE} \theta_{SE}) + \beta_F(x'_F \theta_F)$$
$$+ (d_A (x'_H \theta_H))' \beta_{A \cdot H} + (d_A(x'_{SE} \theta_{SE}))' \beta_{A \cdot SE} + (d_A (x'_F \theta_F))' \beta_{A \cdot F}$$
$$+ (d_{HW}(x'_H \theta_H))' \beta_{HW \cdot H} + (d_{HW}(x'_{SE} \theta_{SE}))' \beta_{HW \cdot SE} + (d_{HW}(x'_F \theta_F))' \beta_{HW \cdot F}$$
$$+ (d_{HW} \cdot d_A (x'_H \theta_H))' \beta_{HW \cdot A \cdot H} + (d_{HW} \cdot d_A(x'_{SE} \theta_{SE}))' \beta_{HW \cdot A \cdot SE}$$
$$+ (d_{HW} \cdot d_A(x'_F \theta_F))' \beta_{HW \cdot A \cdot F} + u.$$

Note that the resulting model is a nonlinear in its parameters. We normalize the coefficients defining the three indices by setting one of the coefficients to 1; for the health index the variable corresponding to the normalized coefficient is the CES-D scale depression measure, for the socioeconomic index it is the dummy variable indicating high education level (more than two-year college), and for the family index it is whether the person is married or not in 2007.

We refer to the males' and females' regression results for 2007 workers as Regression 1 and results for 2007 nonworkers as Regression 2. For nonworkers, there is no conditioning on the hours-worked dummy variables. We also conduct the same regression analysis for the working hours given the same set of regressors for males and females who worked in 2007. We refer to the results as Regression 3.

ESTIMATION METHOD

We estimate all models in Regressions 1–3 by the nonlinear least squares method using the model specified.

In carrying out the estimation, we faced some difficulty due to item nonresponse in certain regressors. In order to keep as many samples as possible in the estimation, we "impute" the missing data for three variables: total assets, grip strength, and word recall, before estimating each specification. We apply the method of Arellano and Meghir (1992) in our context of missing regressors assuming that the nonresponses occur randomly.

First, we regress total assets on all the regressors in the estimation as well as additional variables (information on the job at age 54) for those whose asset data is available. Then, we obtain a "total asset hat" using the actual values if not missing and the estimated values if missing. Second, we perform the similar procedure for word recall using "total asset hat" and obtain "word recall hat." Third, we again perform the similar procedure for grip strength using "total asset hat" and "word recall hat" and obtain "grip strength hat." Finally, we estimate "total asset hat hat" using "word recall hat" and "grip strength hat." We use those three estimated variables in the estimation. We performed those steps separately for each estimation.

EMPIRICAL RESULTS

Table 8-2 presents the summary statistics of the variables used in the regressions. The sample size of those whose work status was available in 2009 and were aged between 50–74 in 2007 are 1,481 for males and 1,430 for females, respectively.

We review the statistics below, comparing males and females. First, the proportion of retired respondents in 2009 is 36% for males and 58% for females. The averages of weekly working hours are reduced from 30.1 hours to 25.4 hours for males, and from 13.3 hours to 12.1 hours for females between the two years. Second, the age structure is similar for both sexes: about 40% in their 50s, with a slightly higher proportion for males. Third, the proportion of the depressed, which is measured in the Center for Epidemiological Studies Depression Scale (CES-D Scale), or the number of words recalled are slightly higher for females, while grip strength is higher for males. A smaller proportion of both sexes have ADL limitations in terms of six basic activities. Fourth, the proportion of having a spouse is close to 90% for males and three-quarters for females, while that of having a working spouse is more than 50% for males and 60% for females. About 10% are engaged in family care of their own or spousal parents. The proportion of those who do not have a child is less than 10% and the age of the youngest child is higher for females. Fifth, educational attainment is higher for males, which is observed in the higher proportion of graduates of two-year colleges or more (including university graduates). The share of EPI or MAI beneficiaries is higher for males. The amount of net assets is also larger for males. The amount is defined as the sum of current stock of assets, either financial or real, minus any debts, either mortgage or nonmortgage, labor income before retirement (expected retirement age as available if not yet retired), Social Security benefits between retirement and the timing of death (expected survival age as available) and expected (or realized) bequests, subtracting expected expenditure (including imputed rents) between now to death. In the regression analysis, four categorical dummy variables are created by dividing the asset level into four groups depending on thresholds of net assets: 1 million, 15 million, and 35 million yen.

Table 8-3 reports the estimated coefficients in Regressions 1–3 for males. The third column reports the result of Regression 2, which explores the factors affecting probability of retirement in 2009 given the respondent reported being retired in 2007. The result indicates that most males are still retired with probability close to 1, except for those in their 50s who

TABLE 8-2 Summary Statistics

Variables	Male			Female		
	# Obs.	Mean	S.D.	# Obs.	Mean	S.D.
Retirement in 2009	1,481	0.36	0.48	1,430	0.58	0.49
Working hours in 2009 [#]	1,388	25.36	23.57	1,363	12.06	18.40
Working hours in 2007 [#]	1,929	30.07	24.65	1,957	13.25	19.01
Working hours	1,929			1,957		
Working hours = 0		0.31	0.46		0.58	0.49
0 < Working hours ≤ 30		0.11	0.31		0.18	0.38
30 < Working hours ≤ 40		0.06	0.23		0.08	0.26
40 < Working hours		0.52	0.50		0.17	0.37
Age	2,032			2,031		
Age 50-59		0.39	0.49		0.35	0.48
Age 60-64		0.20	0.40		0.20	0.40
Age 65-69		0.21	0.41		0.20	0.40
Age 70-74		0.19	0.39		0.22	0.41
Depressed	1,903	0.23	0.42	1,905	0.27	0.44
Memory (word recall) [#]	1,768	4.94	1.59	1,860	5.33	1.58
ADL limitations (any)	2,022	0.05	0.22	2,029	0.06	0.24
Grip strength [#]	1,898	35.73	6.96	1,959	22.71	4.73
Spouse	2,032	0.88	0.32	2,031	0.75	0.44
Working spouse	1,785	0.53	0.50	1,516	0.60	0.49
Providing care	2,032	0.14	0.45	2,031	0.11	0.37
No child	2,032	0.09	0.29	2,030	0.08	0.28
Minimum child age [#]	1,833	30.30	8.33	1,847	34.11	8.27
Education	2,032			2,031		
Education_ high		0.26	0.44		0.15	0.36
Education_middle		0.41	0.49		0.50	0.50
Education_low		0.33	0.47		0.35	0.48
EPIMAI	1,878	0.75	0.43	1,876	0.45	0.50
Net asset in million yen	1,468			1,374		
Asset ≥ 35		0.33	0.47		0.26	0.44
15 ≤ Asset < 35		0.28	0.45		0.25	0.43
1 ≤ Asset < 15		0.19	0.39		0.22	0.42
Asset < 1		0.20	0.40		0.26	0.44

NOTE: [#] means the variable is not a dummy variable.
SOURCE: Data from JSTAR (2007).

have a point estimate of being in the retired status with probability 46.8% when health, family, and socioeconomic indices are held at 0. None of these indices is statistically significant for any age group, although point estimates are sometimes nontrivial.

For males who worked in 2007, we examine the retirement decision depending on different hours worked in that year: less than 30 hours per week, greater or equal to 30 but less than 40 hours per week, and greater

TABLE 8-3 Male Estimation

Column	1	2	3	4
	Working Hours in 2007 > 0		Working Hours in 2007 = 0	
	Retirement in 2009	Working hours in 2009	Retirement in 2009	Working hours in 2009
Constant	-1.259 (0.285)***	-76.53 (54.34)	0.468 (0.392)	33.08 (18.81)
H index (health index)	-0.0558 (0.0421)	-21.38 (9.266)*	-0.0689 (0.0863)	2.635 (3.346)
F index (family index)	0.592 (0.179)***	3.102 (4.785)	-0.230 (0.151)	4.028 (5.070)
E index (economic index)	-0.0871 (0.0743)	-0.374 (1.325)	-0.00554 (0.0387)	1.656 (3.399)
Age 60–64	1.467 (0.578)*	76.61 (54.78)	0.473 (0.491)	-40.90 (21.85)
Age 65–69	3.314 (0.757)***	48.44 (51.94)	0.541 (0.464)	-35.54 (20.99)
Age 70–74	-0.0264 (1.415)	50.38 (47.26)	0.423 (0.404)	-32.79 (19.33)
H3040 (30 ≤ working hours ≤ 40)	1.038 (0.430)*	109.4 (55.34)*		
Hm40 (40 < working hours)	1.387 (0.291)***	107.3 (52.99)*		
Age 60–64 * H3040	0.636 (0.817)	-95.01 (61.26)		
Age 65–69 * H3040	-2.141 (0.969)*	-92.96 (61.59)		
Age 70–74 * H3040	0.247 (1.404)	-98.20 (58.55)		
Age 60–64 * Hm40	-1.348 (0.659)*	-48.81 (52.54)		
Age 65–69 * Hm40	-3.061 (0.798)***	-20.31 (52.06)		
Age 70–74 * Hm40	0.805 (1.597)	-31.41 (65.37)		
H3040 * H index	0.214 (0.165)	21.20 (9.770)*		
Hm40 * H index	0.0522 (0.0439)	18.90 (9.102)*		
H3040 * F index	-0.356 (0.237)	-2.131 (3.836)		
Hm40 * F index	-0.632 (0.188)***	-2.499 (4.079)		
H3040 * E index	0.0324 (0.0624)	0.471 (1.571)		
Hm40 * E index	0.0899 (0.0765)	0.593 (1.530)		
Age 60–64 * H index	0.0236 (0.0658)	15.60 (9.024)	0.112 (0.130)	-5.106 (5.709)
Age 65–69 * H index	0.167 (0.0954)	15.82 (9.215)	0.0846 (0.102)	-2.742 (3.450)
Age 70–74 * H index	-0.185 (0.128)	16.38 (9.258)	0.0306 (0.0553)	-2.405 (3.152)

continued

Variable	(1)	(2)	(3)
Age 60–64 * H3040 * H index	−0.140 (0.166)	−18.06 (9.968)	−3.550 (4.741)
Age 65–69 * H3040 * H index	−0.236 (0.213)	−22.93 (10.84)*	−4.918 (6.310)
Age 70–74 * H3040 * H index	0.0264 (0.189)	−29.52 (13.33)*	−4.411 (5.580)
Age 60–64 * Hm40 * H index	−0.0721 (0.0786)	−11.85 (9.224)	
Age 65–69 * Hm40 * H index	−0.136 (0.0869)	−9.005 (9.356)	
Age 70–74 * Hm40 * H index	0.256 (0.156)	−12.78 (13.52)	
Age 60–64 * F index	−0.591 (0.267)*	−4.773 (6.977)	0.199 (0.151)
Age 65–69 * F index	−1.123 (0.355)**	0.667 (2.622)	0.276 (0.177)
Age 70–74 * F index	−0.258 (0.408)	4.447 (5.520)	0.275 (0.179)
Age 60–64 * H3040 * F index	−0.283 (0.338)	6.348 (9.350)	
Age 65–69 * H3040 * F index	0.676 (0.409)	−0.734 (3.282)	
Age 70–74 * H3040 * F index	0.021 (0.441)	−6.343 (7.892)	
Age 60–64 * Hm40 * F index	0.574 (0.288)*	3.026 (4.906)	
Age 65–69 * Hm40 * F index	1.077 (0.357)**	0.278 (2.974)	
Age 70–74 * Hm40 * F index	0.0816 (0.441)	−5.333 (6.935)	
Age 60–64 * E index	0.134 (0.114)	0.315 (1.406)	0.0218 (0.150)
Age 65–69 * E index	0.108 (0.0977)	−0.961 (1.950)	0.00228 (0.0166)
Age 70–74* E index	−0.0431 (0.0937)	2.248 (3.877)	0.00291 (0.0207)
Age 60–64 * H3040 * E index	−0.0349 (0.0794)	0.0960 (1.836)	
Age 65–69 * H3040 * E index	0.0571 (0.107)	−0.281 (1.917)	
Age 70–74 * H3040 * E index	0.0978 (0.129)	−1.890 (3.602)	
Age 60–64 * Hm40 * E index	−0.196 (0.163)	2.041 (3.660)	
Age 65–69 * Hm40 * E index	−0.158 (0.135)	2.990 (4.880)	
Age 70–74 * Hm40 * E index	−0.00848 (0.0952)	−1.133 (2.677)	
Memory (word recall)	0.129 (0.137)	−0.218 (0.122)	−0.762 (0.891)
ADL limitations (any)	−6.325 (2.875)*	1.323 (0.734)	−0.780 (1.153)
Grip strength	−0.0618 (0.0489)	−0.0905 (0.0404)*	−0.0347 (0.0566)
Working spouse	−0.0918 (0.126)	2.533 (3.487)	1.370 (1.986)
Providing care	−0.159 (0.228)	−1.773 (2.796)	−1.384 (1.850)

TABLE 8-3 Continued

Column	1	2	3	4
	Working Hours in 2007 > 0		Working Hours in 2007 = 0	
			Working Hours in 2009	
	Retirement in 2009	Working hours in 2009	Retirement in 2009	Working hours in 2009
No child	1.883 (0.535)***	−2.920 (5.221)	−0.783 (1.670)	−3.465 (6.541)
Minimum child age	0.0594 (0.0186)**	0.0760 (0.123)	−0.0521 (0.0499)	−0.131 (0.200)
Education_middle	1.993 (1.419)	2.706 (3.942)	−16.28 (117.7)	−2.279 (5.561)
EPI/MAI beneficiaries	−1.126 (1.052)	−5.819 (9.023)	−3.620 (27.15)	−1.572 (3.138)
Asset_m3500 (Asset ≥ 35 million yen)	−1.379 (1.382)	−3.143 (5.088)	14.36 (104.7)	2.844 (6.771)
Asset_15003500 (15 ≤ Asset < 35 million yen)	−1.126 (1.244)	−2.095 (3.658)	11.95 (87.75)	1.538 (3.804)
Asset_1001500 (1 ≤ Asset < 15 million yen)	1.018 (1.145)	−1.923 (3.523)	0.0979 (8.954)	−0.763 (2.258)
Number of observations	847	793	367	361
R-squared	0.188	0.295	0.187	0.21

NOTE: Robust standard errors in parentheses. * denotes $p < 0.1$; ** $p < 0.05$; *** $p < 0.01$.
SOURCE: Data from JSTAR (2007).

or equal to 40 hour per week, for males in their 50s, 60–64, 65–69, and 70 and older. The first column in Table 8-3 summarizes the regression results that we use to predict retirement rates in 2009 by age and hours-worked group below. As described in Table 8-1, those who retired in 2007 remain retired with high probability if they are aged 60 and older. When males work at all, the probability of retiring in two years is significantly less; it is one-quarter without much difference across age groups when they are working less than 30 hours per week. For males who worked 30–40 hours per week, there are differences across age groups. Those who are in their 50s have low probability (5% or less) of retirement in 2009 once they worked at least 30 hours. Interestingly, those who are in their 70s also have low probability of retirement two years later (close to 0%) once they worked 30 hours but below 40 hours per week. While the point estimate of the retirement probability in 2009 goes up for this age group when they worked 40 hours or more per week, the coefficient is not statistically significant (see Table 8-3). On the other hand, the retirement probability does not seem to differ depending on the working hours once they worked for males in their 60s; the retirement probability remains around 10–20%.

This suggests that for those who retire in their 60s, about two-thirds retire via reduced hours, whereas people who are working in their 70s retire mostly after reducing working hours.

Figures 8-5a and 8-5b examine the effects of health, socioeconomic, and family factors on the retirement probability for males. Figure 8-5a shows males whose indices are all above the median values, while Figure 8-5b shows males whose indices are all below the median values. In our construction, the health index is normalized by the CES-D measure so that the health index takes on a higher value when health variables move in the direction indicated by the coefficients in the way analogous to lower the CES-D measure. Similarly, the family index takes on higher value when a variable in the index times its coefficient moves in the same direction as being married, and the socioeconomic index takes on higher value when a variable in the index times its coefficient moves in the same direction as having longer years of education.

For those who retired in 2007, there is no statistically significant difference between the two figures, as discussed earlier, although visually there are some differences. But there is a large and statistically significant difference shown in Figures 8-5a and 8-5b across age groups when they worked in 2007. First, the probability to retire for males in their 50s who work less than 30 hours per week is not affected very much by the three indices, but for those who work 30–40 hours, the probability to retire declines to zero. For those who work more than 40 hours in the higher index values, the probability to retire increases, and for those who work for more than 40 hours in the lower index values, the probability slightly declines to less

A. Top 50th percentile, male

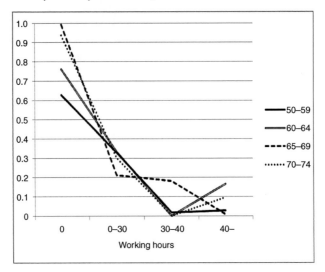

B. Bottom 50th percentile, male

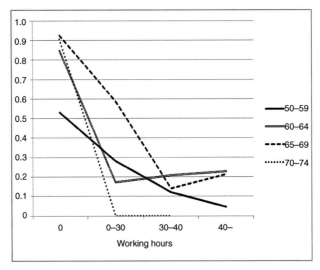

FIGURE 8-5 Predicted retirement rate (male).
SOURCE: Data from JSTAR (2007).

than 10%. Males in their 70s have a similar tendency, though the decline of retirement probability is larger in the lower percentile.

Second, the largest difference is observed for males aged 65–69. Males in this age category who have higher index values retire with much lower probability compared to those who have lower index values (21% versus 59% when they work less than 30 hours and about 0% versus 21% when they work more than 40 hours). The effect of the higher family index is opposite for this age group compared to males in their 50s. Overall, the only index that affects the retirement decision in 2009 is the family index. The health and the socioeconomic indices do not seem to affect the retirement decision with statistical significance.

On the other hand, the health index affected the working hours decision in 2009. The CES-D measure used to normalize the index and the grip strength are statistically significant variables in the health index. This can be seen in the second column of Table 8-3 reporting the results from Regression 3, which we use to predict working hours in 2009 by age and hours-worked group below. First, one can see a clear difference between the age groups. Except for males in their 50s and 70s, on average, working hours seem to be declining. Second, the working hours of males in their 50s rebound from 0 to about 10 hours, but males above 60 seem to stay constant at around 0.

The effect of health index values can be seen clearly in Figures 8-6a and 8-6b. These figures are analogously constructed with Figures 8-5a and 8-5b, except that the vertical axis is the predicted hours worked instead of the predicted retirement probability. For males in their 50s, the predicted working hours for those with the low index values and who worked less than 30 hours per week is about 14 hours per week, whereas for those with high index values, it is more than 34 hours per week. This amount does not differ much from those who worked longer hours per week in 2007. Analogous results hold for those in their 70s. Those with lower index values are predicted to work less hours in 2009 compared to their working hours in 2007, but those with higher index values are predicted to keep working around the same hours per week with the hours worked per week in 2007. Compared with males in their 50s and 70s, the difference between high and low index values are much smaller for males in their 60s.

Table 8-4 reports the estimated coefficients for females in Regressions 1–3. The third column reports the result of Regression 2, which explores the factors affecting probability of retirement in 2009 given the respondent reported being retired in 2007. The result indicates that those in their 50s with a lower health index and higher family index retire with higher probability. The effects of the indices are opposite for females above 70. Those who have a higher health index value and lower family index value retire with higher probability. However, the effect is not so

A. Top 50th percentile, male

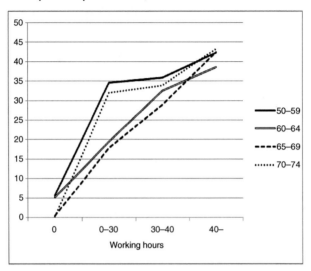

B. Bottom 50th percentile, male

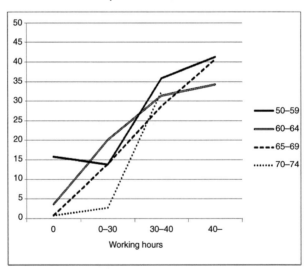

FIGURE 8-6 Predicted working hours (male).
SOURCE: Data from JSTAR (2007).

TABLE 8-4 Female Estimation

Column	1	2	3	4
	Working Hours in 2007 > 0		Working Hours in 2007 = 0	
	Retirement in 2009	Working hours in 2009	Retirement in 2009	Working hours in 2009
Constant	-0.127 (0.135)	15.42 (11.95)	0.832 (0.150)***	1.378 (3.919)
H index (health index)	-0.0686 (0.0760)	-0.0300 (0.261)	-0.152 (0.0692)*	3.800 (1.804)*
F index (family index)	-0.155 (0.0915)	0.0012 (0.00038)**	0.0986 (0.0494)*	-1.932 (1.473)
E index (economic index)	0.203 (0.0937)*	-0.362 (2.063)	-0.0264 (0.0350)	3.213 (1.902)
Age 60–64	-0.0765 (0.226)	-19.48 (16.85)	-0.242 (0.227)	6.538 (5.137)
Age 65–69	-0.151 (0.271)	2.211 (23.79)	-0.0950 (0.188)	2.894 (4.231)
Age 70–74	1.090 (0.494)*	13.35 (39.75)	0.194 (0.175)	-1.931 (4.141)
H3040 (30 ≤ working hours ≤ 40)	0.0699 (0.139)	19.43 (16.55)		
Hm40 (40 < working hours)	0.241 (0.163)	41.63 (15.45)**		
Age 60–64 * H3040	0.680 (0.718)	-35.55 (24.46)		
Age 65–69 * H3040	0.708 (0.554)	-0.677 (34.49)		
Age 70–74 * H3040	0.201 (0.520)	6.217 (203.9)		
Age 60–64 * Hm40	-0.0415 (0.279)	40.96 (25.97)		
Age 65–69 * Hm40	0.486 (0.457)	124.4 (50.22)*		
Age 70–74 * Hm40	2.027 (1.937)	-0.246 (68.71)		
H3040 * H index	-0.104 (0.0979)	0.110 (0.908)		
Hm40 * H index	0.143 (0.106)	0.164 (1.346)		
H3040 * F index	0.0871 (0.0784)	-0.0021 (0.00052)***		
Hm40 * F index	0.164 (0.0992)	-0.00029 (0.00051)		
H3040 * E index	-0.179 (0.119)	2.263 (3.409)		
Hm40 * E index	-0.232 (0.104)*	6.036 (4.156)		
Age 60–64 * H index	0.0880 (0.155)	-0.146 (1.208)	0.0397 (0.0735)	-2.355 (1.720)
Age 65–69 * H index	0.121 (0.200)	0.0352 (0.352)	0.133 (0.0731)	-3.691 (1.868)*
Age 70–74 * H index	0.101 (0.274)	-0.0228 (0.298)	0.160 (0.0708)*	-3.880 (1.820)*

continued

TABLE 8-4 Continued

Column	1	2	3	4
	Working Hours in 2007 > 0		Working Hours in 2007 = 0	
			Working Hours in 2009	
	Retirement in 2009	Working hours in 2009	Retirement in 2009	Working hours in 2009
Age 60–64 * H3040 * H index	0.992 (0.217)***	−0.191 (1.586)		
Age 65–69 * H3040 * H index	−0.111 (0.290)	−0.128 (1.088)		
Age 70–74 * H3040 * H index	−0.536 (0.916)	−1.661 (14.32)		
Age 60–64 * Hm40 * H index	−0.306 (0.183)	0.351 (2.895)		
Age 65–69 * Hm40 * H index	−0.351 (0.250)	0.868 (7.111)		
Age 70–74 * Hm40 * H index	3.364 (4.901)	0.162 (1.421)		
Age 60–64 * F index	−0.0486 (0.0874)	−0.00118 (0.000790)	0.107 (0.0809)	−1.967 (2.063)
Age 65–69 * F index	−0.0666 (0.106)	−0.000843 (0.000607)	−0.0350 (0.0675)	0.492 (1.756)
Age 70–74 * F index	0.412 (0.201)*	0.000677 (0.00156)	−0.118 (0.0591)*	2.352 (1.541)
Age 60–64 * H3040 * F index	0.155 (0.168)	−0.000351 (0.00104)		
Age 65–69 * H3040 * F index	0.297 (0.211)	0.00322 (0.00107)**		
Age 70–74 * H3040 * F index	0.101 (0.139)	0.0154 (0.00980)		
Age 60–64 * Hm40 * F index	0.00244 (0.107)	0.000448 (0.00111)		
Age 65–69 * Hm40 * F index	0.216 (0.175)	0.00557 (0.00117)***		
Age 70–74 * Hm40 * F index	0.109 (0.229)	0.0000363 (0.00284)		
Age 60–64 * E index	−0.402 (0.143)**	−0.535 (4.415)	0.0130 (0.0393)	−3.557 (2.214)
Age 65–69 * E index	−0.486 (0.182)**	−1.098 (3.296)	0.0907 (0.0601)	−4.406 (2.335)
Age 70–74* E index	0.0933 (0.225)	−2.259 (6.260)	0.0138 (0.0321)	−3.152 (1.905)
Age 60–64 * H3040 * E index	0.150 (0.215)	5.103 (6.339)		
Age 65–69 * H3040 * E index	−0.0508 (0.451)	−0.108 (6.097)		
Age 70–74 * H3040 * E index	−1.016 (1.169)	98.69 (.)		
Age 60–64 * Hm40 * E index	0.318 (0.168)	4.908 (6.874)		
Age 65–69 * Hm40 * E index	0.507 (0.204)*	5.825 (8.722)		
Age 70–74 * Hm40 * E index	−1.645 (1.407)	−15.97 (11.82)		

Memory (word recall)	−0.0411 (0.0410)	−4.481 (36.74)	−0.0773 (0.0742)	−0.0970 (0.0797)
ADL limitations (any)	0.372 (0.347)	16.65 (142.0)	−1.339 (0.412)**	−1.505 (0.584)*
Grip strength	−0.0111 (0.0106)	−4.062 (33.36)	0.0454 (0.0327)	0.0436 (0.0340)
Working spouse	−1.266 (0.398)**	7283.6 (.)	−0.409 (0.228)	−0.196 (0.251)
Providing care	1.131 (0.546)*	1021.3 (848.5)	0.280 (0.174)	0.233 (0.165)
No child	−1.706 (1.254)	−6020.0 (4603.5)	1.831 (0.929)*	1.361 (1.055)
Minimum child age	−0.0749 (0.0402)	−308.3 (126.2)*	0.0411 (0.0251)	0.0332 (0.0273)
Education_middle	−0.143 (0.134)	0.775 (0.370)*	−0.665 (0.946)	0.0551 (0.376)
EPI/MAI beneficiaries	−0.220 (0.194)	−0.145 (0.368)	0.133 (0.608)	0.552 (0.463)
Asset_m3500 (Asset ≥ 35 million yen)	−0.194 (0.170)	−0.829 (0.588)	1.487 (1.505)	0.176 (0.517)
Asset_15003500 (15 ≤ Asset < 35 million yen)	0.0916 (0.243)	−1.452 (0.939)	1.327 (1.251)	0.109 (0.404)
Asset_1001500 (1 ≤ Asset < 15 million yen)	0.196 (0.212)	0.543 (0.604)	1.635 (1.346)	0.370 (0.526)
Number of observations	526	500	690	680
R-squared	0.190	0.428	0.113	0.119

NOTE: Robust standard errors in parentheses. * denotes $p < 0.1$; ** $p < 0.05$; *** $p < 0.01$.
SOURCE: Data from JSTAR (2007).

large, as almost everyone stays retired with high probability in any case as seen in Figures 8-7a and 8-7b for working hours set at 0 (discussed below).

For females who worked in 2007, we examine the retirement decision in the same way we did for males using Regression 1. The results are reported in Table 8-4's first column, which we use to predict retirement rates in 2009 by age and hours-worked group below. When females work at all, the probability of retiring in two years is significantly less; it is less than 28% (slightly higher than males' 26%), and there is not much difference across different age groups when they are working less than 30 hours per week. The probability of retirement in 2009 is around 20 to 28%, the same as males' results. However, there is a significant difference across index values. For females, socioeconomic variables affect the retirement decision in a statistically significant way.

Comparing Figures 8-7a and 8-7b, females in their 50s on average are not affected much by the index value. Regardless of the index value, they retire with about 20% probability when they work less than 30 hours per week but retire with about 10% probability when they work more. Those who are above 70 with a higher index value retire with much higher probability, at 55% when they work less than 30 hours. In contrast, for those with a lower index value, the probability of retirement declines to close to zero for females who work at all.

On the other hand, females in their 60s who work less than 30 hours per week retire with less probability when their indices values are high (around 0%) compared to those who have lower indices values, at around (40 to 50%). The difference is still large for the 60–64 age group when females work between 30 to 40 hours per week (about 5% versus 40%).

Turning to the working hours decision in 2009, the health index affected for males, but the family index affected for females. The marital status variable and the minimum child's age (higher age implies less index value) are the statistically significant variables in the family index. This can be seen in the second column of Table 8-4. It reports results from Regression 3, which we use to predict working hours in 2009 by age and hours-worked group in Figures 8-8a and 8-8b. First, unlike males, one cannot see a clear difference between the age groups. Second, all groups seem to be predicted to work less in 2009 than the hours worked per week in 2007. Third, it is observed that females with higher indices values work more hours if they are in their 50s or 60s.

CONCLUSION

We have examined the transition of work status and working hours for Japanese males and females who were between ages 50–75 in 2007 using the JSTAR data. Here we summarize our findings.

A. Top 50th percentile, female

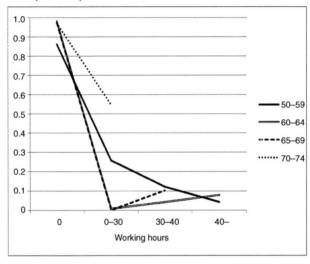

B. Bottom 50th percentile, female

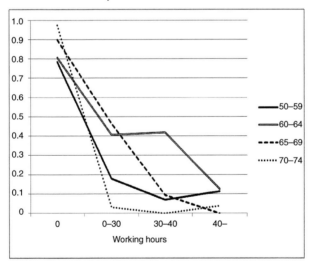

FIGURE 8-7 Predicted retirement rate (female).
SOURCE: Data from JSTAR (2007).

A. Top 50th percentile, female

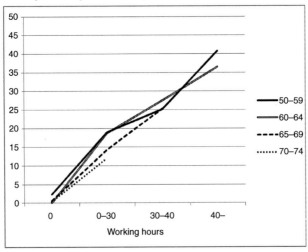

B. Bottom 50th percentile, female

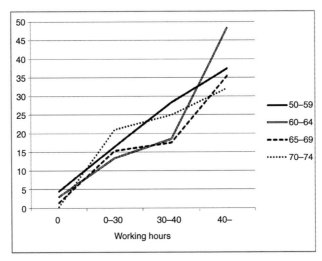

FIGURE 8-8 Predicted working hours (female).
SOURCE: Data from JSTAR (2007).

For males and females, we find strong evidence that those who retire stay retired two years later once they are aged 60 and older for males and for females in general. This decision does not seem to be affected much by the health, family, and socioeconomic indices, although there are statistically significant indices for females. Males in their 50s, on the other hand, do seem to come back to work to some extent. Interestingly, among this age group, it is the unhealthy who are predicted to work longer hours two years later (16 hours per week versus 6 hours per week).

For males and females who were not retired in 2007, retirement probabilities are predicted to be between 20–28% when the three indices are evaluated at the mean values. However, the retirement decisions of males and females seem to be affected by different factors. The important index affecting males' retirement decisions seems to be the family index, whereas the socioeconomic index affects in a statistically significant way the retirement decision for females. Although the sources and the magnitude of the effect of the indices are different, the direction of the effects is the same across males and females. For both males and females, those who are in their 60s retire with lower probability when they have a higher index. The largest effects are observed among males who are aged 65 and older when they work less than 30 hours, females who are aged 60 and older when they work less than 30 hours, and females aged 60–64 when they work between 30–40 hours per week.

In terms of hours worked, the Regression 3 results for males and females show that males and females with a lower index tend to reduce hours worked more quickly than those with a higher index. Overall, higher-index males seem to keep working at current working hours longer than their lower index values counterparts. If their working hours are reduced to 30 hours or less per week when they are in their 50s or above 70, higher index value persons retire with higher probability than those with lower index values. If they reach 30 working hours or less per week when they are in their 60s, they tend to stay in the labor market longer if they have lower index values.

The pattern we have described above is of course tentative to the extent we have assumed stationarity of behavior across different cohorts. To what extent this assumption holds up needs to be examined using longer panel data.

We also need to examine to what extent the pattern described depends on current institutional arrangements. In order to examine this, we need to find some variations in data that can be regarded equivalent to institutional changes.

REFERENCES

Arellano, M., and C. Meghir. (1992). Female labour supply and on-the-job search: An empirical model estimated using complementary data sets. *Review of Economic Studies* 59(3):537-559.

Banks, J., and S. Smith. (2006). Retirement in the UK. *Oxford Review of Economic Policy* 22(1):40-56.

Gustman, A., and T. Steinmeier. (2009). *Integrating Retirement Models.* NBER Working Paper #15607. Cambridge, MA: National Bureau of Economic Research.

Ichimura, H., H. Hashimoto, and S. Shimizutani. (2009). *JSTAR First Results: 2009 Report.* RIETI Discussion Paper Series #09- E-047, Research Institute on Economy, Trade and Industry. Project on Intergenerational Equity and Center for Intergenerational Studies, Hitotsubashi University, Discussion Paper #443-447. Available: http://www.rieti.go.jp/jp/publications/dp/09e047.pdf.

Japanese Study on Aging and Retirement. (2007). Research Institute of Economy, Trade and Industry. Available: http://www.rieti.go.jp/en/projects/jstar/index.html.

Lazear, E. (1986). Retirement from the labor force. Pp. 305-355 (Chapter 5) in *Handbook of Labor Economics, Volume 1,* O.C. Ashenfelter and R. Layard (Eds.). Amsterdam: Elsevier.

Lumsdaine, R., and O.S. Mitchell. (1999). New developments in the economic analysis of retirement. Pp. 3,261-3,307 (Chapter 49) in *Handbook of Labor Economics, Volume 3C,* O.C. Ashenfelter and D. Card (Eds.). Amsterdam: Elsevier.

Organisation for Economic Co-operation and Development). (2008). *Ageing and Employment Policies—Statistics on Average Effective Age of Retirement.* Paris: Organisation for Economic Co-operation and Development.

Oshio, T., and S. Shimizutani. (2011). *Disability Pension Program and Labor Force Participation in Japan: A Historical Perspective.* NBER Working Paper #17052. Cambridge, MA: National Bureau of Economic Research.

Oshio, T., A. Oishi, and S. Shimizutani. (2011). Social security reforms and labor force participation of the elderly in Japan. *Japanese Economic Review* 62(2):248-271.

Rust, J. (1989). Dynamic programming model of retirement behavior. Pp. 359-398 in *The Economics of Aging,* D. Wise (Ed). Chicago: University of Chicago Press.

Shimizutani, S. (2011). A new anatomy of the retirement process in Japan. *Japan and the World Economy* 23(3):141-152.

Shimizutani, S., and T. Oshio. (2011). Claiming Behavior of Public Pension Benefits: New Evidence from Japanese Study on Aging and Retirement (JSTAR). Mimeograph.

Family Roles and Responsibilities

## 9

Patterns and Correlates of Intergenerational Nontime Transfers: Evidence from CHARLS[1]

Xiaoyan Lei, John Giles, Yuqing Hu, Albert Park,
John Strauss, and *Yaohui Zhao*

C hina is now facing an unprecedented aging process, which is rapid, but occurring at a low level of economic development and with few social safety nets. With the introduction of family planning policies in the 1970s that caused a plummet in the birth rate during the past few decades, and with the earlier "baby boom" generation who will soon pass their 60th birthday in the next 15–20 years, it is projected that the old-age dependency ratio will climb from the current 10–40% by 2050.[2] However, unlike the advanced industrialized countries such as the United States and in Europe, which have long experienced aging and whose social safety nets cover the majority of the elder population, China is aging at a relatively low level of development with many times lower per capita income and underdeveloped political and financial institutions.

In comparison with the old-age support system that is operating with fragmented infrastructure and noncomprehensive coverage, informal familial support has long been the most important source of help in low-income countries. As a country with a long-standing history and culture,

[1]The research was supported by the National Institute on Aging (Grant Number R21AG031372), Natural Science Foundation of China (Grant Numbers 70773002 and 70910107022), the World Bank (Contract 7145915), and the Fogarty International Center (Grant Number R03TW008358), as well as the Knowledge for Change Trust Fund at the World Bank. The content is solely the responsibility of the authors and does not necessarily represent the official views of any of the funders.

[2]Authors' calculations based on the numbers provided by the United Nations. Available: http://esa.un.org/wpp/unpp/panel_population.htm.

China has unique traditional family values, especially strong in the rural areas. The deep-rooted Confucian "filial piety," characterized by money and time transfers from children to their parents and the co-residence of multiple generations, has effectively helped sustain an informal old-age security.

The traditional foundation of old-age support is changing today for several reasons. First, economic shifts involving smaller household sizes, greater mobility of the population, and perhaps weakening of ties of kin outside the household are potentially undermining this tradition, making it increasingly difficult for older Chinese to receive support from their adult children. Thus, it is important at this stage to understand the patterns of intergenerational transfers among Chinese families and evaluate to what extent intergenerational transfers still function as a part of elderly support. Second, despite the existence of "filial piety," other Chinese traditional norms may also linger and influence family transfer behaviors. For instance, there is a shared ideal of family continuity through the male line in which the females are considered inferior to the males, so parents tend to favor sons, reflected in the inequitable distribution of transfers (Lee et al., 1994). Therefore, we also try to investigate the correlates of intergenerational transfers, with a hope to better understand the driving forces behind transfer behaviors between elderly parents and their adult children.

In this chapter, we examine incidence and net amount of transfers and their correlations with parental demographics, socioeconomic status (SES), and health status, as well as children's demographics and SES. The main findings include (1) contrary to the situations in most developed countries, transfers are predominantly from children to elderly parents, and are large in magnitude compared with parental pre-transfer income; (2) older people with a larger number of offspring tend to receive more transfers; those residing with other children are less likely to receive transfers from their nonco-resident children; (3) the relationship between parental pre-transfer income and transfers is mixed, depending on the income level of the parents; (4) married children are more able to provide transfers; (5) educated children transfer more frequently and a larger net amount; and (6) oldest sons are less likely to provide transfers.

Our findings reveal that given the insufficient pension system and social safety nets in today's China, children remain the major source of elderly support, implying the traditional social norms still play an important role. The incidence and amount of transfers are responsive to parents' income levels, and affected by the socioeconomic status of children. As China is growing quickly and approaching a graying society, we expect adult children will continue to shoulder the most responsibility for elder support.

LITERATURE REVIEW

Who will pay for the rising army of retirees? Does the government have the resources to meet the challenges? The situation is far from satisfactory. Under the Chinese traditional "pay-as-you-go" (PAYG) pension system, governments collect pension contributions and other taxes to pay current pensions, and each employee gets a promise that he/she will receive a pension paid for by other workers in the future. As China ages rapidly, the number of new workers entering the workforce will decline, and rising longevity will increase the size of the pension-age population. The PAYG system will start to run deficits as the dependency ratio rises, and the value of future net liabilities will start to increase sharply as well.

Although the Chinese government has recently introduced a series of social insurance and new pension programs, it faces great difficulty in implementation due to the rapid demographic transition and urbanization (Cai, Giles, and Meng, 2006). Although the current social insurance system contains three pillars in name (PAYG, funded individual accounts, and voluntary complementary insurance), this system does not differ much from the PAYG system: The money in the individual account is often used to pay for the pensions of existing retirees and is, in large part, an empty account, and the third pillar is very small. It has also been shown that even with the extremely high current payroll tax rate (28%), the pension system, due to its low return rate, would never be able to achieve the promised replacement rate if taking the demographic transition into consideration (Lei, Zhang, and Zhao, 2011a). With this insufficient social insurance, private transfers will continue to be important, at least in the foreseeable future.

A large literature has been devoted to theorizing about the patterns and determinants of private transfers (Altonji, Hayashi, and Kotlikoff, 1997; Becker, 1974; Cox, 1987; Cox and Fafchamps, 2008; Cox and Soldo, 2004; Kotlikoff, 1998; McGarry and Schoeni, 1995). Following the theoretical models, relevant empirical studies have also been conducted. Regarding the patterns of intergenerational transfers, more than one-third of parents give money to children in the United States (Hurd, Smith, and Zissimopoulos, 2007) and parental assistance is important in supporting young men (Rosenzweig and Wolpin, 1993). In Poland, high-income parents transfer to low-income young couples (Cox, Jimenez, and Okrasa, 1997).

In contrast, two or three out of five households provide financial transfers for their aged parents in Korea (Kim, 2010), which is similar to most areas of Asia where children transfer to parents to insure them against low retirement incomes (Cai, Giles, and Meng, 2006; Nugent, 1985). However, multiple transfer patterns between adult children and their parents exist in Malaysian and Indonesian families (Frankenberg, Lillard, and Willis, 2002; Lillard and Willis, 1997). In particular, children are an important source of old-age security, which in part is children's repayment for parental investments in their education; in the meantime, parents and children engage in the exchange of time help for money.

Regarding the determinants of intergenerational transfers, most studies focus on the relationship between transfers and recipients' income with the purpose of exploring the underlying motives. The evidence is mixed, varying across regions. A strong negative correlation has been found in the United States (McGarry and Schoeni, 1995), but a positive one is detected in Peru (Cox, Eser, and Jimenez, 1998).

Studies regarding intergenerational transfers in China are few, possibly because available data are in short supply and not well suited to study this set of questions. In recent years, with China's rapid development and aging, more studies have been done (Cai, Giles, and Meng, 2006; Chou, 2010; Goh, 2009; Lee and Xiao, 1998; Secondi, 1997). For example, Secondi (1997) used data from a large 1988 household survey to test the hypotheses of altruism and exchange and to study the size and direction of transfers in rural China. He found that most of the money flows appeared to be transfers from adult children to elderly parents and remittances from migrants. Cai, Giles, and Meng (2006) addressed how households with elderly members coped when enterprise-based or local public pension systems failed to provide sufficient income. They found evidence that the transfer flow was from children to parents and that private transfers responded to low household income of retired workers when income fell below the poverty line. However, these studies have the same weaknesses in that transfers are defined as a household aggregate for which the donors are unspecified, rendering these studies unable to differentiate between intergenerational and intragenerational transfers.

DATA

We draw on the released 2008 pilot of the China Health and Retirement Longitudinal Study (CHARLS), a survey conducted from July to September in 2008 by the National School of Development at Peking University (Zhao et al., 2009). As one of the sisters of the Health and Retirement Study (HRS)-serial surveys, CHARLS, with its rich information, is ideal for research on transfers. In the interview, the respondents were asked whether they had received transfers from and/or given transfers to each of their children, and if so the corresponding amount.[3] Transfers

---

[3]Amounts are asked if financial transfers occur, and frequencies are asked if time transfers occur. In this chapter, we only focus on financial transfers.

are specified in two categories: financial transfers[4] and in-kind transfers (mostly in the form of goods); both are nontime transfers.

The survey was conducted in Zhejiang and Gansu, representing two very different development levels in China (see the two provinces location on the map in Figure 9-1). Zhejiang, a southeastern costal province, has been enjoying rapid economic growth since the implementation of the reform policies, and now it is one of the richest areas in China. Gansu, located in the hinterland of northwest China, is one of the poorest provinces. Its development has been constrained by its inclement natural environment and insufficient commercial opportunities. The two different economic and natural conditions contribute to different living status of the residents and potentially influence intergenerational transfers. Both provinces had major declines in fertility and mortality, with the fertility decline most rapid starting in the 1970s, when stronger family planning policies began (National Bureau of Statistics of China, 2009).

CHARLS main respondents are a random sample of aged 45 and older. Both the main respondents and their spouses are interviewed in the survey. They are asked for detailed information on themselves and on their families. In this chapter, we are particularly interested in the transfers between the respondents and their adult children.[5] CHARLS has information on all living children of each respondent and spouse, no matter where they live. In order to fully employ the rich information on each of their children, the basic sample of interest are the children of the CHARLS respondents. Specifically we first choose the 789 households with either the main respondent or his/her spouse older than 60.[6] The 2,667 adult children (aged 25 and older[7]) of the 789 respondents are then treated as our study sample.

Several sample restrictions are further applied according to different purposes of the study. For the estimation on transfers, we restrict the analyses to nonco-resident children (2,202 observations) because transfers within the household are not clearly specified conceptually, and CHARLS, like other aging surveys, does not attempt to measure them. For the

---

[4]Financial transfers are further classified into two types: regular financial transfers and nonregular financial transfers. Nonregular transfers are those made at special times of the year, such as Spring Festival or a parent's birthday.

[5]The incidence of transfers between the respondents and their elderly parents are quite small (only 13.4%), so we did not take them into consideration in our analysis. Family transfers can entail interactions among members of three or even four generations, but it is beyond the scope of this chapter to give a comprehensive treatment of this issue.

[6]Only 16 main respondents do not have any children in the sample; they are dropped for the purpose of studying parent-child transfers.

[7]We choose age 25 because many adult Chinese people younger than 25 are full-time college students who are incapable of supporting their parents.

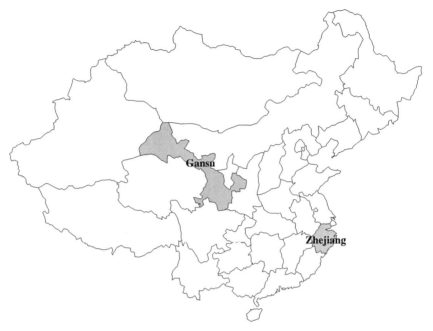

FIGURE 9-1 Location of Zhejiang and Gansu provinces.
SOURCE: China: Outline of Provinces [map]. Daniel Dalet/d-maps.com. Available: http://d-maps.com/carte.php?&num_car=1749&lang=en.

regressions regarding family fixed-effects, only those families with at least two nonco-resident adult children are included (2,068 observations).

In order to use individual information on both parent and child, we need to match individual child and parental characteristics. We choose the information of the main respondent parent because every child has a main respondent parent and, as stated earlier, the main respondents are chosen randomly by the survey.

MEASURES AND SUMMARY STATISTICS

Parent-Level Characteristics

In our analysis, characteristics of parents are mainly concerned with three aspects: demographics, SES, and health.

Demographics include age, age squared, gender, marital status (married and living with his/her spouse/partner, married but not living with spouse, separated, divorced, widowed, or never married), location (urban or rural, Zhejiang or Gansu), the number of children, and living arrangement vis-à-vis their children.

SES has three dimensions: house ownership, education level, and pre-transfer income.[8] Education is classified into five discrete educational groups: (1) illiterate, (2) less than primary education, (3) finished primary, (4) junior high, and (5) senior high and above. In particular, the second category—less than primary education—includes those who did not finish primary school but are capable of reading or writing, or those who reported to have been in "Sishu."[9]

Health-related variables include the Center for Epidemiological Studies Depression Scale (CES-D), a score of cognition using questions from the Telephone Interview of Cognition Status (TICS) used by the HRS and other surveys of the elderly, and dummies indicating whether one has poor general health, has any difficulties performing ADLs (Activities of Daily Living) or IADLs (Instrumental Activities of Daily Living), and has a major diagnosed chronic disease. Following the HRS example, the CHARLS questionnaire asked respondents to assess their general health using a scale of: excellent, very good, good, fair, or poor. Here, we look at whether a respondent reports poor health. ADL or IADL disability is defined as having difficulty in any of the ADL (including physical limitations) and IADL activities.

The cognition of the respondents comprises three questions about time orientation,[10] one question about serial-7 subtraction from 100,[11] and one question concerning picture drawing. These are standard cognition questions from TICS (Smith, McArdle, and Willis, 2010). We differentiate people as those with full marks (11 points), those without full marks but with a score above 8, and those with a score below 8. We choose 8 as the cutoff point because about one-third of the sample have scores below 8.

Respondents are also asked whether they have particular diagnosed diseases. They are coded as having major illness if they have one of the following: (1) cancer or malignant tumor (excluding minor skin cancers); (2) heart attack, coronary heart disease, angina, congestive heart failure, or other heart problems; (3) stroke (including transient ischemic attack or TIA); or (4) chronic lung diseases, such as chronic bronchitis or emphysema (except for asthma, excluding tumors, or cancer). If they have any

---

[8]In our analysis, pre-transfer income with and without public transfers are both conducted, and the results are similar. We only report the results without public transfers included in the pre-transfer income, because public transfers are arguably endogenous in a reasonable economic model.

[9]Sishu is a kind of old-style private Chinese education that mainly taught young children Chinese classics before the 20th century.

[10]Respondents are asked about today's date (year, month, and day), week, and season.

[11]The question is to subtract 7 from 100, then another 7 from that, and so on until the fifth 7.

of the other canvassed diseases,[12] they are considered as having a minor illness. Otherwise, they are defined as having no diseases.

Table 9-1 summarizes parents' characteristics by living arrangement.[13] Among all the main respondent parents of the children studied, 51.8% are co-residing with adult children, 42.6% are fathers, and each has 3.4 children on average, with a mean age of 68.4 years. Overall, our parent sample has low education levels: as many as 54.9% are illiterates, and 21.8% have not graduated from primary school. The annual per capita pre-transfer income is 5.3 thousand RMB on average, with those co-residing with children having slightly lower income than their nonco-residing counterparts (5.1 vs. 5.6 thousand RMB).

Intergenerational transfers seem to play an important role for the Chinese elderly. The sample parents on average receive 2.5 thousand RMB of net transfers from all of their children, amounting to 15.15% of their household pre-transfer income. The amount is much larger for those who are not living with their children (2.9 vs. 2.1 thousand) and the discrepancy in the ratio is especially larger (26.7% vs. 9.7%). This implies that transfers and co-residence are possible substitutes. In addition, more than one-quarter of these Chinese elderly report poor general health, 24% of them have a cognition score lower than 8, nearly 30.4% are diagnosed to have a major chronic illness, and as many as 51.1% have some difficulties in performing ADLs.

The p-values reported in the last column show significant differences between co-resident and nonco-resident parents in their marital status, place of residence, house ownership, and cognition. Specifically, parents living with their children are more likely to be widowed, have more children, be from Gansu, and live in rural areas.

Child-Level Characteristics

Child characteristics are grouped into demographics and SES, the former of which consists of age, the number of their own children (grandchildren of the parents), and five dummies representing whether the child

---

[12]These diseases include hypertension, high cholesterol, diabetes or high blood sugar, liver disease, such as Hepatitis B, or other liver disease (except fatty liver, tumors, and cancer), kidney disease (except for tumor or cancer), stomach or other digestive disease (except for tumor or cancer), emotional, nervous, or psychiatric problems, memory-related disease, and arthritis or rheumatism.

[13]For more detailed information on living arrangement of CHARLS elderly, please see Lei et al. (2011b).

TABLE 9-1 Summary Statistics of Parent Characteristics

Parent Characteristics	All	Co-resident	Nonco-resident	P-values
Age	68.44	68.34	68.54	0.726
Father (%)	42.59	43.52	41.58	0.582
Marital Status (%)				
Married	60.84	54.28	67.89	0.029
Separated	1.14	0.98	1.32	0.657
Divorced	0.51	0.00	1.05	0.045
Widowed	37.01	43.77	29.74	< 0.001
Never married	0.51	0.98	0.00	0.045
# of children	3.40	3.54	3.26	0.016
Zhejiang	52.85	44.01	62.37	< 0.001
Urban	41.95	34.23	50.26	< 0.001
Living with adult children	51.84	100.00	0.00	
House owner	89.48	94.38	84.21	< 0.001
Education (%)				
Illiterate	54.88	57.21	52.37	0.172
Less than primary education	21.80	22.00	21.58	0.885
Primary school	13.43	12.71	14.21	0.539
Middle school	5.83	4.65	7.11	0.144
High school and above	4.06	3.42	4.74	0.353
Pre-transfer income per capita (PTI, 000s)	5.32	5.08	5.58	0.501
Household Pre-transfer income (HPTI, 000s)	16.52	21.68	10.98	< 0.001
Total net amount of transfer (TT, 000s)	2.50	2.10	2.93	0.111
Transfer-income ratio (HPTI/TT, %)	15.15	9.68	26.71	
Self-Reported Health (%)				
Excellent	1.39	1.47	1.32	0.856
Very good	8.75	7.82	9.74	0.344
Good	15.34	15.16	15.53	0.886
Fair	35.23	32.03	38.68	0.051
Poor	26.24	27.87	24.47	0.278
Cognition (%)				
Score = 11	10.27	10.02	10.53	0.817
Score in [8, 11)	32.32	25.18	40.00	< 0.001
Score in [0, 8)	23.95	22.98	25.00	0.508
Disease (%)				
Minor illness	46.51	47.68	45.26	0.498
Major illness	30.42	31.30	29.47	0.579
CES-D score	8.52	8.81	8.21	0.090
ADL or IADL disability	51.08	58.92	42.63	0.090
Observations	789	409	380	

NOTES: (1) Sample are main respondent parents with children no younger than age 25, and older than age 60 or spouse older than age 60. (2) P-values are from t-test of the co-resident and nonco-resident groups.
SOURCE: Data from CHARLS 2008 pilot.

is the oldest son, youngest son,[14] daughter, whether he/she is married, and the highest level of education he/she has attained.[15]

Table 9-2 summarizes child demographic characteristics and SES by living arrangement using the child sample, i.e., those who are aged 25 and older and with at least one parent over 60. Among the 2,667 children, 465 (17.4%) are living with their parents, and this co-residence is highly related to many child characteristics. The average age of those who co-reside is 39.1, significantly less than the mean of 42.5 for those who are nonco-resident. Daughters are less likely to live with parents, and oldest sons and especially youngest sons are more likely to live with their parents. Furthermore, education is also associated with co-residence, but the pattern varies by different level: adult children with low education (those who are illiterate and those with primary school education) and high education (college and above) are not likely to live with parents, but those with intermediate levels (middle school) are significantly more likely to live with parents.

PATTERNS OF TRANSFERS

Transfers are also measured in the family module in the survey. Respondents are asked about the amount and frequency of non-time transfers, and these transfers include financial transfers and in-kind transfers (in the form of goods) received from and given to each child. Financial transfers involve giving money, helping pay bills such as medical care or insurance, schooling, and down payment for a home or rent. These transfers are further divided into regular and irregular financial transfers. Regular transfers were paid on a regular basis, such as monthly payments. Irregular transfers occurred irregularly, such as around a festival, marriage, large medical expenses, and the like. In-kind transfers are nonmonetary gifts provided or given in the past year.

We first separately analyze prevalence of transfers from a child to parents and then examine the amount of net transfers to parents, defined by subtracting the amount given to a particular child from the amount received from the same child.

Table 9-3 summarizes the patterns of transfers. Overall, familial intergenerational transfers are pervasive, with about 60% of the children having provided transfers to their parents. The prevalence of transfers from parents to their adult children is smaller, only 3.3%. The net amounts in terms of financial and in-kind transfers are all positive, toward parents.

---

[14]A son is classified as both the youngest son and the oldest son if he is an only child.

[15]Children's education is classified into five categories: illiterate, primary education, middle school, high school, college and above.

TABLE 9-2 Summary Statistics of Child Characteristics

	All	Co-resident	Nonco-resident	P-values
Child Characteristics				
Age	41.95	39.12	42.54	< 0.001
Oldest son (%)	15.90	22.37	14.53	< 0.001
Youngest son (%)	27.30	61.29	20.12	< 0.001
Daughter (%)	46.04	12.04	53.22	< 0.001
Married (%)	91.38	78.49	94.10	< 0.001
# of children (age < 16)	0.34	0.47	0.31	0.001
Education (%)				
Illiterate	16.91	12.26	17.89	0.001
Primary	34.91	33.12	35.29	0.369
Middle school	28.65	38.06	26.66	< 0.001
High school	13.65	13.55	13.67	0.945
College and above	5.89	3.01	6.49	< 0.001
Co-resident	17.44	100.00	0.00	
Observations	2,667	465	2,202	

NOTES: (1) The sample includes adult children no younger than age 25 with at least one parent who is older than age 60. (2) P-values are from t-test of the co-resident and nonco-resident groups.
SOURCE: Data from CHARLS 2008 pilot.

About 38% of children give financial transfers to their parents, roughly commensurate with in-kind transfers, which have a 42% prevalence rate. Irregular transfers account for the largest part of financial transfers, with prevalence rates roughly three times that of regular financial transfers.

The average net amount of total transfers is about 741 RMB per child, in which financial transfers take up 548 RMB and in-kind transfers take up 192 RMB. The net amount of regular transfers is much smaller than irregular financial transfers (190 RMB compared with 358 RMB).

There exist large disparities between regions: Zhejiang/urban children are more likely to provide transfers to their parents: about 64/68% in general, compared with 55/53% in Gansu/rural. Zhejiang/urban children give 1,140/1,192 RMB per year, while those in Gansu/rural only give 325/421 RMB.

CORRELATES OF TRANSFERS

A series of descriptive results from multivariate analyses of the incidence and magnitude of transfers are discussed in this section, first using ordinary least squares (OLS) models, and then family fixed-effect (FE)

TABLE 9-3 Transfer Patterns

	All	Zhejiang	Gansu	Urban	Rural
Incidence (%)	Children to Parents				
Financial transfer	38.07	47.56	28.19	47.18	31.61
Regular	8.47	13.70	3.01	11.66	6.21
Irregular	30.09	34.74	25.25	36.34	25.66
In-kind transfer	42.23	40.52	44.02	46.27	39.37
Total	59.51	64.15	54.67	68.03	53.46
Incidence (%)	Parents to Children				
Financial transfer	1.93	2.00	1.85	3.55	0.78
Regular	0.42	0.44	0.39	1.00	0.00
Irregular	1.55	1.63	1.47	2.64	0.78
In-kind transfer	1.70	1.11	2.32	1.82	1.62
Total	3.33	2.89	3.78	5.01	2.13
Amount (RMB/year)	Net Transfer				
Financial transfer	548.46	864.78	218.70	894.03	303.18
Regular	190.34	360.96	12.47	339.25	84.65
Irregular	358.12	503.81	206.23	554.78	218.53
In-kind transfer	192.32	275.09	106.04	297.92	117.37
Total	740.78	1139.87	324.75	1191.96	420.55

NOTE: The sample includes nonco-resident adult children aged 25 and older with at least one parent older than age 60.
SOURCE: Data from CHARLS 2008 pilot.

models. Transfers are investigated in two dimensions: the incidence of transfers provided by the child, and the net amount of transfers provided by the child.[16]

Associations with Parent Characteristics

Tables 9-4 and 9-5 report the results from the OLS estimations. Specifically, Table 9-4 reports incidence of gross transfers from children to parents and Table 9-5 examines the net amount of these transfers. We have two specifications, with and without the parental health measures, which can arguably be considered as endogenous.

As is shown in Table 9-4, pre-transfer parental income, number of parents' children, province, and living arrangements are all correlated with the incidence of children giving transfers, while the coefficients of age,

---

[16]An earlier version of this chapter included analyses of gross transfers from parents to children, which as noted is far less common than from children to parents. Results are available upon request.

age squared and gender are not significant.[17] We create a linear spline for pre-transfer income with three linearly connected segments based on two percentile points (1/3 and 2/3) of pre-transfer income. Coefficients for one segment show the slope over that segment. Higher pre-transfer income is correlated with a higher likelihood of a child giving, perhaps because of strategic motives having to do with potential bequests, but, too, perhaps because higher income parents invested more in the child earlier in life and this is an implicit exchange repayment. This relationship is very nonlinear, and at higher levels of income the association becomes flat.

Having more offspring is related to a higher probability of transfers given by children, which is surprising. However, if the parents live with another child, the likelihood of transfers from nonco-resident children declines. Children thus share the burden of support. Interestingly, parental health is not generally associated with transfer incidence, except for CES-D scores, for them having a higher score (so more likely to be depressed) is associated with a lower chance of receiving transfers.

Table 9-5 shows that for the net transfer amounts, pre-transfer parental income has a weakly positive relationship for the bottom one-third income group, but it becomes significantly negative for the top one-third group. We do not have a good explanation for this change in slope. Parental education and health status do not have significant relationships with transfer amount.

Associations with Child Characteristics

Correlates of transfers from the perspective of children are examined by both OLS and family FE models. The OLS models are able to estimate the coefficients of parent characteristics, while the family FE models correct for unobserved family heterogeneity and compare transfer behaviors among different children within the same family. FE results are displayed in Tables 9-6 and 9-7, where the sample is further restricted to those having at least one eligible (i.e., nonco-resident and adult) sibling. Net transfers are classified into three categories: financial transfers, in-kind transfers, and the total of both. In the following, we will discuss the estimation results of child characteristics from both models (Tables 9-4 through 9-7) but will focus mainly on the FE results (Tables 9-6 and 9-7).

Among children's demographic variables, age has a positive, concave relationship with transfer incidence in both the OLS and family FE models. Married children are more likely to transfer to parents, with the effect in the FE model being larger and more significant. The oldest son is less likely to provide transfers, if he lives apart, in the FE models, espe-

---

[17]We have tried interacting age with gender, but none of the coefficients are significant.

TABLE 9-4 OLS Analysis of Gross Transfer Incidence (from children to parents)

		(1)	(2)	(3)	(4)
Parent Characteristics					
Demographics	Age	0.006 (0.034)	0.006 (0.034)	0.009 (0.034)	(0.034)
	Age squared/100	-0.011 (0.024)	-0.011 (0.024)	-0.012 (0.024)	(0.024)
	Father	0.020 (0.035)	0.020 (0.035)	0.017 (0.035)	(0.035)
	Widowed	-0.036 (0.033)	-0.036 (0.033)	-0.029 (0.033)	(0.033)
	Number of children	0.030** (0.013)	0.030** (0.013)	0.029** (0.013)	(0.013)
	Zhejiang	-0.024 (0.106)	-0.024 (0.106)	-0.077 (0.111)	(0.111)
	Urban	0.059 (0.038)	0.059 (0.038)	0.051 (0.039)	(0.039)
	Living with other adult children	-0.180** (0.075)	-0.180** (0.075)	-0.177** (0.074)	(0.074)
SES	House owner	-0.060 (0.043)	-0.060 (0.043)	-0.061 (0.043)	(0.043)
	Education (illiterates omitted)				
	Less than primary education	0.009 (0.039)	0.009 (0.039)	-0.002 (0.041)	(0.041)
	Primary school	0.002 (0.049)	0.002 (0.049)	-0.006 (0.049)	(0.049)
	Middle school	0.068 (0.063)	0.068 (0.063)	0.043 (0.066)	(0.066)
	High school and above	0.050 (0.081)	0.050 (0.081)	0.020 (0.080)	(0.080)
	P-value for education	0.828	0.828	0.958	
	Pre-transfer income (000s)				
	For the lowest 1/3 income group	0.016*** (0.005)	0.016*** (0.005)	0.017*** (0.005)	(0.005)
	For the middle 1/3 income group	-0.010 (0.011)	-0.010 (0.011)	-0.008 (0.011)	(0.011)
	For the highest 1/3 income group	-0.002 (0.002)	-0.002 (0.002)	-0.002 (0.002)	(0.002)
	P-value for pre-transfer income	0.017	0.017	0.008	
Health	Health poor			0.054 (0.037)	(0.037)
	CES-D			-0.009*** (0.003)	(0.003)
	ADL or IADL disability			-0.045 (0.038)	(0.038)
	Cognition score in [8, 11]			-0.029 (0.045)	(0.045)
	Cognition score in [0, 8]			0.001 (0.056)	(0.056)
	Major illness			0.010 (0.033)	(0.033)
	P-value for health			0.089	

Children Characteristics

Demographics	Age	0.043***	(0.011)	0.045***	(0.011)
	Age squared/100	-0.037***	(0.011)	-0.039***	(0.011)
	Oldest son	0.008	(0.035)	0.009	(0.035)
	Youngest son	0.030	(0.032)	0.032	(0.032)
	Daughter	0.016	(0.030)	0.016	(0.030)
	Married	0.086*	(0.050)	0.077	(0.049)
	# of children (age < 16)	0.013	(0.011)	0.012	(0.011)
SES	Education (illiterates omitted)				
	Primary	0.118***	(0.035)	0.119***	(0.035)
	Middle school	0.108**	(0.043)	0.111***	(0.043)
	High school and above	0.229***	(0.045)	0.225***	(0.044)
	P-value for SES	<0.001		<0.001	
County Dummies		Yes		Yes	
Observations		2,202		2,202	
R-squared		0.133		0.142	

NOTES: (1) The sample includes those who are no younger than age 25 and with at least one parent no younger than age 60. (2) Parent characteristics are from main respondents. (3) Clustered standard errors at family level are in parentheses. (4) * denotes $p < 0.1$; ** $p < 0.05$; *** $p < 0.01$.
SOURCE: Data from CHARLS 2008 pilot.

TABLE 9-5 OLS Analysis of Net Transfer Amount

		(1)	(2)	(3)	(4)
Parent Characteristics					
Demographics	Age		-4.397 (103.567)		12.873 (107.494)
	Age squared/100		-14.772 (73.821)		-26.042 (76.321)
	Father		334.428 (206.879)		319.738 (199.056)
	Widowed		-197.960* (117.107)		-171.012 (115.615)
	Number of children		22.342 (45.193)		16.288 (43.332)
	Zhejiang		707.374** (336.641)		557.533* (323.821)
	Urban		248.471 (233.937)		245.186 (239.288)
	Living with other adult children		37.868 (185.181)		68.194 (176.818)
SES	House owner		-563.412 (486.384)		-625.092 (504.109)
	Education (illiterates omitted)				
	Less than primary education		54.473 (188.363)		0.550 (234.450)
	Primary school		82.972 (281.356)		46.336 (281.129)
	Middle school		-83.550 (242.299)		-174.869 (295.173)
	High school and above		-173.389 (427.434)		-312.513 (452.015)
	P-value for education		0.953		0.912
	Pre-transfer income (000s)				
	For the lowest 1/3 income group		24.746* (14.701)		22.020 (14.157)
	For the middle 1/3 income group		14.018 (53.407)		9.771 (53.486)
	For the highest 1/3 income group		-17.654** (8.209)		-17.544** (7.973)
	P-value for pre-transfer income		0.104		0.098
Health	Health poor				229.529 (159.597)
	CES-D				-3.524 (13.107)
	ADL or IADL disability				-232.873 (158.287)
	Cognition score in [8, 11]				-89.988 (420.400)
	Cognition score in [0, 8]				-235.406 (379.792)
	Major illness				49.144 (148.420)
	P-value for pre-transfer income				0.551

Children Characteristics

Demographics					
	Age	45.188	(33.500)	44.621	(33.803)
	Age squared/100	-48.652	(34.362)	-47.573	(34.734)
	Oldest son	269.309	(358.486)	260.596	(351.774)
	Youngest son	13.740	(211.908)	20.508	(224.390)
	Daughter	-207.249	(126.633)	-226.639*	(133.484)
	Married	-26.839	(339.553)	-32.229	(323.768)
	# of children (age < 16)	98.688	(78.154)	102.906	(78.549)
SES	Education (illiterates omitted)				
	Primary	-145.349	(170.049)	-154.430	(172.322)
	Middle school	-5.779	(187.153)	-5.304	(186.350)
	High school and above	859.219***	(264.286)	839.743***	(277.622)

NOTE: Robust standard errors in parentheses. * denotes $p < 0.1$; ** $p < 0.05$; *** $p < 0.01$.
SOURCE: Data from CHARLS 2008 pilot.

TABLE 9-6 Family Fixed Effect of Gross Transfer Probability (from children to parents)

Children's Characteristics	(1)	(2)	(3)	(4)	(5)	(6)
	Transfer		Financial Transfer		In-kind Transfer	
Age	0.060***	(0.011)	0.026***	(0.009)	0.055***	(0.011)
Age squared/100	-0.050***	(0.012)	-0.020**	(0.009)	-0.047***	(0.011)
Oldest son	-0.076**	(0.034)	-0.008	(0.031)	-0.074**	(0.032)
Youngest son	-0.002	(0.030)	0.008	(0.029)	-0.007	(0.028)
Daughter	-0.043	(0.029)	-0.035	(0.028)	0.031	(0.028)
Married	0.143***	(0.055)	0.127**	(0.054)	0.120**	(0.053)
# of children (age < 16)	0.002	(0.016)	0.010	(0.013)	-0.016	(0.010)
Education (illiterate omitted)						
Primary school	0.104***	(0.037)	0.082**	(0.032)	0.075**	(0.037)
Middle school	0.069	(0.047)	0.076*	(0.043)	0.068	(0.044)
High school and above	0.122**	(0.049)	0.140***	(0.047)	0.072	(0.048)
P-value for education	0.011		0.015		0.243	
Observations	2,068		2,068		2,068	
R-squared	0.067		0.033		0.058	

NOTES: (1) The sample includes those who are no younger than age 25, with at least one parent no younger than age 60, and at least one adult sibling who is not living with parents. (2) Clustered standard errors at family level are in parentheses. (3) * denotes $p < 0.1$; ** $p < 0.05$; *** $p < 0.01$. SOURCE: Data from CHARLS 2008 pilot.

TABLE 9-7 Family Fixed Effect of Net Transfer Amount

	(1)	(2)	(3)	(4)	(5)	(6)
	Transfer		Financial Transfer		In-kind Transfer	
Children's Characteristics						
Age	-31.192	(54.853)	-46.214	(53.380)	15.022*	(8.036)
Age squared/100	19.621	(55.265)	36.560	(53.616)	-16.938*	(8.961)
Oldest son	539.203	(453.147)	559.623	(444.135)	-20.421	(35.361)
Youngest son	-16.693	(237.860)	-30.752	(226.217)	14.059	(48.846)
Daughter	-231.014	(141.305)	-225.758*	(124.928)	-5.256	(49.848)
Married	140.903	(228.044)	46.342	(208.387)	94.562	(62.126)
# of children (age < 16)	82.852	(91.813)	81.733	(89.796)	1.119	(9.196)
Education (illiterate omitted)						
Primary school	-143.953	(167.942)	-175.741	(160.958)	31.787	(34.413)
Middle school	-336.365	(336.321)	-362.308	(322.653)	25.943	(55.805)
High school and above	735.808	(449.759)	675.833	(435.832)	59.975	(45.856)
P-value for education	0.251		0.202		0.557	
Observations	2,059		2,059		2,059	
R-squared	0.017		0.018		0.004	

NOTES: (1) The sample includes those who are no younger than age 25, with at least one parent no younger than age 60, and at least one adult sibling who is not living with parents. (2) Clustered standard errors at family level are in parentheses. (3) * denotes $p < 0.1$.

SOURCE: Data from CHARLS 2008 pilot.

cially for in-kind and total transfers. There is no relationship with being the youngest son or daughter.

Regarding the SES of the children, children's educational attainment is significantly associated with the incidence of transfers, even in the more demanding family FE specification, although the magnitude of the coefficients drops substantially in the FE specification.

On the amount of net transfers, oldest sons are more likely to give more financial and total transfers, though the coefficients, while large, are not significant. Daughters, on the other hand, provide less, weakly significant for financial transfers.

Child schooling at the high school or above level is strongly related to the amount of net transfers given in the OLS regressions, but the education dummies as a group become insignificant, and the coefficient magnitudes decline once we take into account fixed family effects.

CONCLUSIONS

The economic literature has studied intergenerational transfers extensively. Most of the research is conducted in developed countries where the direction of transfers mainly goes from parents to children. In China, intergenerational transfers have long been an important source of elderly support. With rapid population aging, shrinking family size, and greater mobility of children, it is possible that the family may be losing its importance in the role of elderly support. In recent years the Chinese government has taken various efforts to develop its old-age support system, which may have further crowded out family support. As yet, we cannot say this with any degree of scientific validity. It is thus necessary to evaluate the current situation of intergenerational transfers first.

With detailed and high-quality data on intergenerational transfers, as well as rich information on both parents and their children, the CHARLS 2008 pilot provides a fine opportunity to achieve this goal. This chapter develops empirical models to explore the patterns and correlates of intergenerational transfers between the elderly parents and adult children in Zhejiang and Gansu provinces.

Contrary to the situations in most developed countries, we find that transfers are predominantly from children to elderly parents and still play important roles in the elderly support of current China. Our results reveal that older people with a larger number of offspring are more likely to receive transfers, a result indicating the potential challenge faced with dwindling number of children. Parental income has a mixed predication depending on how large is the pre-transfer income of the parent. For those among the bottom income group, the relationship is positive but becomes negative for the top income group. Within family, there is responsibility-sharing among children, possibly based on children's capabilities. For example, highly educated children transfer more frequently, as do married children. Although there is no significant difference in amount of transfers, oldest sons appear less likely to provide any transfer, which seems to contradict the conventional impression. Daughters are just as likely to give as other children but are likely to give less on net.

The one caveat about these results is that the older cohorts we studied still had an average of 3.4 children each, so the bite of the more stringent family planning programs that began in the 1970s has not been reached as yet. How transfers will evolve in later cohorts, who have fewer children but with more human capital and higher lifecycle incomes due to China's rapid development, will need to be studied.

REFERENCES

Altonji, J.G., F. Hayashi, and L.J. Kotlikoff. (1997). Parental altruism and inter vivos transfers: Theory and evidence. *Journal of Political Economy* 105(6):1,121-1,166.

Becker, G.S. (1974). A theory of social interactions. *Journal of Political Economy* 82(6):1,063-1,093.

Cai, F., J. Giles, and X. Meng. (2006). How well do children insure parents against low retirement income? An analysis using survey data from urban China. *Journal of Public Economics* 90(12):2,229-2,255.

China Health and Retirement Longitudinal Survey. (2008). China Center for Economic Research, Peking University. Available: http://charls.ccer.edu.cn/charls/data.asp.

Chou, R.J. (2010). Filial piety by contract? The emergence, implementation, and implications of the "family support agreement" in China. *The Gerontologist* 51(1):3-16.

Cox, D. (1987). Motives for private income transfers. *Journal of Political Economy* 95(3):508-546.

Cox, D., and M. Fafchamps. (2008). Extended family, and kinship networks: Economic insights and evolutionary directions. In *Handbook of Development Economics, Volume 4*, T.P. Schultz and J. Strauss (Eds.). Amsterdam: North Holland Press.

Cox, D., and B.J. Soldo. (2004). *Motivation for Money and Care That Adult Children Provide for Parents: Evidence from "Point-Blank" Survey Questions*. CRR Working Paper No. 2004-17. Boston: Center for Retirement Research at Boston College.

Cox, D., E. Jimenez, and W. Okrasa. (1997). Family safety nets and economic transition: A study of worker households in Poland. *Review of Income and Wealth* 43(2):191-209.

Cox, D., Z. Eser, and E. Jimenez. (1998). Motives for private transfers over the life cycle: An analytical framework and evidence for Peru. *Journal of Development Economics* 55(1):57-80.

Frankenberg, E., L. Lillard, and R.J. Willis. (2002). Patterns of intergenerational transfers in Southeast Asia. *Journal of Marriage and Family* 64:627-641.

Goh, E.C.L. (2009). Grandparents as childcare providers: An in-depth analysis of the case of Xiamen, China. *Journal of Aging Studies* 23(1):60-68.

Hurd, M.D., J.P. Smith, and J.M. Zissimopoulos. (2007). *Inter-Vivos Giving Over the Life Cycle*. RAND Working Paper No. WR-524. Santa Monica, CA: RAND Corporation.

Kim, H. (2010). Intergenerational transfers and old-age security in Korea. Pp. 227-278 in *The Economic Consequences of Demographic Change in East Asia*, T. Ito and A. Rose (Eds.). NBER-EASE Volume 19 Book Series East Asia Seminar on Economics. Cambridge, MA: National Bureau of Economic Research.

Kotlikoff, L.J. (1988). Intergenerational transfers and savings. *The Journal of Economic Perspectives 2(2)*:41-58.

Lee, Y., and Z. Xiao. (1998). Children's support for elderly parents in urban and rural China: Results from a national survey. *Journal of Cross-Cultural Gerontology 13(1998)*:39-62.

Lee, Y., W.L. Parish, and R.J. Willis. (1994). Sons, daughters, and intergenerational support in Taiwan. *American Journal of Sociology 99(4)*:1,010-1,041.

Lei, X., C. Zhang, and Y. Zhao. (2011a). Old-Age Support and Protection in China. Unpublished manuscript, China Center for Economic Research, Peking University.

Lei, X., J. Strauss, M. Tian, and Y. Zhao. (2011b). *Living Arrangements of the Elderly in China: Evidence from CHARLS.* RAND Labor and Population Working Paper WR-866. Santa Monica, CA: RAND.

Lillard, L.A., and R.J. Willis. (1997). Motives for intergenerational transfers: Evidence from Malaysia. *Demography 34(1)*:115-134.

McGarry, K., and R.F. Schoeni. (1995). Transfer behavior in the Health and Retirement Study: Measurement and the redistribution of resources within the family. *The Journal of Human Resources, Special Issue on the Health and Retirement Study: Data Quality and Early Results 30(30)*:S184-S226.

National Bureau of Statistics of China (2009). *China's Population and Employment Statistical Yearbook.* Beijing: China Statistics Press.

Nugent, J. (1985). The old-age security motive for fertility. *Population and Development Review 11(1)*:75-97.

Rosenzweig, M.R., and K.I. Wolpin. (1993). Intergenerational support and the life-cycle incomes of young men and their parents: Human capital investments, co-residence, and intergenerational financial transfers. *Journal of Labor Economics 11(1)*:84-112.

Secondi, G. (1997). Private monetary transfers in rural China: Are families altruistic? *Journal of Development Studies 33(4)*:487-509.

Smith, J., J.J. McArdle, and R. Willis. (2010). Financial decision making and cognition in a family context. *The Economic Journal 120 (November)*:F363-F380.

Zhao, Y., J. Strauss, A. Park, Y. Shen, and Y. Sun. (2009). *China Health and Retirement Longitudinal Study, Pilot, User's Guide.* National School of Development, Peking University.

10

Household Dynamics and Living Arrangements of the Elderly in Indonesia: Evidence from a Longitudinal Survey[1]

Firman Witoelar

Like many other developing countries in Asia, Indonesia is experiencing rapid population aging (Kinsella and He, 2009). The average number of children born per women has declined from around 4 in the early 1980s to around 2.5 in 2000, while life expectancy has increased from around 56 to 68 during the same period. In 2005, the percentage of those aged 60 and older was around 7.5% of the total population. While this is a lower percentage than, for instance, Singapore or even Thailand, it still amounts to 16 million people, given Indonesia's population size (Ananta and Arifin, 2009). One of the consequences of these demographic changes over the past few decades is that families are smaller and the number of children from whom parents can draw support at a later age also becomes smaller. This is particularly important in Indonesia and in other developing countries in the region, where social programs and pension schemes to support the elderly are lacking.[2] In Indonesia, as

[1]I gratefully acknowledge the financial support of the World Bank's Research Support Budget (RF-P121879-RESE-BBRSB). Earlier results of the paper were presented at the Conference on Policy Research and Data Needs to Meet the Challenges and Opportunities of Population Aging in Asia, New Delhi, March 14-15, 2011. All errors are mine. These are the views of the author and should not be attributed to the World Bank and its member countries.

[2]See Abikusno (2009) for a discussion on past and recent laws and government policies related to older persons in Indonesia. Although 1966–1998 saw few policies that addressed aging issues, the recognition of the issues and waves of reforms in 1998 brought about laws and policies that are seen to be more favorable to older persons (including one on pension). In 2004, a law on the comprehensive national security system was passed that contains articles written to protect the pension sector.

in other developing countries in the region, support for the elderly has primarily come from networks of families or relatives, with remittances from children living elsewhere and shared residence being the two most important mechanisms.

In addition to demographic pressure, there have also been concerns that pressure from "modernization" would weaken traditional family structures. Moreover, as the population ages, Indonesia is experiencing nutrition and health transitions with the population moving out of undernutrition and communicable diseases and the elderly population increasingly exposed to higher risk factors correlated with chronic health problems (Witoelar, Strauss, and Sikoki, 2009). In Indonesia, early concerns about the implications of population aging, rapid economic changes, and changing health challenges on traditional familial support systems and family structures have been brought up by Hugo (1992) and by Wirakartakusumah et al. (1997). Despite these concerns, a number of empirical studies on aging and living arrangements in Southeast Asia done in the late 1990s suggest that shared living remains common and the decline in co-residency was modest, as was reviewed by Frankenberg, Chan, and Ofstedal (2002) and by Beard and Kunharibowo (2001). One of the aims of this chapter is to revisit the question and see how much the pattern of living arrangements among the elderly has changed.

Data from the National Socioeconomic Survey (the Susenas), the nationally representative survey of households conducted annually in Indonesia, indeed show that the living arrangements among the elderly had not changed considerably between 1993 and 2007. Figures 10-1 and 10-2 show living arrangements by age in 1993 and 2007 for men and women aged 55 and older, respectively. The figures show that, like in many countries in Asia, most older adults in Indonesia co-reside with at least one of their children. There are differences in the living arrangement patterns between males and females, as will be discussed later in this chapter. Overall, the patterns do not seem to have changed over the years. (Similar patterns emerge when we use data from other years of the Susenas between 1993 and 2007.) These figures seem to still be consistent with what some previous studies have found on the patterns of living arrangements of the elderly in Southeast Asia. Frankenberg, Chan, and Ofstedal (2002) found that in Indonesia, Singapore, and Taiwan, the pattern of living arrangements is relatively stable, at least throughout the 1990s.

It is important to note, however, that the Susenas is not particularly well suited for analysis of this kind. First, one could only identify relationships in the household relative to the household head. Second, only limited socioeconomic characteristics were collected. Third and perhaps most importantly, the survey does not collect any information on nonco-resident family members. In addition, cross-sectional analysis may

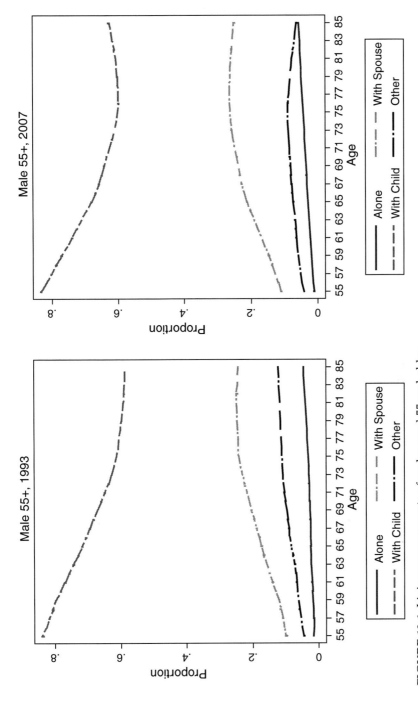

FIGURE 10-1 Living arrangements of males aged 55 and older.
SOURCE: Data from National Socioeconomic Survey (Susenas), 1993 and 2007.

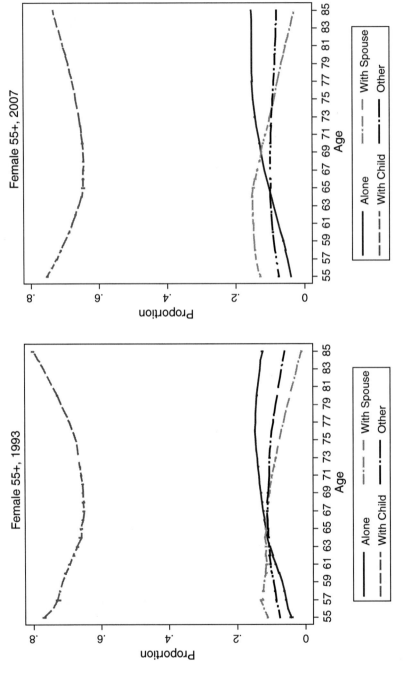

FIGURE 10-2 Living arrangements of females aged 55 and older.
SOURCE: Data from National Socioeconomic Survey (Susenas), 1993 and 2007.

mask what has really been happening to elderly living arrangements over the 14-year period. For example, studies have shown that in the wake of the Asian financial crisis in 1997–1999, one of the mechanisms used to cope with the crisis was to combine households (Frankenberg, Smith, and Thomas, 2003). Such episodes highlight the reality that co-residency and parental home-leaving are not merely lifecycle events.

The Indonesia Family Life Survey (IFLS), a longitudinal household survey that spans 1993 to 2007, does not have these limitations. The four rounds of the survey follow individuals over 14 years. Since the first round of the survey, household rosters listing all household members were completed. In addition to documenting the relationship of household members to the head, the roster also contains information that enables the researcher to link children to their biological parents. Rich information about households and individuals were collected, including socioeconomic variables, such as education, consumption, income, and labor market outcomes, as well as health. In addition, the survey also collects information of nonco-resident family members.[3]

This chapter is descriptive in nature, and its main objectives are straightforward. First, I want to document the pattern of living arrangements of the population aged 55 and older, by gender, over the survey years and see whether there have been significant changes over the 14 years. Second, I want to look at key socioeconomic characteristics that we hypothesize to be correlated with living arrangements. I first look at cross-section correlations between the covariates and living arrangements in the base year 1993 for those aged 55 and older. I also want to know whether relationships that existed in cross-sectional analysis hold in the longitudinal analysis. I use these baseline characteristics and study their correlations with living arrangements 14 years later.

The chapter is organized as follows. The next section will discuss the data and the key socioeconomic variables that we use in the analysis. I then document the living arrangements of individuals aged 55 and older in each of the survey years—1993, 1997, 2000, and 2007—as if they were independent cross-sections. Next, I employ a multivariate framework to look at cross-sectional correlations in the base year of 1993. Finally, I use the longitudinal sample of individuals to look at correlations between those key variables at the baseline year (1993) and living arrangements 14 years later under both the linear probability models (LPM) and multi-nomial logit (MNL) models.

---

[3]See Strauss et al. (2009a) for the overview of the IFLS Wave 4.

DATA AND METHODOLOGY

Data

The Indonesia Family Life Survey is a large-scale, broad-based longitudinal survey of households, individuals, and communities with detailed questions on a vast number of socioeconomic characteristics of the respondents. As noted above, the survey has been fielded four times (1993, 1997, 2000, 2007), covering a span of 14 years. The survey collects detailed questions about household membership, including questions about non-coresident family members, which is crucial for studies that aim to look at issues related to changing household structure and living arrangements. While the IFLS was not originally designed to specifically study aging and its consequences, it was expanded in the last round (IFLS4 2007) to include questions related to aging. The questions added were specifically chosen to be comparable to questions being asked in surveys on aging around the world, such as the Health and Retirement Study (HRS) in the United States; Survey of Health, Ageing and Retirement in Europe (SHARE), Korean Longitudinal Study of Ageing in South Korea (KLoSA), China Health and Retirement Longitudinal Study (CHARLS) in China, and the new Longitudinal Aging Study in India (LASI). IFLS4 has the advantage of having detailed information of the now "elderly" respondents when they were younger.

In this chapter, when the focus is on cross-sectional relationships between living arrangements of the elderly and household as well as individual covariates, I will restrict the sample on those aged 55 and older during the time of the survey (1993, 1997, 2000, and 2007), and the attention will be restricted to those who have at least one living child. In the longitudinal part of the analysis, where the focus is on the relationships between living arrangements in 2007 with covariates in the baseline year, 1993, we will restrict the sample to those who were 55 and older in 2007. The covariates come from 1993, when the individuals were 41 and older. One reason to look at the sample of those who were 55 and older in 2007, rather than focusing on those who were 55 and older in 1993 and see what happened 14 years later, is that I will not have to worry as much about mortality selection. Also, defining the sample in this way allows us to work with a significantly larger sample (around 3,800 individuals) as opposed to using the sample consisting of individuals 55 years and older who were also interviewed in 1993.

As in any longitudinal household survey, attrition becomes a concern, especially for a survey that spans over long period of time. IFLS has maintained a relatively low attrition rate, with around 90% of IFLS1 households and around 80% of IFLS1 household members re-contacted in

IFLS4. The low attrition rate was not due to low mobility; in fact, almost one-third of those interviewed in 1993 had moved by 2007. However, the survey managed to lower the attrition rate by tracking down some of the movers (see Thomas et al., forthcoming). For the older age group, the main cause of attrition is death. Of the household members aged 40 to 80 in 1993 (the main sample in this paper), the re-contact rate in 2007 was 95% with the following breakdown: around 70% were found, 25% had died, and 5% were not found (see Table 2.5 in Strauss et al., 2009b). To address this concern, I employ attrition-corrected person-weights when I look at living arrangement patterns in Tables 10-1 and 10-2.

Methodology

As the framework for this analysis, I considered four types of mutually exclusive and exhaustive living arrangements: (1) elderly living alone, where the household does not contain anyone but elderly; (2) elderly living with a spouse, where the household consists of only the elderly person and the spouse (who may or may not be elderly); (3) elderly living with at least one adult child, when the household contains at least one adult child of the elderly;[4] and (4) other form of living arrangement, a residual category that includes households where the elderly live with siblings' family, with immediate family of his/her children but not with any of one his/her children, and so forth.

The analysis focuses on adult children since one of main reasons one cares about co-residence is to look at elderly support. Only biological children are considered as children in the analysis. Therefore, an older adult who lives only with his/her daughter-in-law will not be categorized as living with a child, but will be indicated as living in the "other" category. An older adult who lives with a servant will be counted as living in the "other" category rather than "living alone."

Multivariate Analysis

Using the sample of those aged 55 and older in 1993, I first look at cross-sectional correlations between individual characteristics and living arrangement using a simple linear probability model (LPM) with the dependent variable equal to 1 if the individual co-resided with at least one biological child in 1993. Still using the LPM and the 1993 covariates,

---

[4]Adult child here is defined as aged 15 and older. Note that as long as an adult child lives in the household, the elderly will be included in this category, including those who live with or without a spouse or with other people.

we then look at the probability of co-residence in 2007 for individuals who were aged 55 and older in 2007.

I follow the literature in this area by adopting a multinomial logit model of living arrangements. While there exist a large number of studies in the literature using this approach with cross-sectional data, the use of detailed panel data in this kind of analysis has so far been limited, especially for developing countries, due to the availability of the data. I set those living alone as the base group and then examine the relative risks of living only with a spouse, co-residing with a child, or living in another arrangement, as well as the marginal effects of changing one of the covariates. The usual assumption of the multinomial logit, the independence from irrelevant alternatives (IIA), applies. It implies that the relative probabilities for any of two available alternatives depend only on the attributes of those alternatives. In particular, it assumes that the unobservables in each alternative are not correlated with each other.

Covariates

In the multivariate analyses, I first put a focus on a limited number of variables at the baseline that are likely to have already been determined during the time of the survey. I use the individual's own age, education, and the total number of surviving sons and daughters in the basic specification. For age, we use dummy variables indicating whether the individuals are aged 60–64, or 65 and older, with the group aged 55–59 being the omitted category. The non-linearity of the relationship between own age and living arrangements is apparent from the figures, which we want to capture in the multivariate context.

I created dummy variables indicating whether individuals have some primary education, completed primary education, or completed junior high school, using the group of those without schooling as the base category. The total number of living children at the time of the survey provides us with the potential number of sources of support for the elderly. I expect this variable to be positively correlated with co-residency. Here, it is crucial that I include not only children who are listed in the household rosters, but also other children living elsewhere.[5]

I use separate variables to indicate sons and daughters since anthropological literature on Indonesia suggests that gender is an important factor determining who will take care of the parents in old age, and it varies between ethnicities in Indonesia. I include a variable indicating

---

[5]Because of this requirement, I only include individuals aged 55 or older who were individually interviewed in 1993 since we only have information for these individuals regarding nonco-resident family members.

the age of the oldest child. In results not shown, I also include per capita expenditure—a proxy of income—as one of the covariates.[6] Well-known studies from developed countries, such as the study by Costa (1997), have shown that income plays an important role enabling elderly to live alone. Privacy of both parents and children as a normal good has been modeled in studies of living arrangements in developed countries (see, for example, Ermisch, 1999). In the current study, the results show that per capita expenditure (*pce*) did not have statistically significant relationships with living arrangements of the elderly.

I then add information about the marital status of the elderly, and for those who are married, age of the spouse and the spouse's education. In some specifications, I also consider several variables that we usually do not want to include as explanatory variables in cross-sectional analysis of living arrangements, such as information about labor participation of the individuals, their spouses, and their co-resident children. Employment decisions may very well be determined jointly with living arrangement decisions, although in Indonesia, Cameron and Cobb-Clark (2002) find little evidence that old-age support from children through financial transfer and co-residence affects the labor supply decisions of the elderly.

Finally, I use two variables measuring (subjectively) the health conditions of the individuals at the baseline year. First, I use self-assessment of basic physical functioning and Activities of Daily Living (ADLs). ADLs provide useful information about a person's functional status and have been shown to be correlated with socioeconomic status (SES) measures (see, for instance, National Socioeconomic Survey, 1993, 2007). The second measure I use is General Health Status (GHS). In all four waves of IFLS, respondents were asked the question, "In general, how is your health?" with the following options: very healthy, somewhat healthy, somewhat unhealthy, and unhealthy. Those who answered somewhat unhealthy and unhealthy were coded to have poor health.

LIVING ARRANGEMENT PATTERNS

This section begins by going back to Figures 10-1 and 10-2 that show the patterns of living arrangement of adults aged 55 and older using the Susenas data from 1993 and 2007.[7] The pattern that emerges from the fig-

---

[6]Per capita consumption is constructed from the household consumption expenditure module of IFLS, which reports the market expenditures as well as own production of households on food and nonfood items including on durable and nondurable goods.

[7]Note that the Susenas does not separate biological and nonbiological children in categorizing relationship to the head of the households. The Susenas also does not separate parent and parent-in-law of the head of the households. Numbers used to create Figures 10-1 and 10-2 thus combine biological with non-biological children, parent with parent-in-law.

ures also shows, in contrast to women, as men age, they seem to rely less on their children but more on their spouses. For women, the likelihood of sharing residence with a child decreases with age before it increases again. At all ages, the percentage of men co-residing with a spouse is always higher than the percentage of those living alone or in other living arrangements. Figures created using other years of the Susenas between 1993 and 2007 (not shown) have a similar pattern. As mentioned, other than being available for every year, the Susenas is not well suited for this analysis.

Figures 10-3 and 10-4 use data from the IFLS1 and IFLS4 to look at living arrangements of IFLS respondents who are aged 55 and older.[8] The majority of elderly men live with their adult child, and the age patterns do not seem to change between 1993 and 2007. The figures show, as in the Susenas data, a declining line describing the proportion of men aged 55 and older who live with at least a child by age, respectively. As they age, men are less likely to live with their adult children and more likely to live only with their spouses. From the figures alone, there does not seem to be a movement into co-residence as men age. The proportion living alone increases as men age, but it is well below 2% even for the oldest of the elderly.

The patterns for women show that in 1993, as in the Susenas, the proportion of elderly women living with a child decreases with age before increasing sharply at older age. For 2007, however, the U-shaped line is much less apparent. At the same time, the proportion of elderly women living alone increases with age. The U-shaped pattern is particularly interesting since the upturn suggests that as elderly women age they tend to move into shared living arrangements with their adult children, either by moving into the children's households or by taking in the children who have left their households earlier. This pattern is consistent with the pattern of old-age support of elderly women by the children. Both for men and women, "other" living arrangements do not change with age.

Table 10-1 presents the distributions of living arrangements in each of the four waves of IFLS of individuals aged 55 and older. The table treats each wave of IFLS as if it were an independent, cross-sectional sample. The sample is weighted using cross-section person-weight that accounts for attrition.[9] The table shows that living arrangement patterns seem to

---

[8]For the figures from IFLS to be comparable to the Susenas figures, biological and non-biological children are both included in the calculation. Parent and parent-in-law are also combined. In the analysis, however, only biological child and parent are used when we define parent-child shared living arrangement.

[9]The estimates using the cross-sectional person-weights will be representative of the Indonesian population living in the IFLS provinces in 1993 (for IFLS1), 1997 (IFLS2), 2000 (IFLS3), and 2007 (IFLS4). See Strauss et al. (2009b) for a discussion of how the person-weights are constructed.

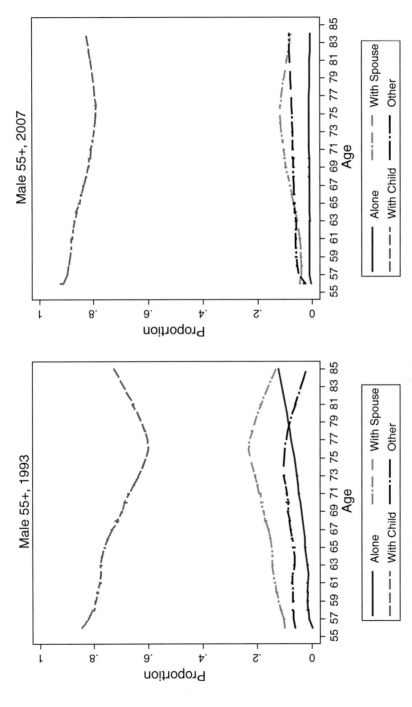

FIGURE 10-3 Living arrangements of males aged 55 and older.
SOURCE: Data from Indonesia Family Life Survey, IFLS 1 and IFLS4.

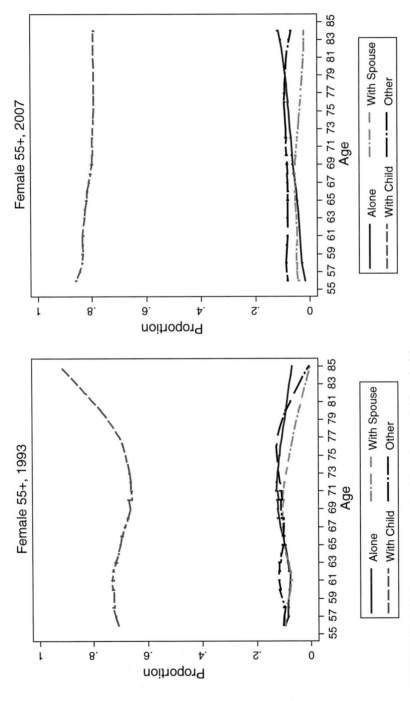

FIGURE 10-4 Living arrangements of females aged 55 and older.
SOURCE: Data from Indonesia Family Life Survey, IFLS 1 and IFLS4.

TABLE 10-1 Cross-Sectional Living Arrangement Patterns: 1993, 1997, 2000, and 2007 (IFLS)

55 + Older at Time of Survey		1993	1997	2000	2007
Male	# of observations	1,743	2,004	2,479	2,879
	% alone	2.3	1.7	2.1	3.0
	% with spouse	16.0	17.1	14.1	19.5
	% with ≥ 1 child	70.3	68.9	72.4	66.2
	% other	11.4	12.3	11.9	12.4
Female	# of observations	2,015	2,392	3,039	3,430
	% alone	9.8	9.1	7.5	11.1
	% with spouse	9.7	10.6	8.8	12.5
	% with ≥ 1 child	60.8	63.2	66.6	61.4
	% other	19.6	16.9	17.5	15.9

NOTE: The numbers were estimated using cross-sectional attrition-corrected person-weights for the corresponding year.
SOURCE: Author's calculation based on data from Indonesia Family Life Survey—IFLS1, IFLS2, IFLS3, and IFLS4.

be relatively stable over the 14 years, with lower percentage of men living alone (around 3%) than women (7–10%), and the majority of the elderly living with at least one of their children. This seems to confirm the findings of previous studies that find modest if any decrease in co-residency. The table shows decreasing percentages of elderly living alone between 1993 and 2000, which then increased again in 2007. During the same period, co-residency with adult children increased and then decreased by 2007. Further study needs to be done to support this claim, but the pattern is consistent with the fact that during the period of economic crisis in 1997–1999 after the Asian financial crisis (which came right after a drought brought about by El Niño), one coping mechanism was to combine households (Frankenberg, Smith, and Thomas, 2003).

Table 10-2 shows the marital status of the elderly and their living arrangements in 1993, 1997, 2000, and 2007, again weighted using the cross-sectional person-weights. It is clear that in each of the survey years, among those aged 55 and older, most of the men (close to 90%) are married while only around 40% women are. The table also shows that almost 90% of men who co-reside with an adult child are married; only a small fraction of men live with their adult children without their wives being present.

MULTIVARIATE ANALYSES

Tables 10-3a and 10-3b present the descriptive statistics of the analytical samples for the multivariate analyses: individuals aged 55 and older in

TABLE 10-2 Marital Status and Living Arrangements: 1993, 1997, 2000, and 2007

	Living Arrangements				
	Living Alone	With Spouse Only	With an Adult Child	Other Living Arr.	All Living Arr.
Male Aged 55+					
1993					
Married	11.8	99.9	93.4	93.0	92.5
Divorced/separated	72.5	0.1	6.1	4.1	6.3
Never married	15.7	0.0	13.7	23.1	52.6
1997					
Married	2.7	100.0	90.7	89.9	90.7
Divorced/separated	68.6	0.0	8.8	6.7	8.0
Never married	28.7	0.0	0.4	3.3	1.4
2000					
Married	10.1	100.0	88.8	88.4	88.8
Divorced/separated	60.6	0.0	10.3	6.0	9.1
Never married	29.2	0.0	0.9	5.7	2.1
2007					
Married	16.3	100.0	86.9	83.8	87.0
Divorced/separated	65.1	0.0	11.9	11.6	11.0
Never married	18.6	0.0	1.2	4.6	2.0
Female Aged 55+					
1993					
Married	3.8	100.0	45.9	35.3	44.9
Divorced/separated	82.8	0.0	48.4	53.5	48.1
Never married	13.4	0.0	5.7	11.2	7.0
1997					
Married	1.7	100.0	43.7	39.6	45.1
Divorced/separated	85.4	0.0	52.0	51.3	49.4
Never married	12.9	0.0	4.3	9.1	5.5
2000					
Married	3.5	100.0	45.9	35.8	45.6
Divorced/separated	83.8	0.0	49.3	51.7	48.0
Never married	12.7	0.0	4.7	12.5	6.3
2007					
Married	3.0	100.0	43.8	35.2	44.7
Divorced/separated	87.4	0.0	52.6	52.7	50.1
Never married	9.6	0.0	3.6	12.1	5.2

NOTE: The numbers were estimated using cross-sectional attrition-corrected person-weights for the corresponding year.
SOURCE: Author's calculation based on data from Indonesia Family Life Survey—IFLS1, IFLS2, IFLS3, and IFLS4.

TABLE 10-3a Analytical Sample: Living Arrangements in 1993 and 2007

	Male (N = 1,782)		Female (N = 2,016)	
	1993	2007	1993	2007
Living Alone	0.4	2.5	3.0	11.1
Living with Spouse Only	5.5	20.5	6.5	14.4
Co-reside with an Adult Child	68.7	65.1	75.2	63.8
Other Living Arrangements	25.4	11.9	15.4	10.7

SOURCE: Data from Indonesia Family Life Survey—IFLS1, IFLS2, IFLS3, and IFLS4.

2007 for whom we have data in 1993 and who have at least one surviving adult child. These restrictions bring down the number of eligible samples to around 3,800 observations. Table 10-3a shows the living arrangements in 1993 and 2000 of these individuals, and the Table 10-3b shows the 1993 covariates.

On average, the sample individuals were around 51 years old in 1993. Almost all of the men and most of the women were married in 1993, and on average they have around four surviving children. Most marriages in Indonesia are between older men and younger women, which are shown by the means of spouse's age and also by the fact that the children of elderly women in the sample are older than that of men (14–31 years for women, 12–27 years for men). Higher incidence of poor GHS and ADL problems among women are consistent with recent findings on health of the elderly in Indonesia (Witoelar et al., 2009).

Cross-Sectional Relationships

Tables 10-4 and 10-5 show the cross-sectional relationships between the 1993 covariates and the probability of co-residing with an adult child in 1993 for elderly men and women, separately. The first columns of these tables include only variables that are more or less predetermined and exogenous to living arrangement. The next specifications then add some variables that are less exogenous, including those that are very likely to be determined jointly with living arrangements.

In Table 10-4, the negative coefficient on males aged 70 and older suggests that the decline in the proportion of elderly men who co-reside occurs at an older age when the men are likely to be more vulnerable. Own education seems to predict higher likelihood of co-residency and so does age of the oldest child. The number of living sons and daughters are positively correlated with higher probability of co-residency, unsurprisingly. However, as we add the variables that are related to having a

TABLE 10-3b Analytical Sample: Baseline Characteristics, 1993

Covariates (1993 variables)	Male (N = 1,782)					Female (N = 2,016)				
	Living Alone	With Spouse	With Adult Child	Other Living Arr.	All Males	Living Alone	With Spouse	With an Adult Child	Other Living Arr.	All Female
Own age (years)	54.00	57.50	51.50	48.20	51.00	58.70	55.10	51.00	49.70	51.30
Education (years)	4.90	2.80	5.50	5.80	5.38	1.60	1.80	3.30	2.90	3.10
# surviving children	4.00	3.00	4.70	3.50	4.30	3.10	3.50	4.80	3.50	4.40
# of sons	2.40	1.40	2.40	1.70	2.15	1.50	1.90	2.40	1.70	2.30
# of daughters	1.60	1.50	2.30	1.80	2.15	1.60	1.70	2.30	1.80	2.20
Age of oldest child (years)	21.60	29.00	27.40	23.10	26.50	34.30	32.50	31.00	28.60	30.90
Married = 1	0.71	1.00	0.98	0.99	0.98	0.07	1.00	0.78	0.70	0.78
Spouse's age (years)	0.00	51.30	43.90	38.60	42.80	0.00	61.80	42.10	41.40	42.00
Spouse's education (years)	0.00	1.96	3.74	4.22	3.75	0.00	2.67	3.90	3.40	3.63
Max. yrs education of children (years)	0.00	0.00	8.84	0.00	6.07	0.00	0.00	8.69	0.00	6.53
Working = 1	1.00	0.92	0.90	0.94	0.91	0.65	0.59	0.49	0.58	0.52
Spouse working = 1	0.00	0.59	0.45	0.50	0.47	0.00	0.82	0.64	0.68	0.64
Co-resident child working = 1	0.00	0.00	0.47	0.00	0.33	0.00	0.00	0.57	0.00	0.43
Any ADL problem = 1	0.00	0.16	0.11	0.08	0.11	0.50	0.31	0.27	0.22	0.27
GHS poor = 1	0.00	0.12	0.11	0.09	0.11	0.22	0.14	0.14	0.11	0.14
Rural = 1	0.14	0.74	0.55	0.63	0.58	0.62	0.74	0.53	0.72	0.57

SOURCE: Data from Indonesia Family Life Survey—IFLS1, IFLS2, IFLS3, and IFLS4.

TABLE 10-4 Cross-Sectional Analysis: LPM of Living with a Child, Male, Aged 55+, in 1993

Variables in 1993	(1)	(2)	(3)	(4)
Aged 60–69	−0.026	−0.015	−0.018	−0.019
	(0.98)	(0.86)	(1.05)	(1.09)
Aged 70+	−0.132	−0.037	−0.045	−0.046
	(3.59)***	(1.34)	(1.80)*	(1.81)*
Completed primary	0.037	−0.042	−0.027	−0.028
	(1.14)	(1.86)*	(1.36)	(1.41)
Completed junior high	0.107	−0.081	−0.051	−0.050
	(3.10)***	(3.36)***	(2.31)**	(2.27)**
Completed senior high	0.117	−0.153	−0.118	−0.116
	(2.87)***	(5.16)***	(4.00)***	(3.94)***
# of living sons	0.034	0.003	−0.007	−0.006
	(4.66)***	(0.59)	(1.47)	(1.41)
# of living daughters	0.040	0.015	0.014	0.014
	(5.13)***	(2.88)***	(2.83)***	(2.90)***
Age of oldest child	0.439	0.162	0.105	0.105
	(4.45)***	(2.40)**	(1.47)	(1.48)
Rural	−0.118	0.054	0.046	0.045
	(4.40)***	(3.04)***	(2.68)***	(2.64)***
Spouse aged 60–69		−0.020	−0.025	−0.026
		(0.87)	(1.22)	(1.26)
Spouse aged 70+		0.009	−0.002	−0.005
		(0.15)	(0.04)	(0.10)
Spouse, some primary sch.		0.001	0.010	0.010
		(0.04)	(0.47)	(0.47)
Spouse, compl. junior high		−0.113	−0.090	−0.089
		(4.71)***	(3.88)***	(3.82)***
Spouse, compl. senior high		−0.140	−0.099	−0.097
		(4.54)***	(2.92)***	(2.86)***
Divorced/widowed/never married		0.018	−0.005	−0.006
		(0.46)	(0.15)	(0.18)
Max. education of children		0.073	0.061	0.061
		(42.09)***	(34.43)***	(34.40)***
Working			−0.017	−0.012
			(0.92)	(0.63)
Spouse working			−0.010	−0.010
			(0.62)	(0.64)
Child working			0.268	0.267
			(16.78)***	(16.79)***
Poor GHS				0.031
				(1.46)
Any problem with ADLs				−0.003
				(0.16)
Constant	0.173	0.054	0.096	0.088
	(1.66)*	(0.79)	(1.30)	(1.20)
Observations	1,343	1,343	1,343	1,343
R-squared	0.11	0.62	0.68	0.68

NOTES: The sample consists of males aged 55–84 in 1993 with at least one living child. Dependent variable = 1 if the elderly was living with an adult child in 1993, 0 otherwise. Dummy variables for province of residence in 1993 are included in the regressions. Robust t statistics are in parentheses with significance at 10% (*), 5% (**), and 1% (***) indicated. Standard errors are corrected for clustering at the household level.
SOURCE: Author's calculation based on data from Indonesia Family Life Survey—IFLS1.

spouse, the number of sons becomes not statistically significant, while the number of daughters is still statistically significant. Coefficients on own and spouse's education are negative, but the coefficient on education of the child is positive. If own and spouse's education is associated with income, the negative coefficients are consistent with the notion that privacy is a normal good: Elderly with higher household incomes tend to be less likely to co-reside with their children. Education of the children is positively associated with co-residency, perhaps suggesting that educated children are more equipped to support their elderly parents. This point is somewhat reinforced with the inclusion of the dummy variable indicating whether any of the co-resident children are working. The coefficient on this is positive. In the last specification, we include the measures for ADL and GHS, both of which are not statistically significant for men.

Turning to the results for women presented in Table 10-5, many of the correlations for men also exist women. One notable difference is that the number of sons is associated *negatively* with the probability of co-residence. Also, women having "poor health" is positively associated with co-residence, although having any problem with ADL has the opposite sign.

The results discussed thus far are based on cross-sectional relationships. For variables indicating labor participation, health status, and even marital status, making inference based on these cross-sectional correlations is problematic, given that labor market participation decisions and living arrangement decisions could are taken jointly.

Longitudinal Evidence

I next look at the longitudinal evidence, where the focus is on how the same covariates correlate with living arrangements 14 years later. The results of linear probability estimation of co-residency with a child in 2007 for men and women aged 55 and older are presented in Tables 10-6 and 10-7, respectively. The explanatory variables and the specifications are exactly the same as the cross-sectional analysis. Overall, the relationships are qualitatively similar to those we saw in the cross-sectional analysis.

For both men and women, own age correlates negatively with the probability of co-residing with a child. Note that these relationships differ from the one we have seen in the figures, in which for women, the probability of living with a child seems to be increasing with age. Controlling for other factors, the U-shape relationship between age and probability of co-residency for women is not evident. As in the cross-sectional results, for men, both the number of sons and daughters seem to correlate positively with future co-residency. However, for women, beyond the basic specification, the number of sons does not have statistically significant correlations with the probability of co-residency. The number of

TABLE 10-5 Cross-Sectional Analysis: LPM of Living with a Child, Female, Aged 55+, in 1993

Variables in 1993	(1)	(2)	(3)	(4)
Aged 60–69	–0.057	–0.012	–0.017	–0.013
	(2.02)**	(0.58)	(0.93)	(0.74)
Aged 70+	–0.210	–0.037	–0.035	–0.022
	(5.17)***	(1.24)	(1.31)	(0.80)
Completed primary	0.084	–0.022	–0.021	–0.020
	(2.56)**	(0.91)	(1.00)	(0.96)
Completed junior high	–0.044	–0.170	–0.143	–0.138
	(0.97)	(6.93)***	(6.53)***	(6.30)***
Completed senior high	0.020	–0.202	–0.175	–0.174
	(0.33)	(6.21)***	(5.09)***	(5.07)***
# of living sons	0.018	–0.012	–0.013	–0.013
	(2.28)**	(2.21)**	(2.73)***	(2.71)***
# of living daughters	0.040	0.006	0.012	0.013
	(4.90)***	(1.12)	(2.33)**	(2.52)**
Age of oldest child	0.625	0.334	0.267	0.273
	(9.64)***	(9.14)***	(9.14)***	(9.14)***
Rural	–0.120	0.028	0.014	0.009
	(4.28)***	(1.39)	(0.77)	(0.50)
Spouse aged 60–69		–0.021	–0.026	–0.027
		(0.69)	(0.93)	(0.96)
Spouse aged 70+		–0.036	–0.038	–0.038
		(0.94)	(1.10)	(1.12)
Spouse, some primary sch.		–0.045	–0.042	–0.038
		(1.43)	(1.52)	(1.37)
Spouse, compl. junior high		–0.069	–0.043	–0.042
		(2.13)**	(1.47)	(1.44)
Spouse, compl. senior high		–0.179	–0.106	–0.105
		(4.67)***	(2.79)***	(2.85)***
Divorced/widowed/never married		–0.030	–0.031	–0.028
		(0.86)	(0.96)	(0.86)
Max. education of children		0.073	0.054	0.054
		(40.20)***	(28.00)***	(28.10)***
Working			–0.020	–0.022
			(1.13)	(1.29)
Spouse working			0.020	0.018
			(0.87)	(0.80)
Child working			0.352	0.352
			(19.48)***	(19.58)***
Poor GHS				0.040
				(1.97)**
Any problem with ADLs				–0.051
				(2.87)***
Constant	0.032	–0.014	–0.016	–0.015
	(0.55)	(0.35)	(0.43)	(0.42)
Observations	1,277	1,277	1,277	1,277
R–squared	0.09	0.57	0.67	0.67

NOTES: The sample consists of females aged 55–84 in 1993 with at least one living child. Dependent variable = 1 if the elderly was living with an adult child in 1993, 0 otherwise. Dummy variables for province of residence in 1993 are included in the regressions. Robust t statistics are in parentheses with significance at 10% (*), 5% (**), and 1% (***) indicated. Standard errors are corrected for clustering at the household level.
SOURCE: Author's calculation based on data from Indonesia Family Life Survey—IFLS1.

TABLE 10-6 LPM of Living with an Adult Child 14 Years Later, Male, Aged 55+, in 2007

Variables in 1993	(1)	(2)	(3)	(4)
Aged 60–69	0.011	−0.005	−0.009	−0.009
	(0.41)	(0.23)	(0.48)	(0.50)
Aged 70+	−0.163	−0.041	−0.014	−0.018
	(1.30)	(0.40)	(0.15)	(0.19)
Completed primary	0.024	−0.030	−0.025	−0.025
	(0.77)	(1.39)	(1.29)	(1.27)
Completed junior high	0.067	−0.070	−0.048	−0.047
	(2.11)**	(3.14)***	(2.26)**	(2.25)**
Completed senior high	0.004	−0.131	−0.094	−0.093
	(0.12)	(5.45)***	(3.99)***	(3.95)***
# of living sons	0.065	0.015	0.006	0.006
	(9.79)***	(3.52)***	(1.53)	(1.52)
# of living daughters	0.057	0.011	0.009	0.009
	(7.82)***	(2.49)**	(2.17)**	(2.16)**
Age of oldest child	0.465	0.123	0.104	0.104
	(11.35)***	(5.07)***	(4.42)***	(4.42)***
Rural	−0.090	0.046	0.047	0.047
	(3.88)***	(3.45)***	(3.67)***	(3.65)***
Spouse aged 60–69		−0.064	−0.075	−0.076
		(1.63)	(2.12)**	(2.12)**
Spouse aged 70+		−0.103	−0.093	−0.090
		(0.97)	(1.00)	(0.98)
Spouse, some primary sch.		−0.057	−0.049	−0.049
		(3.27)***	(3.06)***	(3.03)***
Spouse, compl. junior high		−0.113	−0.099	−0.098
		(5.83)***	(5.26)***	(5.22)***
Spouse, compl. senior high		−0.128	−0.104	−0.104
		(5.75)***	(4.60)***	(4.56)***
Divorced/widowed/never married		0.087	0.047	0.044
		(1.46)	(0.85)	(0.80)
Max. education of children		0.077	0.072	0.072
		(54.49)***	(51.24)***	(51.27)***
Working			0.021	0.023
			(0.97)	(1.05)
Spouse working			−0.024	−0.025
			(1.99)**	(2.03)**
Child working			0.171	0.171
			(12.55)***	(12.57)***
Poor GHS				0.021
				(0.97)
Any problem with ADLs				−0.004
				(0.17)
Constant	0.033	0.105	0.087	0.082
	(0.60)	(3.17)***	(2.24)**	(2.09)**
Observations	1,782	1,782	1,782	1,782
R-squared	0.16	0.71	0.74	0.74

NOTES: The sample consists of males aged 55–84 in 2007 of whom 1993 data are available and who had at least one living child in 1993. Dependent variable = 1 if the elderly was living with an adult child in 2007, 0 otherwise. Dummy variables for province of residence in 1993 are included in the regressions. Robust t statistics are in parentheses with significance at 10% (*), 5% (**), and 1% (***) indicated. Standard errors are corrected for clustering at the household level.
SOURCE: Author's calculation based on data from Indonesia Family Life Survey—IFLS1 and IFLS4.

TABLE 10-7 LPM of Living with an Adult Child 14 Years Later, Female, Aged 55+, in 2007

Variables in 1993	(1)	(2)	(3)	(4)
Aged 60–69	–0.074	–0.012	–0.024	–0.023
	(2.64)***	(0.57)	(1.27)	(1.24)
Aged 70+	–0.154	0.045	0.047	0.049
	(1.37)	(0.51)	(0.56)	(0.59)
Completed primary	0.017	–0.050	–0.044	–0.042
	(0.72)	(2.97)***	(2.79)***	(2.72)***
Completed junior high	0.021	–0.145	–0.129	–0.127
	(0.77)	(8.03)***	(7.41)***	(7.30)***
Completed senior high	0.050	–0.174	–0.132	–0.130
	(1.63)	(8.42)***	(6.21)***	(6.11)***
# of living sons	0.048	0.005	–0.003	–0.003
	(8.58)***	(1.24)	(0.86)	(0.83)
# of living daughters	0.044	0.015	0.014	0.014
	(7.24)***	(3.64)***	(3.65)***	(3.76)***
Age of oldest child	0.481	0.163	0.124	0.127
	(5.59)***	(3.31)***	(2.37)**	(2.35)**
Rural	–0.113	0.035	0.037	0.036
	(5.56)***	(2.55)**	(2.84)***	(2.75)***
Spouse aged 60–69		–0.020	–0.024	–0.026
		(1.17)	(1.55)	(1.65)*
Spouse aged 70+		–0.055	–0.053	–0.056
		(1.60)	(1.74)*	(1.84)*
Spouse, some primary sch.		–0.013	–0.012	–0.013
		(0.62)	(0.63)	(0.67)
Spouse, compl. junior high		–0.032	–0.008	–0.009
		(1.48)	(0.40)	(0.46)
Spouse, compl. senior high		–0.091	–0.061	–0.062
		(4.01)***	(2.73)***	(2.80)***
Divorced/widowed/never married		–0.007	0.010	0.008
		(0.29)	(0.38)	(0.31)
Max. education of children		0.070	0.061	0.061
		(44.91)***	(41.68)***	(41.64)***
Working			–0.030	–0.029
			(2.39)**	(2.30)**
Spouse working			0.024	0.024
			(1.40)	(1.39)
Child working			0.216	0.215
			(18.61)***	(18.55)***
Poor GHS				0.048
				(2.52)**
Any problem with ADLs				–0.020
				(1.38)
Constant	0.197	0.155	0.152	0.148
	(2.16)**	(2.89)***	(2.59)***	(2.46)**
Observations	2,016	2,016	2,016	2,016
R-squared	0.12	0.60	0.65	0.65

NOTES: The sample consists of females aged 55–84 in 2007 of whom 1993 data are available and who had at least one living child in 1993. Dependent variable = 1 if the elderly was living with an adult child in 2007, 0 otherwise. Dummy variables for province of residence in 1993 are included in the regressions. Robust t statistics are in parentheses with significance at 10% (*), 5% (**), and 1% (***) indicated. Standard errors are corrected for clustering at the household level. SOURCE: Author's calculation based on data from Indonesia Family Life Survey—IFLS1 and IFLS4.

daughters, on the other hand, is positively correlated with co-residency in all specifications. Elderly women who co-reside with their children are significantly more likely to co-reside with a daughter than with a son.

Finally, neither the ADL nor the GHS in 1993 seems to be correlated with the probability of elderly men co-residing 14 years later. For women, however, poor GHS in 1993 has a positive correlation with the probability to co-reside with their children in 2007.

The multinomial logit results add some insights. For each male and female, results from two specifications were presented. The first specification includes only the basic specification without the characteristics of the spouse. The second specification includes spouse's characteristics and variables indicating work status of the respondent, the spouse, and the child, as well as health status of the elderly. Tables 10-8 and 10-9 show how predicted probabilities change with a change in a covariate, holding other variables at their means. These tables are based on regression results presented in Appendix Tables 10-A1 and 10-A2.[10] Table 10-8 shows, for example, that an additional son would increase the probability of co-residence by 0.061, while an additional daughter would increase it by 0.042. Note, however, that from Appendix Table 10-A1, most of the coefficients for males are not statistically significant. For women, similar to the LPM results, the likelihood of co-residency with a child is higher, the more educated the children are. Table 10-8 shows that an increase of 1 year of maximum education of the children at the baseline year increases the probability of living with a child 14 years later by 0.010. For men, the coefficient is not significant and the marginal effect is negative. For women, having a spouse who works in the baseline year increases the likelihood of living with the spouse and decreases the likelihood of living with an adult child (see Appendix Table 10-A2). Again, this is consistent with the possibility that an elderly couple may value privacy and will tend to choose not to co-reside with a child if they have adequate resources. The results on age are consistent with what we have seen from the LPM results, and the U-shaped relationship between age and the likelihood of co-residency of elderly women is not evident. In fact, both older age groups show lower odds for co-residency compared to the age group 55–59 for both men and women.

---

[10]The marginal effects is defined as $\dfrac{\partial \Pr(y=j|\mathbf{x})}{\partial x_k} = \Pr(y=j|\mathbf{x})\left\{\beta_{jk} - \sum_{h=1}^{j} \Pr(y=j|\mathbf{x})\right\}$ where j represents the possible outcomes ($j = 0,1,2,3$) and $\mathbf{x}$ is the vector of covariates. The discrete change (for example from $x_k = 0$ to $x_k = 1$) is defined as $\dfrac{\Delta \Pr(y=j|\mathbf{x})}{\Delta x_k} = \Pr(y=j|\mathbf{x}, x_k = 1) - \Pr(y=j|\mathbf{x}, x_k = 0)$.

CONCLUSIONS

In the 14 years between 1993 and 2007, there does not seem to be much change in living arrangements. The first thing to note from the descriptive results is that by focusing on age 55 and above for both men and women, we may be focusing on different lifecycle stages of the individuals. Because men tend to marry later and marry younger women, the sample of men consists of a much larger fraction of married men compared to women in the same age group. Mortality selection may play a role in the differences across groups, too, where relatively healthier men are observed in the sample. Own education and whether or not the elderly or his/her spouse is working in the base year are negatively correlated with the probability of living with an adult child, suggesting that elderly with more human capital (and household resources) may prefer living by themselves to living in a shared residence with their children.

There are gender differences in how own, spouse, or child's characteristics at the baseline correlate with living arrangements. In particular, children's potential earning (as measured by years of education) and work status seem to increase likelihood of co-residency for women, but not as much for men.

Further examination may tell us how much lifecycle variables such as age play a role in influencing a transition between living arrangements. More work should be done in looking at the transition, in particular since the four waves of IFLS would permit looking at transition between four different points in time (for respondents who were interviewed in all waves). More insights could be gained by such an exercise.

While the pattern of living arrangements seems to stay constant for now, demographic pressure will likely affect living arrangements as the population ages further. One important caveat of this paper is that the analysis excludes elderly who have no surviving children at the time of the survey—around 6 to 8%. This selected sample could include those who would be most vulnerable in old age.

TABLE 10-8 Changes in Predicted Probabilities from MNL:
Living Arrangements of Males, Aged 55+, in 2007

		Pr (y | x)
	x	sd(x)
Marginal Effect		
Number of sons	2.151	1.499
± 1 standard deviation		
Marginal effect		
Number of daughters	2.149	1.434
± 1 standard deviation		
Marginal effect		
Max. years of children's educ.	6.060	5.073
± 1 standard deviation		
Marginal effect		
Discrete Change from 0 to 1		
Own age		
Aged 60–69	0.418	0.493
Age 70	0.275	0.447
Own education		
Completed primary	0.313	0.464
Completed junior high	0.267	0.442
Completed senior high	0.238	0.426
Maximum age of child > 15	0.945	0.228
Divorced/widowed/never married	0.017	0.131
Spouse's age		
Aged 60–69	0.043	0.202
Age 70	0.003	0.058
Spouse's education		
Completed primary	0.334	0.472
Completed junior high	0.206	0.405
Completed senior high	0.136	0.343
	0.576	0.494
Rural labor participation		
Working	0.912	0.283
Spouse working	0.467	0.499
Any child working	0.325	0.469
Health status		
Any problem with ADLs	0.106	0.308
"Poor" GHS	0.107	0.309

NOTE: This table is based on regressions in Appendix Table 10-A1, Specification 2.
SOURCE: Author's calculation based on data from Indonesia Family Life Survey, IFLS1
and IFLS4.

Living Alone	With Spouse	With Adult Child	Other Living Arr.	
0.209	0.659	0.124	0.008	
Ave. |Change|	With Spouse	With Adult Child	Other Living Arr.	Living Alone (base)
0.023	−0.018	0.043	−0.027	0.002
0.031	−0.034	0.061	−0.026	−0.001
0.023	−0.015	0.046	−0.005	−0.026
0.021	−0.034	0.042	−0.009	0.000
0.011	0.022	−0.006	−0.014	−0.014
0.002	0.004	−0.001	−0.003	0.000
0.039	0.057	−0.078	0.012	0.010
0.087	0.131	−0.174	0.029	0.014
0.032	−0.060	0.050	0.015	−0.005
0.044	−0.076	0.088	−0.008	−0.003
0.090	−0.135	0.179	−0.038	−0.007
0.042	0.085	−0.037	−0.045	−0.003
0.088	−0.176	0.125	0.011	0.039
0.017	0.010	−0.032	0.023	−0.002
0.346	0.059	−0.692	0.569	0.064
0.016	0.000	−0.033	0.030	0.002
0.005	−0.003	0.009	−0.006	−0.001
0.025	0.018	−0.046	0.031	−0.003
0.030	0.048	−0.053	0.011	−0.006
0.018	−0.018	−0.018	0.035	0.001
0.034	0.067	−0.067	0.000	0.001
0.032	−0.051	0.065	−0.013	−0.001
0.005	0.010	−0.005	−0.003	−0.002
0.015	−0.030	0.020	0.008	0.002

TABLE 10-9 Changes in Predicted Probabilities from MNL:
Living Arrangements of Females, Aged 55+, in 2007

	Pr (y|x)	
	x	sd(x)
Marginal Effect		
Number of sons	2.262	1.565
± 1 standard deviation		
Marginal effect		
Number of daughters	2.189	1.544
±1 standard deviation		
Marginal effect		
Max. years of children's educ.	6.513	5.085
± 1 standard deviation		
Marginal effect		
Discrete Change from 0 to 1		
Own age		
Aged 60–69	0.448	0.497
Age 70	0.269	0.444
Own education		
Completed primary	0.266	0.442
Completed junior high	0.170	0.375
Completed senior high	0.117	0.321
Maximum age of child > 15	0.988	0.111
Divorced/widowed/never married	0.221	0.415
Spouse's age		
Aged 60–69	0.197	0.398
Age 70	0.057	0.231
Spouse's education		
Completed primary	0.231	0.421
Completed junior high	0.191	0.393
Completed senior high	0.154	0.361
	0.577	0.494
Rural labor participation		
Working	0.516	0.500
Spouse working	0.641	0.480
Any child working	0.426	0.495
Health status		
Any problem with ADLs	0.275	0.447
"Poor" GHS	0.140	0.347

NOTE: This table is based on regressions in Appendix Table 10-A2, Specification 2.
SOURCE: Author's calculation based on data from Indonesia Family Life Survey, IFLS1
and IFLS4.

Living Alone	With Spouse	With Adult Child	Other Living Arr.	
0.209	0.659	0.124	0.008	
Ave. |Change|	With Spouse	With Adult Child	Other Living Arr.	Living Alone (base)
0.014	−0.011	0.028	−0.017	0.001
0.023	−0.018	0.043	−0.027	0.002
0.023	−0.015	0.046	−0.005	−0.026
0.015	−0.010	0.030	−0.004	−0.017
0.026	−0.006	0.052	−0.021	−0.025
0.005	−0.001	0.010	−0.004	−0.005
0.046	0.028	−0.092	0.035	0.029
0.080	0.039	−0.160	0.091	0.030
0.011	0.001	−0.011	0.022	−0.012
0.011	0.007	−0.021	0.000	0.015
0.016	0.016	0.017	−0.022	−0.011
0.059	0.006	−0.117	0.051	0.061
0.091	−0.167	0.149	−0.015	0.032
0.038	−0.014	−0.039	−0.023	0.075
0.066	−0.045	−0.050	−0.036	0.131
0.010	−0.004	0.020	−0.002	−0.014
0.027	0.003	0.050	−0.009	−0.044
0.021	−0.024	0.041	−0.005	−0.013
0.013	0.015	−0.015	0.010	−0.010
0.025	0.023	−0.017	−0.034	0.028
0.031	0.039	0.010	0.013	−0.062
0.053	−0.030	0.107	−0.036	−0.041
0.008	0.005	−0.016	0.011	0.000
0.028	−0.013	−0.042	0.014	0.041

APPENDIX TABLE 10-A1 MNL of Living Arrangements, 1993–2007, Males, Aged 55+, in 2007 (living alone is the base outcome)

	Specification 1					
	with spouse		with an adult child		other	
	RRR	Z	RRR	Z	RRR	Z
Aged 60–69	0.467	−1.52	0.323*	−2.33	0.384	−1.88
Age 70+	0.540	−1.16	0.236**	−2.79	0.381	−1.78
Some primary school	1.584	1.04	2.220	1.84	2.311	1.81
Completed primary	1.519	0.90	2.310	1.85	1.781	1.18
Completed junior high	2.330	1.44	5.384**	2.96	3.081	1.84
# of living sons	1.022	0.19	1.341	2.58	0.955	−0.37
# of living daughters	0.861	−1.30	1.085	0.74	0.918	−0.71
Age of oldest child	2.497	1.30	1.451	0.57	1.019	0.03
Spouse aged 60–69						
Spouse aged 70+						
Spouse, some primary sch.						
Spouse, compl. primary						
Spouse, compl. junior high						
Divorced/widowed/never married						
Max. education of children						
Working						
Spouse working						
Child working						
Any ADL problem						
Poor GHS						
Rural	2.349	2.27	1.693	1.45	2.120	1.92
Number of observations	1,783					
Likelihood ratio (Chi-squared)	245.4					
p-value	0.000					
Pseudo R-squared	0.073					

NOTES: The sample consists of males aged 55–84 in 2007 of whom 1993 data are available and who had at least one living child in 1993. Relative risk ratios are reported. Province dummy variables are included in the regressions but not reported. * denotes $p < 0.05$; ** $p < 0.01$.

SOURCE: Author's calculation based on data from Indonesia Family Life Survey, IFLS1 and IFLS4.

| Specification 2 | | | | | |
| with spouse | | with an adult child | | other | |
RRR	Z	RRR	Z	RRR	Z
0.460	−1.53	0.155*	−2.35	0.389	−1.83
0.500	−1.26	0.116**	−2.85	0.358	−1.81
1.459	0.80	0.976	1.65	2.224	1.64
1.046	0.09	0.901	1.14	1.458	0.69
1.333	0.40	2.593	1.95	2.101	1.01
0.963	−0.31	0.148	1.84	0.919	−0.65
0.831	−1.53	0.121	0.36	0.913	−0.73
2.231	1.11	0.865	0.36	0.982	−0.03
1.324	0.35	0.954	0.23	1.500	0.48
0.135	−1.48	0.000	−0.00	0.627	−0.36
0.773	−0.60	0.309	−0.73	0.976	−0.05
1.137	0.23	0.645	0.28	1.102	0.16
1.608	0.56	1.121	0.39	1.857	0.71
0.030**	−2.81	0.154*	−2.09	0.184	−1.87
1.056	1.31	0.042	0.79	1.012	0.26
0.814	−0.35	0.493	−0.26	1.213	0.30
1.226	0.56	0.285	−0.61	0.891	−0.31
0.933	−0.17	0.523	0.72	1.086	0.19
1.342	0.48	0.760	0.40	1.246	0.34
0.711	−0.63	0.443	−0.30	0.885	−0.22
2.601	2.41	0.726	1.67	2.238	1.96
1,783					
299.08					
0.000					
0.089					

APPENDIX TABLE 10-A2 MNL of Living Arrangements, 1993–2007, Females, 55+, in 2007 (living alone is the base outcome)

	Specification 1					
	with spouse		with an adult child		other	
	RRR	Z	RRR	Z	RRR	Z
Aged 60-69	0.588*	−2.10	0.465***	−3.43	0.654	−1.52
Aged 70+	0.237***	−5.04	0.294***	−5.22	0.632	−1.56
Some primary school	1.699	2.19	1.474	1.91	1.696*	2.09
Completed primary	1.402	1.18	1.237	0.90	1.110	0.34
Completed junior high	2.148*	2.05	1.902*	2.01	1.299	0.61
# of living sons	0.908	−1.54	1.123*	2.35	0.875*	−2.01
# of living daughters	1.098	1.39	1.327***	5.09	1.202**	2.68
Age of oldest child	0.386	−0.85	0.448	−0.76	0.695	−0.29
Spouse aged 60–69						
Spouse aged 70+						
Spouse, some primary sch.						
Spouse, compl. primary						
Spouse, compl. junior high						
Divorced/widowed/never married						
Max. education of children						
Working						
Spouse working						
Child working						
Any ADL problem						
Poor GHS						
Rural	1.536	2.03	0.908	−0.57	1.128	0.54
Number of observations	2,018					
Likelihood ratio (Chi-squared)	585.1					
p-value	0.000					
Pseudo R-squared	0.138					

NOTES: The sample consists of females aged 55–85 in 2007 of whom 1993 data are available and who had at least one living child in 1993. Relative risk ratios are reported. Province dummy variables are included in the regressions but not reported. * denotes $p < 0.05$; ** $p < 0.01$; *** $p < 0.001$.

SOURCE: Author's calculation based on data from Indonesia Family Life Survey, IFLS1 and IFLS4.

| Specification 2 | | | | | |
| with spouse | | with an adult child | | other | |
RRR	Z	RRR	Z	RRR	Z
1.081	0.28	0.156	−1.82	0.998	−0.01
1.183	0.49	0.157	−2.05	1.462	1.10
1.160	0.56	0.245	0.57	1.394	1.24
0.897	−0.33	0.208	−0.85	0.825	−0.56
1.382	0.70	0.441	0.38	0.918	−0.17
0.836**	−2.65	0.054	0.37	0.835**	−2.60
1.058	0.80	0.073***	4.13	1.179*	2.34
0.313	−1.01	0.268	−1.29	0.557	−0.46
0.404***	−3.34	0.112**	−3.16	0.394**	−3.14
0.155***	−4.34	0.117**	−3.14	0.256**	−3.20
1.152	0.50	0.307	0.85	1.179	0.54
2.002	1.94	0.646*	2.26	1.733	1.42
0.813	−0.48	0.451	0.61	1.124	0.25
0.010	−4.39	0.252	−0.50	0.597	−1.36
1.042	1.73	0.021***	3.66	1.019	0.74
0.982	−0.09	0.116*	−2.16	0.524**	−3.07
3.544***	4.42	0.440**	2.97	2.176**	2.63
1.075	0.31	0.354	3.58	1.180	0.71
1.069	0.27	0.191	−0.12	1.104	0.40
0.540	−2.01	0.145	−2.04	0.748	−0.99
1.437	1.56	0.207	0.64	1.254	0.96

2,016

590.2

0.000

0.139

REFERENCES

Abikusno, N. (2009). Evaluation and implementation of ageing-related policies in Indonesia. In *Older Persons in Southeast Asia: An Emerging Asset,* E.N. Arifin and A. Ananta (Eds.). Singapore: ISEAS.

Ananta, A., and E.N. Arifin. (2009). Older persons in Southeast Asia: From liability to asset. In *Older Persons in Southeast Asia: An Emerging Asset,* E.N. Arifin and A. Ananta (Eds.). Singapore: ISEAS.

Beard, V.A., and Y. Kunharibowo. (2001). Living arrangements and support relationships among elderly Indonesians: Case studies from Java and Sumatra. *International Journal of Population Geography* 7:17-33.

Cameron, L., and D. Cobb-Clark. (2002). Old age labour supply in the developing world. *Applied Economic Letters* 9(10):649-652.

Costa, D.L. (1997). Displacing the family: Union army pensions and elderly living arrangements. *Journal of Political Economy* 105:6.

Ermisch, J. (1999). Prices, parents, and young people's household formation. *Journal of Urban Economics* 45(1):47-71.

Frankenberg, E., A. Chan, and M.B. Ofstedal. (2002.) Stability and change in living arrangements in Indonesia, Singapore, and Taiwan, 1993-99. *Population Studies* 56(2):201-213.

Frankenberg, E., J.P. Smith, and D. Thomas. (2003). Economic shocks, wealth and welfare. *Journal of Human Resources* 38(2):280-321.

Hugo, G. (1992). Aging in Indonesia: A neglected area of policy concern. Pp. 207-229 (Chapter 12) in *Aging in East and Southeast Asia,* D.R. Phillips (Ed). London: Edward Albert.

Indonesia Family Life Survey, Wave 1. (1994). Available: http://www.rand.org/labor/FLS/IFLS.html.

Indonesia Family Life Survey, Wave 2. (1997). Available: http://www.rand.org/labor/FLS/IFLS.html.

Indonesia Family Life Survey, Wave 3. (2000). Available: http://www.rand.org/labor/FLS/IFLS/ifls3.html.

Indonesia Family Life Survey, Wave 4. (2008). Available: http://www.rand.org/labor/FLS/IFLS/ifls4.html.

Kinsella, K., and W. He. (2009). *An Aging World: 2008.* U.S. Census Bureau, International Population Reports #PS95/09-1. Washington, DC: U.S. Government Printing Office.

National Socioeconomic Survey. (1993). Available: http://www.rand.org/labor/bps/susenas/1993.html.

National Socioeconomic Survey. (2007). Available: http://www.rand.org/labor/bps/susenas/2007.html.

Strauss, J., F. Witoelar, B. Sikoki, and A.M. Wattie. (2009a). *The Fourth Wave of the Indonesia Family Life Survey: Overview and Field Report, Volume 1.* Working Paper #WR-675/1-NIA/NICHD, Labor and Population Program. Santa Monica, CA: RAND Corporation.

Strauss, J., F. Witoelar, B. Sikoki, and A.M. Wattie. (2009b). *User's Guide for the Indonesia Family Life Survey: Wave 4, Volume 2.* Working Paper #WR-675/1-NIA/NICHD, Labor and Population Program. Santa Monica, CA: RAND Corporation.

Thomas, D., F. Witoelar, E. Frankenberg, B. Sikoki, J. Strauss, C. Sumantri, and W. Suriastini. (Forthcoming). Cutting the costs of attrition: Results from the Indonesia Family Life Survey. *Journal of Development Economics.*

Wirakartakusumah, A., M. Djuhari, H. Sirait, and Z. Hidayat. (1997). Some problems and issues of older persons in Asia and the Pacific. *Asian Population Studies* 144:21-43.

Witoelar, F., J. Strauss, and B. Sikoki. (2009). *Socioeconomic Success and Health in Later Life: Evidence from the Indonesia Family Life Survey.* RAND Labor and Population Working Paper #WR-704. Santa Monica, CA: RAND Corporation.

11

Social Networks, Family, and Care Giving Among Older Adults in India

Lisa F. Berkman, T.V. Sekher,
Benjamin Capistrant, and Yuhui Zheng

Social networks and family ties are among the core institutions providing support and opportunities for engagement to older adults around the world (Berkman, 2000; Bloom et al., 2010; Bongaarts and Zimmer, 2002; Wachter, 1997). Social networks are defined by the web of associations and the structure of ties that surround a person (Berkman and Glass, 2000; McPherson, Smith-Lovin, and Cook, 2001; Wellman and Berkowitz, 1988). The network has several functions including the provision of emotional, instrumental, appraisal, and financial support. At the same time, it is important to acknowledge that social networks may involve both negative and positive interactions, with resulting health impacts (Berkman, 2009; Berkman and Glass, 2000; Seeman et al., 2001). Furthermore, the contribution of support provided by older adults to their families and communities is important and often not well recognized. As societies undergo demographic transitions with rising life expectancy and decreases in fertility, societies as a whole "age" (Kirk, 1996). India, while early in this transition, has started to experience the growing pains associated not only with population growth but also an aging society. Over the next decades, the demographic and health transition will challenge core institutions to adapt and to develop innovative approaches to work, family life, caregiving, and education across the life course (Lee, 2003; Lloyd-Sherlock, 2010). Globally, somewhere around 2020, there will be more people aged 65 and older than children under 5. In India, this crossover will happen later, but not so much later. Furthermore as women continue to join the paid labor force, integrating care needs of older and younger family members while remaining in the labor force will pose challenges to both women and men in most societies (Budlender, 2008; Das et al., 2010; Sabates-Wheeler and Roelen, 2011). The changing older dependency ratios for world regions for 2000, 2020, and 2040 suggest that in Asia (excluding the Near East), the number of people aged 65 and older for every 100 people 20–64 will grow from 11 to 28 in this time period (United Nations, 2008). In this regard, India is no exception. Thus, it is critical that data regarding the family and network dynamics of older people in India be understood so that both formal and informal sectors can develop and plan effectively to maintain health, well-being, and productivity in the growing population of older adults and their families.

As in many countries, the family is a cherished institution in India and often provides important nonformal social security for the older population (Bloom et al., 2010). Most older men and women in India live with their families, and it is the most preferred living arrangement of older people (Gupta, 2009). Families continue to be the central organizing unit for economic support and for providing care for those physically unable to care for themselves (Kozel and Parker, 2000; Samuel and Thyloth, 2002). In the absence of institutions that provide social insurance (Barrientos, Gorman, and Heslop, 2003; Lloyd-Sherlock, 2002), we suspect that India's older populations will continue to rely on the family and social networks (Gupta, 2009; Gupta, Rowe, and Pillai, 2009). Social networks comprised of both family and friends are an important resource in the older person's life (Cohen and Wills, 1985; Shanas, 1973, 1979), although there is little evidence in India of the impacts of social networks on physical and mental well-being. As the nature of family, intergenerational relationships, and the role of women in the family are changing, these transitions may well impact the care and welfare of older people (Lloyd-Sherlock, 2000, 2002). In some instances, the family in the 21st century may be unable to meet the needs of the aged, thereby creating a need to look for other support services. India's National Policy on Older Persons (Government of India, 1999) emphasizes that programs will be developed to promote family values and sensitize the young to the necessity and desirability of intergenerational bonding and continuity.

The aim of this chapter is to provide a description of family and network ties among older men and women in India and to illustrate the dynamic interplay between caregiving and receiving among older people. In this chapter, we present findings from the Longitudinal Aging Study in India (LASI) pilot study, a cross-sectional survey of men and women over the age of 45 and their spouses in four states in India. In all our analysis, we will only include participants aged 45 and older: spouses younger than 45 were excluded because they were a representative sample of the population of their ages.

METHODS

Sample

LASI is a panel survey representing persons at least 45 years of age in India. Its pilot study is funded by the National Institute on Aging and samples individuals in four states (Karnataka, Kerala, Punjab, and Rajasthan). The survey instrument has been designed to collect information that is conceptually comparable to the U.S. Health and Retirement Study (HRS) and its sister surveys in Asia, and includes variables on demographics; family structure and social network; health and health behaviors; health care utilization; work and pension; housing and environment; and income, assets, debts, and consumption. The LASI survey instrument captures local characteristics of India. To capture regional variation, we will include two northern states (Punjab and Rajasthan) and two southern states (Karnataka and Kerala). Karnataka and Rajasthan were included in the Study on Global AGEing and Adult Health (SAGE), which will enable us to compare our findings with the SAGE data. The inclusion of Kerala and Punjab will demonstrate our ability to obtain a broader representation of India, where geographic variations accompanied by socioeconomic and cultural differences call for careful study and deliberation, especially when preparing for the nationally representative sampling for the subsequent baseline study. Punjab is an example of an economically developed state, while Rajasthan is relatively poor. Rajasthan is also one of the states with the highest ratio of males to females and is the capital of the practice of *sati*; thus, the well-being of widows may be particularly low in this state. Kerala, which is known for its relatively efficient healthcare system, has undergone rapid social development and is included as a potential harbinger of how the situation might evolve in other Indian states. The sampling frame for LASI is drawn from the *2001 Census Primary Census Abstract*. We use listing directories of villages and towns to select sample areas within each state for the pilot project. The primary sampling units (PSUs) are the randomly selected villages in rural areas and census enumeration blocks in urban areas that typically consist of 100–150 households. Basic distributions by gender are shown in Tables 11-1A and 11-1B.

Three Measures of Family and Social Networks

Social networks are comprised of multiple ties with family, friends, and links to more formal and informal social institutions. These ties form a web that provides resources to its members, often in the form of social support. Social support itself takes a number of forms, including emotional, instrumental, appraisal, and financial support. Social ties need not be positive but can also lead to negative outcomes including conflict and abuse. In this section, we explore some of the basic kinds of ties with spouse or partner, friends, and social activities often involving weaker ties and their social patterning in terms of social, economic, and demographic characteristics. We start with an exploration of three different aspects of social networks: ties with spouse, ties with close friends, and participation in social activities. These ties range from the most intimate and close ties with a partner to more extended and weaker ties with those who engage in social activities. There is little information currently available on these types of ties in India so basic information is essential.

We examined three measures of family and social networks. The first measure is closeness with spouse. The question asks "How close is your relationship with your spouse or partner?" The response categories include "Very close/Quite close/Not very close/Not at all close." We generated a binary variable about closeness with spouse, which takes a value of 1 if reporting "Very close" and 0 for reporting other categories.

The second measure is related to ties outside of the household. It indicates whether a respondent reported having any close friends. This measure was generated based on two questions in LASI. The first was "Do you have any friends?" If the answer is yes, then a second question was: "How many of these friends would you say you have a close relationship with?" If a respondent reported having any friend, and had a close relationship with one or more friends, then the measure of "having any close friend" takes the value of 1. Otherwise, it is 0.

The third measure is related to participation in social activities. LASI asks about how frequently a person participates in each of the following seven activities: (1) Go to the cinema, (2) eat out of the house, (3) go to a park/beach, (4) play cards or games, (5) visit relatives / friends, (6) attend cultural performances/shows, and (7) attend religious functions /events (outside home). The response categories are as follows: Twice a month or more / About once a month / Every few months / About once or twice a year / Less than once a year. Since activity 7, attending religious events, is strongly correlated with religion, we decided to exclude this activity for the measure of participation in social activities. The measure takes the value of 1 if for one or more of the other six activities, a person reported participating "Twice a month or more" or "About once a month."

Analysis

Since all three outcomes are binary, we applied a logit model to examine how social ties are associated with various sociodemographic characteristics and economic positions. Demographic characteristics include age group, gender, living in urban area, marital status, and living with a child or not. Economic positions are measured by education and per capita consumption. Per capita consumption is preferred over income for low-income regions and rural areas. LASI collected detailed data on household consumption. We used the variable of per capita consumption on Organisation for Economic Co-operation and Development equivalence, which takes into account not only number of household members, but also different consumption burden by age. The household adult was assigned a weight of 1, additional adults each were assigned a weight of 0.5, and each child was assigned a weight of 0.3. The per capita consumption measure was generated by adding all weights of the household members, and dividing the total household consumption by this summed value. Since LASI provides imputed data for missing values using a hot deck method, we control for imputed consumption in the models to adjust for any systematic bias due to missing data for some components of household consumption. We recoded the per capita consumption measure into terciles: low, middle, and high. The cutoff values for the terciles were 31,100 (RPs) and 57,033 (RPs). Finally, we control for region, caste, and state.

RESULTS

Sociodemographic Characteristics of LASI Participants

Sample characteristics of LASI are shown in Tables 11-1A and 11-1B. The pilot survey was done in selected states including Karnataka, Kerala, Punjab, and Rajasthan. Table 11-1A shows the distribution of the three social tie measures of interest, and Table 11-1B shows the other demographic conditions. Seventy-one percent of women and 75% of men lived in rural areas. Women were much less likely to be currently married: 65% versus 91% among men. This is not due to differences in age structure in our sample: Table 11-1B shows that for female participants, 61% were aged between 45–59, 30% aged between 60–74, and 9% were 75 and older. The corresponding percentages for male participants were 58%, 33%, and 9%, respectively.

In LASI, 32% of women are currently widowed. There is a growing concern about the increasing proportion of widows among older persons. The two main reasons for the significant gender disparity in widowhood are the longer life span of women compared to men and the general tendency in India for women to marry men older than themselves. Adjustment to widowhood can be difficult for women in all societies, particularly in India. Widows often face restrictions and social stigma. Lack of inheritance rights and property, and insufficient incomes and earnings expose elderly widows to deprivation and social isolation. As has been noted, "Widowhood is more than the loss of a husband—it may mean the loss of a separate identity" (United Nations Population Fund, 1998, p. 42).

TABLE 11-1A Distribution of Outcomes by Gender (in percentage)

	Men	Women
Very close to spouse if married		
No	22	20
Yes	78	80
Total	100	100
Any social activities		
No	33	40
Yes	67	60
Total	100	100
Any close friend		
No	44	66
Yes	56	34
Total	100	100

NOTE: Data are weighted by individual all-state representative sampling weight.
SOURCE: Data from LASI pilot study, respondents aged 45 and older.

Living arrangements are an important component of analysis of welfare of elderly. In other words, the care and support experienced by the elderly are commonly linked to the place of their residence. Table 11-1B shows that among women, 51% were living with spouse and children, 12% living with spouse only, 28% living with children only, and 8% living with neither spouse nor child. For men, 77% were living with both spouse and child, 13% were living with spouse only, 6% were living with spouse only, and 4% were living with neither spouse nor child. However, the large numbers of women surviving their spouses as compared to men may create increasing economic vulnerability of older Indians. One of the main social effects of extension of life is the extended period of widowhood for many women. According to the 2001 Census of India, 51% of the women aged 60 years and older are widowed, compared to only 15% among men. Men commonly have wives to care for them into older ages, but spouses may not be the major source of care for the majority of older women in India. Finally, in LASI, we have created a measure of economic status of the households by categorizing into them into five wealth quintiles: The lowest quintile constitutes the poorest households, and the highest quintile represents the richest households.

Distribution of Outcome Measures

Table 11-1A shows the distributions of the three outcome measures by gender. Men and women reported similar level of closeness to spouses, if married: 78% among men and 80% among women. However, women

TABLE 11-1B Distributions of Demographic and Socioeconomic Variables by Gender (in percentage)

	Men	Women
Age Group		
45–59	58	61
60–74	33	30
75 and older	9	9
Residence		
Rural	75	71
Urban	25	29
Marital Status		
Married	91	65
Never married/divorced/separated	3	4
Widowed	6	32
Living Arrangement		
Live with spouse and child	77	51
Live only with spouse, not child	13	12
Live only with child, not spouse	6	28
Live with neither spouse nor child	4	8
Education		
Illiterate	40	56
Primary	27	23
Secondary	11	8
High school or more	22	14
Per capita Consumption Terciles		
Low	33	33
Middle	33	34
High	34	32
Consumption Values Imputed	18	18
Religion		
Other	2	1
Hindu	75	76
Muslim	9	8
Christian	6	7
Sikh	8	7
Caste		
Other/none	32	32
Scheduled caste/scheduled tribe	27	28
Other backward class	41	40
State		
Karnataka	32	32
Kerala	21	25
Punjab	14	13
Rajasthan	33	30

NOTE: Data are weighted by individual all-state representative sampling weight.
SOURCE: Data from LASI pilot study, respondents aged 45 and older.

were less likely to participate in any social activities: 60% among women versus 67% among men. Finally, only 34% of women reported having any close friend, while 56% of men did. The gender distributions across the four regions in LASI are very similar.

Regression Analysis

Closeness with Spouse

We first assess the relationship quality between the spouse and the participant in LASI. A set of questions was included in the survey to measure the extent of satisfaction with life and current situations. One question is about a respondent's relationship with a spouse. The responses were categorized into three levels: completely/very satisfied, somewhat satisfied, and not satisfied. Table 11-2 shows the odds ratios for "feeling very close to your spouse" among men and women who were married in LASI. Respondents who are somewhat satisfied or not satisfied are contrasted with those who are completely or very satisfied.

The results of this analysis suggest that there is little difference in marital satisfaction with age. While those aged 60 and older are slightly less likely to report being close to their partners, these results are not significant. Gender differences are also not substantial in these analyses once we control for covariates. Those living in urban areas were likely to be close to their spouses but the association was not significant (OR 0.77, 95% CI 0.45–1.30). When comparing educational levels with terciles of consumption, some important differences emerge. Within educational levels, relative to the illiterate group, those with any education, primary, secondary, or high school and above were twice or more likely to report being close to their spouses. In contrast, those in the middle and high tercile of consumption were more likely to report being close to a spouse, but the associations were not significant. Those with imputed consumption values were more likely to report being close to spouses. Finally, religion, caste, and state were not associated with closeness to spouse.

Ties with Close Friends

Ties with close friends are a potential source of support, friendship, and intimacy. Even in countries where close ties are often kinship based, close friends turn out to have a critical role in social networks. Table 11-3 shows the association of close friendships with the same set of social and demographic characteristics we examined previously in a multiple logistic analysis looking at the independent association of each variable.

TABLE 11-2 Odds Ratios of Logistic Regression for the Outcome of "Very Close to Spouse," if Married

Covariates	Odds Ratio	95% CI
Age Group		
60–74	0.86	[0.59,1.24]
75 and older	0.76	[0.35,1.63]
Gender		
Female	1.23	[0.92,1.66]
Residence		
Urban	0.77	[0.45,1.30]
Living Arrangement		
Live with child	1.34	[0.76,2.38]
Education		
Primary	2.58**	[1.60,4.16]
Secondary	1.85	[0.93,3.69]
High school or more	2.05*	[1.15,3.65]
Per Capita Consumption Terciles		
Middle	1.13	[0.71,1.81]
High	1.48	[0.84,2.59]
Consumption Values Imputed	1.82*	[1.06,3.12]
Religion		
Muslim	0.83	[0.35,1.98]
Christian	2.19	[0.84,5.75]
Sikh	1.42	[0.69,2.89]
State		
Kerala	1.62	[0.76,3.44]
Punjab	1.17	[0.52,2.59]
Rajasthan	1.02	[0.51,2.04]
Observations	1,110	

NOTES: Data are weighted by individual all-state representative sampling weight. Complex sample design is taken into account for estimating standard errors. * denotes $p < 0.05$; ** $p < 0.01$.

SOURCE: Data from LASI pilot study, respondents aged 45 and older and reported being currently married.

The results of this analysis contrast in some significant ways with those related to spousal relationships. Age, for instance, is strongly associated with friendship patterns, with older men and women much less likely to have close friends. Younger respondents are more than three times as likely to have close friends compared to older people. Surprisingly, since women are often thought of as caregivers and social "connectors," in this analysis, they are much less likely to report close friends than are men (OR .35, 95% CI .24–.51). There is a hint, though not statistically significant, that widowed, divorced, and single respondents are more likely to have close friends than their married counterparts, suggestive of

TABLE 11-3 Odds Ratios of Logistic Regression for the Outcome of "Any Close Friend"

Covariates	Odds ratio	95% CI
Age Group		
60–74	0.70*	[0.52,0.95]
75 and older	0.29***	[0.18,0.45]
Gender		
Female	0.35***	[0.24,0.51]
Residence		
Urban	0.99	[0.58,1.69]
Marital Status		
Never married/divorced/separated	1.34	[0.56,3.19]
Widowed	1.2	[0.82,1.77]
Living Arrangement		
Live with child	0.69**	[0.52,0.91]
Education		
Primary	1.55*	[1.02,2.36]
Secondary	2.63***	[1.64,4.22]
High school or more	2.43***	[1.53,3.84]
Per Capita Consumption Terciles		
Middle	1.3	[0.90,1.88]
High	1.80*	[1.12,2.88]
Consumption Values Imputed	1.66*	[1.12,2.46]
Religion		
Muslim	0.45**	[0.26,0.78]
Christian	1.02	[0.59,1.76]
Sikh	2.79*	[1.24,6.26]
Caste		
Scheduled caste/scheduled tribe	1.1	[0.69,1.73]
Other backward class	1.08	[0.78,1.50]
State		
Kerala	1.94*	[1.11,3.41]
Punjab	0.54	[0.24,1.20]
Rajasthan	0.82	[0.46,1.45]
Observations	1,420	

NOTES: Data are weighted by individual all-state representative sampling weight. Complex sample design is taken into account for estimating standard errors. * denotes $p < 0.05$; ** $p < 0.01$; *** $p < 0.001$.
SOURCE: Data from LASI pilot study, respondents aged 45 and older.

some level of substitution among types of ties. These odds ratios, however, are relatively small. Finally, increasing education and consumption were associated with an increasing likelihood of having close friends. Respondents living in Kerala were more likely to report having close friends than those living in other regions.

Social Activities and Social Participation

The LASI pilot survey included questions about social participation. Specifically, a question asked about social activities including going to the cinema, eating out of the house, going to the park/beach, playing cards or games, visiting relatives/friends, attending cultural performances/shows, and attending religious functions/events (outside home). In a multivariate logistic regression analysis, we examined the associations between demographic and economic conditions and participation in social activities. Table 11-4 shows the results of the analysis with odds ratios and 95% confidence intervals.

The results from this analysis indicate the participation in social activities is substantially lower among those aged 75 and older than those at younger ages. Women are less likely to engage in social activities than are men. The strongest associations, however, are in relation to socioeconomic position. Both men and women with high levels of education and in middle and high consumption terciles are more likely to engage in social activities. In these analyses, respondents living in Rajasthan were much less likely to participate in social activities than those in other regions.

Positive and Negative Aspects of Social Relationships

Social networks may be positive and enriching as well as negative and conflict-laden. While a deep analysis of these dimensions is beyond the scope of this chapter, here we present some preliminary findings with regard to the quality of different types of social ties. Our aim was to explore both positive and negative aspects of ties, including ill treatment of older men and women, patterns of communication among friends, and patterns of financial support in terms of support both given and received by participants. We describe these findings in the text. The data are available from the authors upon request.

Ill Treatment of Elderly within the Family

Elder abuse and neglect are increasingly acknowledged as a social problem internationally (Acierno et al., 2010; Cooper, Selwood, and Livingston, 2008; Dong et al., 2009), and India is no exception. The responsibility of caring for the elderly in India is traditionally borne by the immediate family (Gupta, 2009). However, with a changing trend toward nuclear family set-ups, the vulnerability of the elderly is considerably increasing. The intersection of high care demands and competing time-use priorities can result in low-quality care and high caregiver burden (Boggatz et al., 2007; Dias and Patel, 2009; Navaie-Waliser, Spriggs, and

TABLE 11-4 Odds Ratios of Logistic Regression for the Outcome of "Any Social Activities"

Covariates	Odds ratio	95% CI
Age Group		
60–74	0.75	[0.54,1.03]
75 and older	0.30***	[0.19,0.48]
Gender		
Female	0.70*	[0.51,0.96]
Residence		
Urban	1.56	[0.92,2.64]
Marital Status		
Never married/divorced/separated	0.59	[0.29,1.19]
Widowed	0.85	[0.60,1.22]
Living Arrangement		
Live with child	1.12	[0.74,1.70]
Education		
Primary	1.57	[0.98,2.52]
Secondary	2.32*	[1.10,4.86]
High school or more	2.77***	[1.56,4.91]
Per Capita Consumption Terciles		
Middle	1.56*	[1.08,2.26]
High	1.66*	[1.11,2.50]
Consumption Values Imputed	1.05	[0.63,1.76]
Religion		
Muslim	0.74	[0.40,1.38]
Christian	1.2	[0.72,1.99]
Sikh	2.72**	[1.33,5.56]
Caste		
Scheduled caste/scheduled tribe	0.76	[0.52,1.12]
Other backward class	0.9	[0.67,1.22]
State		
Kerala	0.61	[0.33,1.11]
Punjab	0.88	[0.37,2.05]
Rajasthan	0.12***	[0.07,0.22]
Observations	1,422	

NOTES: Data are weighted by individual all-state representative sampling weight. Complex sample design is taken into account for estimating standard errors. * denotes $p < 0.05$; ** $p < 0.01$; *** $p < 0.001$.
SOURCE: Data from LASI pilot study, respondents aged 45 and older.

Feldman, 2002), which may manifest in continued unmet needs/neglect and, in the most extreme cases, even direct abuse. Even though there is a general perception about the mistreatment perpetrated on older adults (Cooper et al., 2008; Newman, 2006), the exact magnitude and nature of abuse is still unknown in India. A recent study (Sebastian and Sekher, 2010) observed that female elderly, especially widows, those in the oldest-old age group (80+ years), and the physically immobile, are more vulnerable to abuse than others. Not only the poor, but also the rich are susceptible to neglect and abuse in many families. Chokkanathan and Lee (2005) found that the prevalence of mistreatment was 14% among older adults in an urban setting in India. The mistreatment of elderly is multidimensional and multilayered, emerging from differences in gender, economic position, and physical condition (Selwood, Cooper, and Livingston, 2007; World Health Organizagiton, 2008). The general perception that families are the safest place for the aged in India has been questioned by micro-level studies in recent years (Chokkanathan and Lee, 2005; Selwood, Cooper, and Livingston, 2007; Srinivasan, 2009).

The question "How often do you feel ill-treated within your family?" was posed to all respondents in the LASI pilot survey. This question is not an explicit question about abuse but taps a more general domain related to perceptions of being treated poorly. About 7% stated "often" and 19% responded by stating "some of the time." However, no significant difference was observed between males and females and also between rural and urban areas. It is also important to note that about three-fourth of respondents stated that they never/hardly ever felt ill-treated within the family. Reporting being ill-treated often is higher among lower-income groups and also among the less educated. The findings of this survey are in tune with prevalence estimates of earlier studies (Chokkanathan and Lee, 2005).

Communication with Friends

Frequency of communication is often identified as an indicator of closeness among social ties. In LASI, if the respondent has friends, the question was asked, "On average, how often do you do each of the following (meet up, speak on phone) with any of your friends?" This section describes how often the older respondents maintain close relationships with their friends through meeting with them or speaking over the phone. The responses given were grouped into three categories: frequently, sometimes, and rarely. Nearly 85% of elderly meet up with a friend frequently. Only 7% responded "rarely." Meeting with a friend frequently is relatively less common among urban residents and among females. Nearly half of the older respondents (47%) talk with their friends over the phone frequently. Among the older population, speaking over the phone is not as frequent as meeting their friends. Half of the males and 42% of the females speak with their friends frequently. Speaking frequently over the phone is more common among higher economic groups and those with better education.

Financial Support Given to or Received from Family and Friends

LASI asked questions about household financial help given to or received from family members and friends. Financial help includes giving money, helping pay bills, covering the cost of medical care or insurance, schooling, marriages, religious events, rent for housing, and other expenses. Only 5.5% of respondents (N = 81) received any financial help from family; and only 7.4% (N = 110) gave any financial help to family. While financial help is a relatively rare occurrence in this cohort, it is of interest to note that support was given about as much as it was received among older men and women and their families.

CONCLUSIONS

Social networks, family dynamics, and both positive and negative aspects of these relationships are central to the well-being and functioning of men and women across the globe. In this chapter, we have described the basic relationships of older Indian men and women across four states from the LASI pilot study. In this study, the vast majority of both men and women are well connected both in terms of their intimate family ties as well as to more extended, weaker social networks. While 4% of men and 8% of women lived with neither spouse nor children, about 32% of women were widowed. As India continues to experience demographic and health transitions, it will be critical to monitor the ways in which informal social networks from both family and friends will continue to support Indians well into old age.

Another important aspect of these analyses points out that older men and women *both* give and receive support. In our present analyses, this is particularly true with regard to financial support. One critical aspect of an aging society is the recognition that with increases in life expectancy and healthier functioning into older ages, older men and women will be able to contribute to the well-being of their families and communities (Hughes et al., 2007; Verbugge and Chan, 2008). Older men and women are not only on the receiving end of support, but also contribute to the dynamic and interdependent aspects of social institutions (Cong and Silverstein, 2011; Silverstein et al., 2002). This bidirectional force is often less recognized as societies begin to have larger older populations with a resultant undue emphasis on the burden of older people in rapidly evolving societies such as India.

Socioeconomic conditions, as well as rural versus urban geography, may also shape patterns of social networks and perceptions about the quality of social relations (Pinquart and Sörensen, 2000; Yen and Syme, 1999). In the LASI data, increasing education and income are associated with a greater likelihood of social participation and having close friends. This pattern is often found in Western industrialized countries, particularly the United States (Berkman and Glass, 2000). In other studies, participation in religious activities and ties with close family are not socio-economically stratified as much as other types of contacts (Berkman and Glass, 2000). Among both indicators on socioeconomic position, those who are most disadvantaged are least likely to be satisfied with their spouses. Within educational levels, those with primary-level education are most likely to be satisfied with the relationship with their spouse. Interestingly, rural residents are about twice as likely as urban residents to report being satisfied with their spousal relationships. These differences suggest more subtle processes of either experience or evaluation of social relationships (Gerstel, Riessman, and Rosenfield, 1985; Goldman, Korenman, and Weinstein, 1995; Julien and Markman, 1991). It is important to note, of course, that this is a cross-sectional study and that the relationship between social networks and socioeconomic and geographic locale is likely to be bidirectional with selection processes going in both senses: that is, that social ties shape both socioeconomic opportunities and geographic mobility.

Our initial analyses are descriptive; however, the next phases of analyses will be aimed at gaining a more nuanced understanding of the social networks of older men and women in India and the social and economic forces that shape them. With more longitudinal data, we will be able to understand the ways in which such social ties and the positive and negative aspects of these ties shape health outcomes and are, in turn, shaped by them.

REFERENCES

Acierno, R., M.A. Hernandez, A.B. Amstadter, H.S. Resnick, K. Steve, W. Muzzy, and D.G. Kilpatrick. (2010). Prevalence and correlates of emotional, physical, sexual, and financial abuse and potential neglect in the United States: The National Elder Mistreatment Study. *American Journal of Public Health* 100(2):292-297. doi:10.2105/AJPH.2009.163089.

Barrientos, A., M. Gorman, and A. Heslop. (2003). Old age poverty in developing countries: Contributions and dependence in later life. *World Development* 31(3):555-570.

Berkman, L.F. (2000). Social support, social networks, social cohesion and health. *Social Work in Health Care* 31(2):3-14. doi:doi: 10.1300/J010v31n02_02.

Berkman, L.F. (2009). Social epidemiology: Social determinants of health in the United States. *Annual Review of Public Health* 30(30):27-41.

Berkman, L.F., and T.A. Glass. (2000). Social integration, social networks, social support and health. In *Social Epidemiology,* L.F. Berkman and I. Kawachi (Eds.). New York: Oxford University Press.

Bloom, D.E., A. Mahal, L. Rosenberg, and J. Sevilla. (2010). Economic security arrangements in the context of population ageing in India. *International Social Security Review* 63(3-4): 59-89.

Boggatz, T., A. Dijkstra, C. Lohrmann, and T. Dassen. (2007). The meaning of care dependency as shared by care givers and care recipients: A concept analysis. *Journal of Advanced Nursing 60(5)*:561-569.

Bongaarts, J., and Z. Zimmer. (2002). Living arrangements of older adults in the developing world. *The Journals of Gerontology Series B: Psychological Sciences and Social Sciences 57(3)*:S145-S157.

Budlender, D. (2008). *The Statistical Evidence on Care and Non-Care Work across Six Countries* (No. 4) (pp. 1-61). Geneva: National Research Institute for Social Development.

Chokkanathan, S., and A. Lee. (2005). Elder mistreatment in urban India: A community based study. *Journal of Elder Abuse and Neglect 17(2)*:45-61.

Cohen, S., and T.A. Wills. (1985). Stress, social support and the buffering hypothesis. *Psychological Bulletin 8*:310-357.

Cong, Z., and M. Silverstein. (2011). Intergenerational time-for-money exchanges in rural China: Does reciprocity reduce depressive symptoms of older grandparents? *Research in Human Development 5(1)*:6-25. doi:doi:10.1080/15427600701853749.

Cooper, C., A. Selwood, and G. Livingston. (2008). The prevalence of elder abuse and neglect: A systematic review. *Age and Ageing 37(2)*:151-160. doi:10.1093/ageing/afm194.

Das, S., A. Hazra, B.K. Ray, M. Ghosal, T.K. Banerjee, T. Roy, A. Chaudhuri et al. (2010). Burden among stroke caregivers: Results of a community-based study from Kolkata, India. *Stroke 41(12)*:2,965-2,968. doi:10.1161/STROKEAHA.110.589598.

Dias, A., and V. Patel. (2009). Closing the treatment gap for dementia in India. *Indian Journal of Psychiatry 51(5)*:93-97.

Dong, X., M. Simon, C. Mendes de Leon, T. Fulmer, T. Beck, L. Hebert, C. Dyer et al. (2009). Elder self-neglect and abuse and mortality risk in a community-dwelling population. *JAMA: The Journal of the American Medical Association 302(5)*:517-526. doi:10.1001/jama.2009.1109.

Gerstel, N., C.K. Riessman, and S. Rosenfield. (1985). Explaining the symptomatology of separated and divorced women and men: The role of material conditions and social networks. *Social Forces 64(1)*:84-101.

Goldman, N., S. Korenman, and R. Weinstein. (1995). Marital status and health among the elderly. *Social Science & Medicine 40(12)*:1,717-1,730. doi:doi: 10.1016/0277-9536(94)00281-W.

Government of India. (1999). *National Policy for Older Persons*. New Delhi: Ministry of Social Justice and Empowerment.

Gupta, R. (2009). Systems perspective: Understanding care giving of the elderly in India. *Health Care for Women International 30(12)*:1,040-1,054.

Gupta, R., N. Rowe, and V.K. Pillai. (2009). Perceived caregiver burden in India. *Affilia 24(1)*:69-79. doi:10.1177/0886109908326998.

Hughes, M.E., L.J. Waite, T.A. LaPierre, and Y. Luo. (2007). All in the family: The impact of caring for grandchildren on grandparents' health. *The Journals of Gerontology Series B: Psychological Sciences and Social Sciences 62(2)*:S108-S119.

Julien, D., and H.J. Markman. (1991). Social support and social networks as determinants of individual and marital outcomes. *Journal of Social and Personal Relationships 8(4)*:549-568. doi:10.1177/026540759184006.

Kirk, D. (1996). Demographic transition theory. *Population Studies 50(3)*:361-387. doi:10.1080/0032472031000149536.

Kozel, V., and B. Parker. (2000). Integrated approaches to poverty assessment in India. In *Integrating Quantitative and Qualitative Research in Development Projects*, M. Bamberger (Ed.). Washington, DC: World Bank.

Lee, R. (2003). The demographic transition: Three centuries of fundamental change. *The Journal of Economic Perspectives 17(4)*:167-190. doi:10.1257/089533003772034943.

Lloyd-Sherlock, P. (2000). Old age and poverty in developing countries: New policy challenges. *World Development 28(12):*2,157-2,168.

Lloyd-Sherlock, P. (2002). Formal social protection for older people in developing countries: Three different approaches. *Journal of Social Policy 31(04):695.*

Lloyd-Sherlock, P. (2010). *Population Ageing and International Development: From Generalisation to Evidence.* Portland, OR: Policy. Available: http://hollis.harvard. edu/?itemid=%7Clibrary/m/aleph%7C012264681.

Longitudinal Aging Study in India, Pilot Wave (2011). Harvard School of Public Health; International Institute of Population Sciences, Mumbai, India, and RAND Corporation. Available: https://mmicdata.rand.org/megametadata/?section=study&studyid=36.

McPherson, M., L. Smith-Lovin, and J.M. Cook. (2001). Birds of a feather: Homophily in social networks. *Annual Review of Sociology 27:*415-444.

Navaie-Waliser, M., A. Spriggs, and P.H. Feldman. (2002). Informal caregiving: Differential experiences by gender. *Medical Care 40(12):*1,249-1,259.

Newman, M. (2006). International/cultural perspectives on elder abuse. In *Elder Abuse: A Public Health Perspective,* R.W. Summers and A.M. Hoffman (Eds.). Washington, DC: American Public Health Association.

Pinquart, M., and Sörensen, S. (2000). Influences of socioeconomic status, social network, and competence on subjective well-being in later life: A meta-analysis. *Psychology and Aging 15(2):*187-224.

Sabates-Wheeler, R., and K. Roelen. (2011). Transformative social protection programming for children and their carers: A gender perspective. *Gender & Development 19(2):*179-194. doi:10.1080/13552074.2011.592629.

Samuel, M., and M. Thyloth. (2002). Caregivers' roles in India. *Psychiatric Services 53(3):*346-347.

Sebastian, D., and T.V. Sekher. (2010). Abuse and neglect of elderly in Indian families: Findings of elder abuse screening test in Kerala. *Journal of the Indian Academy of Geriatrics 6:*54-60.

Seeman, T.E., T.M. Lusignolo, M. Albert, and L. Berkman. (2001). Social relationships, social support, and patterns of cognitive aging in healthy, high-functioning older adults: MacArthur Studies of Successful Aging. *Health Psychology 20(4):*243-255.

Selwood, A., C. Cooper, and G. Livingston. (2007). What is elder abuse—who decides? *International Journal of Geriatric Psychiatry 22(10):*1009-1012. doi:10.1002/gps.1781.

Shanas, E. (1973). Family-kin networks and aging in cross-cultural perspective. *Journal of Marriage and Family 35(3):*505-511.

Shanas, E. (1979). The family as a social support system in old age. *The Gerontologist 19(2):*169-174. doi:10.1093/geront/19.2.169.

Silverstein, M., S.J. Conroy, H.Wang, R. Giarrusso, and V.L. Bengtson. (2002). Reciprocity in parent–child relations over the adult life course. *The Journals of Gerontology Series B: Psychological Sciences and Social Sciences 57(1):*S3-S13. doi:10.1093/geronb/57.1.S3.

Srinivasan, C. (2009). Resources, stressors and psychological distress among older adults in Chennai, India. *Social Science & Medicine 68(2):*243-250. doi:10.1016/j.socscimed.2008.10.008.

United Nations. (2008). World Population Prospects: The 2008 Revision Population Database. *World Population Prospects: The 2008 Revision Population Database. Medium Variant Projections.* Available: http://esa.un.org/unpp/.

United Nations Population Fund. (1998). *The State of the World Population, 1998.* New York: United Nations Population Fund.

Verbugge, L.M., and A. Chan. (2008). Giving help in return: Family reciprocity by older Singaporeans. *Ageing & Society 28(01):5.*

Wachter, K.W. (1997). Kinship resources for the elderly. *Philosophical Transactions of the Royal Society of London.Series B: Biological Sciences 352(1363):*1,811-1,817.

Wellman, B., and S.D. Berkowitz. (1988). *Social Structures: A Network Approach*. Structural
    Analysis in the Social Sciences (vol. 2). New York: Cambridge University Press. Avai-
    lable: http://discovery.lib.harvard.edu/?itemid=%7Clibrary/m/aleph%7C001338800.
World Health Organization. (2008). *A Global Response to Elder Abuse and Neglect*. Geneva:
    World Health Organization.
Yen, I.H., and S.L. Syme. (1999). The social environment and health: A discussion of the
    epidemiologic literature. *Annual Review of Public Health 20(1)*:287-308. doi:doi: 10.1146/
    annurev.publhealth.20.1.287.

12

Effects of Social Activities on Cognitive Functions: Evidence from CHARLS[1]

Yuqing Hu, Xiaoyan Lei, James P. Smith, and *Yaohui Zhao*

C ognitive function is a key dimension of the quality of life for the elderly in all countries. It is closely related to the ability to process information in daily life and helps shape overall well-being over the life course (McArdle, Smith, and Willis, 2011). Cognitive function involves operations such as perception, memory, creation of imagery, and thinking, and it declines sharply as people approach advanced age (Levy, 1994; Tilvis et al., 2004). With population aging, more people will begin to suffer from cognitive impairment. The situation is especially severe in China because of its extraordinary speed of population aging, accompanied by the eventual decline of families as a source of eldercare and the lack of long-term care facilities. It is thus important to study determinants of cognitive function to understand how to best postpone and slow down its eventual decline.

Social activities are of particular interest to us as they play a significant role in the daily lives of most Chinese elderly. Social-emotional Selec-

[1]This research was supported by grants from the National Institute on Aging to CCER at Peking University and the RAND Corporation, and grants from the Natural Science Foundation of China. It was also supported by the National Institute on Aging (Grant Number R21AG031372), Natural Science Foundation of China (Grant Numbers 70773002 and 70910107022), the World Bank (Contract 7145915), and the Fogarty International Center (Grant Number R03TW008358). The content is solely the responsibility of the authors and does not necessarily represent the official views of any of the funders. We appreciate the helpful comments received at the National Academy of Sciences meeting in New Delhi, India, and from the NAS reviewers.

tivity Theory (SST) argues that as people age, they become increasingly selective by investing greater resources in emotionally meaningful goals and activities. Present-oriented goals with emotional meaning are prioritized over future-oriented goals aimed at acquiring information about future decisions and expanding horizons (Löckenhoff and Carstensen, 2004). Due to a gradual decline in cognitive functioning and the ability to deal with complex cognitive tasks, the elderly seek out more emotional goals. Such motivations further limit their ability to seek information as well as their attention, memory, and cognition processing. However, cognitively stimulating social activity is hypothesized to benefit cognitive functions by providing resistance to mental diseases, such as dementia, and by reducing rates of cognitive decline (Hsu, 2007; Wang et al., 2002). The effects of different social activities on cognitive functions of the old warrant more exploration, especially for China where little research currently exists in part due to the lack of high-quality micro data.

A large volume of literature has investigated the relationship between cognition and social activities or social engagement among the elderly (Allaire and Marsiske, 1999; Wang et al., 2002; Zunzunegui et al., 2003). These studies confirm a positive relationship between the two. Among these studies, Zunzunegui et al. (2003), using data from a longitudinal survey of community-dwelling people over age 65, analyzed causal effects of social networks, social integration, and social engagement on cognitive decline of community-dwelling older Spanish adults with social variables measured at baseline, and cognitive change and decline measured after four years of follow-up. They were unable to determine whether the observed effect of social relations on cognitive function was the result of cumulative lifelong exposure to extensive social networks or a consequence of an abrupt change from an extensive network to a more limited one.

Similar studies on the relation between cognition and social activities in developing countries such as China are more fragmentary, primarily due to the lack of relevant data and a concentration on the young relative to health of the elderly. Asian populations are of particular interest because their elderly people are more likely to reside with their children and social activities may play different roles in their lives than in the western world. Glei et al. (2005) and Hsu (2007) are two exceptions that used longitudinal data from a survey of elderly in Taiwan and explored the effects of social participation on cognitive function. Hsu (2007) focused on regular social group participation and ignored leisure activity. He found that participating in any of these social groups has no significant correlation with cognitive function. Glei et al. (2005) used a broader definition of social interaction that includes more recreational activities and found that participating in these social activities may play an important role on delaying cognitive decline. In our study, we employ a similar definition of social activity as in Glei et al. and investigate data from mainland China, which has the same tradition of living arrangements but is at a different stage of economic development under a different institutional background than Taiwan. In addition to what has been done in Hsu (2007) and Glei et al. (2005), we will try to seek a causal explanation through exploring the community-level facilities and organizations that enable more social interactions among Chinese elderly.

More specifically, this chapter attempts to address three questions. First, what is the relationship between social activity and different dimensions of cognitive function for Chinese elderly? Second, what are the differences among effects of alternative social activities on different dimensions of cognitive abilities? Instead of directly identifying the causal relationship, we test in an ordinary least squares (OLS) reduced form setting whether community facilities, which are strongly correlated with social activities, are correlated to cognitive function. To address these issues, we will use the recently collected data from the 2008 pilot survey of the China Health and Retirement Longitudinal Study (CHARLS). In addition to OLS estimates of association, we present OLS reduced form estimates that include some arguably exogenous determinants of individuals' social activities.

The chapter is organized as follows. The next section presents a summary of CHARLS data, including a description of variables and summary statistics. The following section shows the principal relationships between cognitive functions and social activities emerging from the CHARLS data. We then present OLS reduced form estimations showing the relationship between cognitive functions and community facilities. The final section highlights our main conclusions.

DATA, VARIABLES, AND SUMMARY STATISTICS

Data and Variables

The 2008 CHARLS pilot was conducted in Zhejiang and Gansu provinces. Zhejiang, located in the developed coastal region, is a dynamic province with fast economic growth, a private sector, small-scale industrialization, and an export orientation. In contrast, Gansu, located in the less developed western region, is one of the poorest, most rural provinces in China. These two provinces were selected in part due to their economic diversity. Among all provinces in 2008, Zhejiang had the highest rural and urban incomes per capita after Shanghai and Beijing, while Gansu had the second lowest rural per capita income and fourth lowest urban per capita income. The target population of CHARLS is individuals aged 45 and older and their spouses/partners irrespective of age.

The sampling design of the 2008 wave of CHARLS aimed to be representative of residents aged 45 and older in these two provinces. Within each province, CHARLS randomly selected 13 county-level units by PPS (Probability Proportional to Size), stratified by regions and urban/rural. Within each county-level unit, CHARLS randomly selected three village-level units (villages in rural areas and urban communities in urban areas) by PPS as primary sampling units (PSUs). Within each PSU, CHARLS randomly selected 25 dwellings in rural and 36 in urban areas from a complete list of dwelling units generated from a mapping/listing operation. In situations where more than one age-eligible household lived in a dwelling unit, CHARLS randomly selected one. Within each household, one person aged 45 and older was randomly chosen as the main respondent, and the spouse was automatically included. Based on this sampling procedure, one or two individuals in each household were interviewed depending on marital status of the main respondent. The total sample size was 2,685 individuals in 1,570 households. The CHARLS pilot experience was very positive. Overall response rate was 85%: 79% in urban areas and 90% in rural areas. Response rates were about the same in the two provinces, 83.9% in Zhejiang and 85.8% in Gansu. The high response rates reflected detailed procedures put in place to ensure a high response to the survey.[2]

In the CHARLS sample, people for the most part do not choose the community in which they live, but instead they mostly live where they were born. CHARLS respondents who are by design aged 45 and older are relatively immobile and did not participate in the great Chinese migration patterns. About 9 in 10 CHARLS respondents are living in the same county in which he or she was born and less than 1 in every 20 is living in a different province in which he or she was born (Smith et al., 2012).

Following protocols of the Health and Retirement Studies (HRS) international surveys, the 2008 CHARLS main questionnaire consists of seven modules: (1) demographic background, (2) family, (3) health status and functioning, (4) healthcare and insurance, (5) work, retirement and pension, (6) income, expenditure and assets, and (7) interviewer observation (Zhao et al., 2009). All data were collected in face-to-face, computer-aided personal interviews (CAPI).

Rich information makes CHARLS well suited for research on cognitive abilities and social activities. Our study sample includes respondents

---

[2]Letters to respondents were delivered (often by the village leader) to households to inform them of the significance of the study, contents of questionnaires, provision of a free physical examination, and compensation, as well as the expected date of arrival of the interviewers. On the day of the interview, interviewers were often introduced to the households by community leaders to confirm the authenticity of their identity. When refused, multiple attempts were made to persuade respondents to participate and the team leader was required to go and make a final attempt before declaring the household a refusal.

45 years and older, representing Zhejiang and Gansu provinces. After discarding 109 individuals younger than 45 years old (spouses of the main respondents), 1 with missing age, and 282 with missing cognition due to proxy,[3] we are left with a sample of 2,293 observations, among which 1,131 are men and 1,162 are women, 850 (37.1%) are younger than 50 years old, 768 (33.5%) are 50–60 years old, 461 (20.1%) are 60–70 years old, and 214 (9.3%) are aged 70 and older.

Social Activity (SA)

In CHARLS, questions on social activities are in the "health status and function" module, where interviewees are asked whether they have taken part in 10 specifically listed activities in the past month. The 10 activities are (1) volunteer or charity work; (2) caring for a sick or disabled adult who does not live with the respondent and who does not pay for the help; (3) providing help to family, friends, or neighbors who do not live with the respondent and who do not pay for the help; (4) attending an educational or training course; (5) interacting with friends; (6) playing Mahjong, chess, or cards, or going to a community club; (7) attending a sporting event or other kind of club; (8) taking part in a community-related organization; (9) investing in stocks; and (10) surfing the Internet. Seven out of these 10 are considered social activities, while the remaining three activities—3, 9, and 10—are not.[4]

Table 12-1 depicts participation rates in each of these social activities. Interacting with friends and playing table games such as Mahjong have much higher participation rates than other activities (34.5% interacted with friends and 17.1% played Mahjong, chess, or card games), so we put each of them into a distinct group and grouped the rest into a category called "other social activities." We define a variable called "any activity" to indicate if a respondent was involved in at least one social activity. Forty-six percent participated in at least one activity.

Table games, especially the traditional Chinese game of Mahjong, play an important role in many Chinese seniors' lives. When relatives live far away, Mahjong helps form a sense of belonging by providing a chance to interact with those with whom one shares interests and personalities. The effort to win games—remembering rules, learning skills, and observing and reacting to others' behavior—forces the brain to work and is hypothesized to enhance people's cognitive functioning through such

---

[3]Missing values of the control variables are imputed by multiple imputation method.

[4]Options 9 and 10 are obviously not social activities. We do not consider option 3 as a social activity, as the wording is very likely to be understood as providing economic help to family and friends, which seems different from social activities in the Chinese context.

TABLE 12-1 Description of Social Activities and Cognitive Function

Social Activity and Other Activity Variables	All	Gender	
		Male	Female
Interacted with friends	0.345	0.317	0.371
Played Mahjong, chess, or cards	0.171	0.236	0.108
Other social activities	0.086	0.076	0.095
Done voluntary or charity work	0.012	0.016	0.009
Cared for sick or disabled as volunteer	0.040	0.039	0.040
Attended education or training course	0.006	0.007	0.005
Gone to sport, social, or other club	0.027	0.014	0.039
Taken part in community-related organization	0.016	0.016	0.016
Attended any activity above	0.457	0.470	0.444
Number of activities attended	0.616	0.645	0.588
Number of observations	2,293	1,131	1,162
Cognitive function			
Mental intactness (0-11)	8.621	9.046	8.167
	[2.14]	[1.89]	[2.30]
Number of observations	1,873	968	905
Episodic memory	2.986	3.103	2.862
	[2.02]	[1.99]	[2.05]
Number of observations	1,901	979	922

NOTE: For cognitive function, standard errors are below coefficients in brackets.
SOURCE: Data from CHARLS 2008 Pilot.

activities. Provided that sufficient infrastructure and services in the community exist, playing Mahjong or chess at home or in the neighborhood is a common way for older Chinese to spend leisure time by interacting with friends and neighbors.

Cognitive Ability (CA)

Cognitive function of respondents is also measured in the "health status and function" module in the CHARLS questionnaire, which tests orientation, calculation, word recall, and other cognitive dimensions. Cognitive ability can be generally categorized into fluid cognitive ability (FCA) and crystallized cognitive ability (CCA). The former concerns learning

Region		Province		Age Group			
Urban	Rural	Zhejiang	Gansu	< 50	50–60	60–70	> 70
0.385	0.313	0.405	0.271	0.400	0.311	0.323	0.290
0.229	0.125	0.230	0.101	0.195	0.175	0.141	0.131
0.129	0.051	0.104	0.064	0.118	0.073	0.067	0.042
0.020	0.006	0.011	0.014	0.019	0.009	0.004	0.014
0.047	0.034	0.041	0.039	0.059	0.038	0.024	0.005
0.011	0.002	0.007	0.005	0.011	0.004	0.002	0.005
0.056	0.003	0.039	0.012	0.037	0.023	0.020	0.014
0.020	0.013	0.022	0.008	0.022	0.009	0.017	0.009
0.535	0.394	0.556	0.338	0.514	0.419	0.451	0.374
0.767	0.496	0.756	0.448	0.742	0.569	0.532	0.467
1,017	1,276	1,253	1,040	850	768	461	214
9.153	8.140	9.144	7.979	9.032	8.593	8.156	7.687
[1.93]	[2.21]	[1.92]	[2.23]	[1.95]	[2.13]	[2.31]	[2.26]
889	984	1032	841	741	648	353	131
3.411	2.608	3.083	2.869	3.498	3.022	2.388	1.544
[1.97]	[1.99]	[2.07]	[1.96]	[2.03]	[1.97]	[1.82]	[1.63]
895	1,006	1,041	860	750	661	354	136

performance and processing of new material, which tends to decline substantially in adulthood (Schaie, 1994; Verhaegen and Salthouse, 1997). The latter includes knowledge and skills accumulated in the past, which are not as easily lost.

In this research, for simplicity, we classify cognitive abilities into two categories: mental intactness (MI) and episodic memory (EM). As shown in Table 12-2, three items are used to measure mental intactness: a serial-7 number subtraction question, time orientation, and picture drawing. The scores range from 0–5, 0–5, and 0–1, respectively. Orientation in time consists of three questions about the interview date (day, month, year), day of the week, and season, which were coded as dummies to indicate whether answers are correct. To measure episodic memory, we use imme-

TABLE 12-2 Definition of Cognitive Abilities

Types	Items	Survey Questions	Score
Mental intactness (0–11)	Numerical ability	What does 100 minus 7 equal? And 7 from that?..	0~5
	Time orientation	Please tell me today's date (year, month, day).	0~3
		Please tell me the day of the week.	0~1
		What is the current season (among Spring, Summer, Fall, or Winter)?	0~1
	Picture drawing	Do you see this picture? Please draw that picture on this paper.	0~1
Episodic memory (0–10)	Immediate word recall	Try to remember the words I just read to you. I'll ask you to recall them later.	0~10
	Delayed word recall	A little while ago, I read you a list of words and you repeated the ones you could remember. Please tell me any of the words that you remember now.	0~10

NOTES: Scores have been adjusted so that higher values indicate better cognitive function
Episodic memory is the mean of scores of immediate and delayed word recalls.
SOURCE: Data from CHARLS 2008 Pilot.

diate and delayed word recall. In the recall test, respondents are read a list of 10 simple nouns, then immediately asked to repeat as many of those words as possible in any order. After 20 questions concerning CESD, they are again asked to recall as many of the original words as possible. The item is coded as 1 if recalled by the interviewee, and as 0 if not. Scores for immediate and delayed recall both vary from 0 to 10. We follow the approach by McArdle, Smith, and Willis (2011), using the mean of scores in immediate and delayed word recall as the measure of episodic memory. Figure 12-1 depicts the different downward trends of mental intactness and episodic memory, where original average scores have been smoothed. Clearly both cognitive measures steadily decline with age, with the age pattern becoming more erratic as sample sizes in CHARLS 2008 become thinner at older ages. One caution in reading this graph is that the number of observations over aged 80 in the CHARLS data is relatively small (only 69 in total), so that the patterns start to become erratic at these ages.

Episodic memory is a very general measure of an important aspect of fluid intelligence since access to memory is basic to any type of cognitive ability. Most of the variation in this measure is picking out the low end—people with bad memory so social activities of the sort analyzed here may have noticeable impacts. Intact mental status, however, contains elements of both fluid and crystallized intelligence, needed for many cognitive tasks but not specific to any particular domain (see McArdle et al., 2011).

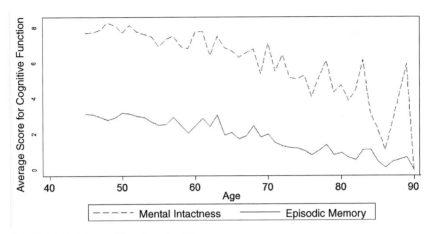

FIGURE 12-1 Cognition trend with age.
SOURCE: Data from CHARLS 2008 Pilot.

Other Variables

Other control variables are mainly concerned with demographics, socio-economic status, and community-level variables. Demographics include a quadratic in age to capture any nonlinear effect of age, sex (female = 1), marital status of the respondent (married = 1), location of household (urban or rural [urban = 1]), province of residence (Zhejiang or Gansu), number of children, and number of siblings. Number of children, including both biological and non-biological daughters and sons, serves as one measure for family support.

Socioeconomic status has two dimensions: education and log household expenditure per capita (log PCE). Education is classified into five discrete educational groups: illiterate, able to write or read, finished primary school, finished junior high school, finished senior high school or above. In the second category, "able to write or read" includes those not finishing primary school but capable of reading or writing, or those reported to have been in *Sishu*.[5] The category of "high school or above" includes those completing a senior high school, vocational school, college, or graduate level education. We also control log PCE to capture effects of financial resources. In rural developing economies, consumption expenditures represent the best measure of the economic resources available to the family (Strauss and Thomas, 2008).

---

[5]*Sishu* is an old-style private Chinese education that mainly taught young children Chinese classics before the 20th century.

Lastly, we include community demographics and socioeconomic status, since we believe that cognition may be affected by one's surrounding environment (Engelhardt et al., 2010; Hauser, 2009). Three aspects of the community are considered: demographics, public services, and a general community evaluation. For demographics, we include the sex ratio (the percentage female) and the number of big surnames (a surname shared by large numbers of people in the village). The latter is included since the possibility exists that some unobserved genetic factors systematically affect people's cognitive functions, and the number of big surnames may indicate relatives in the community with whom the respondent may interact so it may serve as a measure of social connectedness.

Community-level variables generated from the CHARLS community survey are used to capture public services. These community-level variables are derived from a separate survey of community leaders that describes current facilities and histories of the community. For example, the number of libraries and the distance from the community/village office to the most commonly used library are both used. Similarly, number and distance are asked for kindergartens, primary schools, middle schools, senior high schools, theatres, nursing homes, bus lines, and train station. We include a variable measuring percentage of people with one or more telephones and percentage with one or more mobile phones in the community. Accessibility and availability of public services is a reflection of social and economic capital in a society that is effective in improving people's health (Yip et al., 2007). For evaluation of community, we have three measures: (1) log public expenditure during the past year, (2) community log per capita expenditures, and (3) interviewer rating of whether community medical service is poor. Community log PCE is an average of individual respondents' log PCEs in each community.

Summary Statistics

Table 12-1 presents summary statistics for participation in social activities by sex, region, province, and age group. Fewer than half of respondents engaged in any kind of social activities, with 44% of women and 47% of men taking part. Interacting with friends is the most popular activity, with a participation rate of 34.5%, followed by Mahjong, chess, cards, or a club (17.1%), and only 8.6% participating in "other social activities."[6] Men are more active in playing Mahjong, chess, cards, or going to a club, doing voluntary or charity work, or attending an educational or training course, while women are more inclined to interact with friends.

Regional disparity is more pronounced than gender differences. Liv-

---

[6]There is some overlap among the various social activities.

ing in an urban area or in Zhejiang province has a great advantage in participation in social activities: 53.5% of urban people took part in social activities, compared with only 39.4% for those in rural areas. In Zhejiang, 55.6% of residents are involved in social activities, compared to only 33.8% of Gansu residents. Urban residents have a 7.4% higher participation rate in interacting with friends, and a 10.4% higher rate in playing Mahjong, chess, or cards. This rural-urban difference may be due partly to the urban elderly having more leisure time than rural elderly who are busy trying to make a living. One factor that likely impacts participation is accessibility and availability of activating facilities in the village/community, as discussed below.

The last four columns in Table 12-1 list social activity participation across four age groups. People become less engaged as they age, which may be partly due to declining health with age.[7] However, there are two exceptions: participation rates for interacting with friends drop sharply between ages 50–60 (from 40 to 31.1%). But then it bounces back up in the 60–70 age group (32.3%), indicating that while retirement may reduce interactions with work-related social networks, after a period of adjustment, people are able to socialize with friends outside of their former jobs. Taking part in a community-related organization demonstrates a similar pattern. This may be explained by the possibility that retirement detaches people from occupational positions in community-related organizations, but they once again become involved in such organizations as participants rather than staff.

Table 12-3 summarizes the distribution of test scores on the MI and EM of respondents, where large differences exist across sex, region, and age. The mean score for MI is 8.62 and for EM is 2.99. The description illustrates that women are on average much more cognitively impaired. Rural Gansu elderly are also more disadvantaged in both aspects of cognitive abilities. Comparing people of different age groups, the older group is associated with lower cognitive ability, which is consistent with cognition declining with aging.

Table 12-4 provides a summary of demographic and SES attributes across sex, region, province, and age groups. Our analytical sample has a mean age of 59.4, is about half female, 44.4% urban residents, and 54.6% Zhejiang residents. Age, sex, and location of residence do not significantly differ among these groups. Respondents have an average of 2.74 children and 3.21 siblings. Female, rural, and Gansu elderly have more

---

[7]These age patterns may reflect cohort effects as well, and cohort effects are plausible given the large changes in China over time. With only cross-sectional data, we cannot distinguish between age and cohort effects. The use of 10-year age groups centered on ages 50 and 60 reflects the fact that the official retirement age for urban women is 50 and for urban men is 60.

TABLE 12-3 Social Activity and Cognition

| | Interacting with Friends | | | | | |
| | Yes | | | No | | |
	All	Female	Male	All	Female	Male
Intactness score	8.9	8.47	9.37	8.47	7.971	8.88
	[1.994]	[2.162]	[1.668]	[2.210]	[2.370]	[1.973]
Memory score	3.33	3.17	3.51	2.79	2.666	2.9
	[2.001]	[2.021]	[1.965]	[2.01]	[2.053]	[1.967]
	Other Activities					
	Yes			No		
	All	Female	Male	All	Female	Male
Intactness score	9.59	9.382	9.83	8.53	8.034	8.98
	[1.694]	[1.808]	[1.522]	[2.160]	[2.312]	[1.905]
Memory score	3.89	4.044	3.71	2.9	2.733	3.05
	[1.934]	[1.815]	[2.065]	[2.009]	[2.038]	[1.971]

NOTE: Standard errors in brackets.
SOURCE: Data from CHARLS 2008 Pilot.

TABLE 12-4 Description of Other Characteristics: Demographics and SES

		Sex		Region	
Attributes	All	Male	Female	Urban	Rural
Demographics					
Age (45+)	59.44	60.10	58.80	59.32	59.53
Female	0.507	0	1	0.533	0.486
Urban	0.444	0.420	0.466	1.000	0.000
Zhejiang	0.546	0.544	0.549	0.666	0.451
No. of children	2.74	2.60	2.87	2.59	2.85
No. of siblings	3.21	3.05	3.37	3.24	3.19
SES					
Education					
Illiterate	0.425	0.247	0.598	0.332	0.498
Sishu/home school and below	0.189	0.233	0.145	0.187	0.190
Elementary school	0.171	0.231	0.112	0.190	0.155
Middle school	0.127	0.168	0.088	0.156	0.104
High school and above	0.088	0.119	0.057	0.133	0.052
Log PCE	8.408	8.429	8.388	8.689	8.185
Number of observations	2,293	1,131	1,162	1,017	1,276

SOURCE: Data from CHARLS 2008 Pilot.

Playing Mahjong, Chess, or Cards

Yes			No		
All	Female	Male	All	Female	Male
9.43 [1.587]	9.25 [1.739]	9.51 [1.506]	8.43 [2.214]	8.008 [2.333]	8.89 [1.980]
3.84 [1.923]	4.044 [1.882]	3.75 [1.938]	2.79 [1.994]	2.697 [2.024]	2.89 [1.957]

Any Activities

Yes			No		
All	Female	Male	All	Female	Male
9.02 [1.916]	8.596 [2.136]	9.41 [1.599]	8.25 [2.273]	7.785 [2.376]	8.7 [2.075]
3.39 [1.965]	3.282 [1.996]	3.49 [1.933]	2.62 [2.003]	2.496 [2.035]	2.74 [1.967]

Province		Age Group			
Zhejiang	Gansu	<50	50~60	60~70	>70
59.88	58.912	49.55	59.12	69.09	79.05
0.509	0.504	0.546	0.500	0.449	0.500
0.540	0.327	0.466	0.419	0.423	0.486
1	0	0.540	0.543	0.508	0.668
2.55	2.96	2.02	2.62	3.54	4.25
3.15	3.28	3.81	3.45	2.44	1.62
0.372	0.489	0.326	0.412	0.523	0.654
0.250	0.115	0.139	0.244	0.197	0.173
0.194	0.142	0.171	0.207	0.139	0.108
0.110	0.148	0.206	0.087	0.091	0.037
0.074	0.104	0.159	0.051	0.048	0.023
8.695	8.064	8.651	8.341	8.230	8.070
1,253	1,040	850	768	461	214

children and siblings than their male, urban, and Zhejiang counterparts. People of older ages have more children, but have fewer siblings.

The highest attained education level for these older Chinese respondents is generally low, and its distribution is skewed with more than 60% having failed to finish primary school, 42.5% are illiterate, and 18.9% can read or write. Only a small portion (11.9% of men and 5.7% of women) have reached a senior high school level education or above. A large sex discrepancy exists: 59.8% of women are illiterate, approximately twice the rate among men. Among men, 11.9% have attained a high school education or above, while only 5.7% of women have done the same.[8] Residents of Zhejiang and urban areas have a greater advantage in educational resources, leading to higher education levels for those residents. Not surprisingly given the rapid secular increase in education in China, education levels decline with age with people over 70 the most disadvantaged: as many as 65% are illiterate.

Disparities in log PCE are large between these two Chinese provinces, selected in part for their economic diversity. On average, log PCE is 8.69 for urban people, 8.19 for those living in rural areas, 8.70 for Zhejiang province, and 8.06 for Gansu province. Table 12-5 tabulates community characteristics by region and province. As shown, urban areas have a larger percentage of women, while the difference between Zhejiang and Gansu is much smaller. In addition, the table implies that urban regions and Zhejiang have better public services. Schools, libraries, theatres, and other places are more accessible (shorter distances indicate they are closer together). They also enjoy better economic status, with larger fractions of the population having telephones and mobile phones, and more expenditure and income per capita.

The Association of Social Activities and Cognitive Function

Table 12-3 displays the two-way association between participation in social activities and our two cognitive function measures—MI and EM. Those who participate in social activities uniformly have higher scores in mental intactness and episodic memory for both men and women, particularly sharp for episodic memory.

To go beyond a simple two-way association, we estimated OLS association regressions that control for other confounding factors in Tables 12-6 (for mental intactness) and 12-7 (for episodic memory). In each table, Models (1) and (2) display the results from two models with different

---

[8]In Lei et al. (2011), we found that Chinese women were less cognitively able than Chinese men with most but not all of that difference being explained by the lower education level of Chinese women in these generations.

TABLE 12-5 Description of Other Characteristics: Community

| Community-Level Variables | Overall | Region | | Province | |
		Urban	Rural	Zhejiang	Gansu
% of female	0.501	0.533	0.486	0.501	0.504
# of big surnames	1.615	1.476	1.679	1.428	1.831
# of kindergartens	1.098	1.479	0.719	1.168	0.979
distance from kindergarten	2.551	0.893	0.675	1.932	3.436
# of primary school	0.651	0.444	0.815	0.358	1.003
distance from primary school	0.772	1.991	4.150	2.998	0.129
# of middle schools	0.188	0.291	0.106	0.191	0.185
distance from middle school	3.190	1.993	3.106	1.305	3.590
# of senior high schools	0.045	0.101	0.000	0.066	0.019
distance from senior high school	11.461	5.848	15.789	8.129	15.588
# of post offices	0.181	0.313	0.076	0.163	0.203
distance from post office	4.224	2.057	6.000	2.809	5.989
# of libraries	0.438	0.657	0.264	0.629	0.209
distance from the library	8.726	3.363	12.765	2.552	16.255
# of theatres	0.085	0.170	0.017	0.073	0.099
distance from the theatre	13.367	5.469	19.875	7.347	21.004
# of nursing homes	0.081	0.128	0.043	0.095	0.064
distance from nursing home	9.491	6.668	11.619	3.848	18.530
# of bus lines	2.123	3.306	1.194	2.880	1.197
distance from bus line	2.253	0.886	3.313	0.434	4.502
distance from train station	81.811	81.665	81.915	84.846	78.399
% of people having telephones	64.714	73.178	60.800	74.218	53.716
% of people having cellphones	77.013	88.549	71.679	88.815	63.355
Whether the medical care is poor	0.017	0.023	0.013	0.000	0.036
Log public expenditure during the past year	8.514	10.469	7.621	11.936	4.560
Log per capita income	8.124	8.584	7.791	8.905	7.253
Observations	2,293	1,017	1,276	1,253	1,040

SOURCE: Data from CHARLS 2008 Pilot.

measures for social activities. In the first model, three separate social activities "interacting with friends," "playing Mahjong, chess, or attending a
club," and "taking part in other social activities" are included together
as the key explanatory variables; in the second model, we use instead the
variable "taking part in any of the social activities." In addition to these
cognitive measures, both models include standard demographic controls
(a quadratic in age, female, urban, Zhejiang residence, and the number of
children and number of siblings), economic controls (education and log
PCE), as well as detailed measures of the community in which the respondent lived. These variables are described in detail above.

Table 12-6 reports OLS association estimates on MI. When each type
of social activity is included in the model together, all coefficients on social
activities are positively related to MI but are statistically insignificant. MI
is positively associated but only at the 10% level with "any social activity."
Some of the lack of statistical significance on these individual measures of
social activity may well be due to the relatively small sample size in the
CHARLS pilot compared to other HRS surveys. While our main interest
lies in the associations between cognition and social activity, we briefly
discuss estimated relationships with the other variables in the model. For
demographics, an older age and female are associated with a worse mental status. Both associations are statistically significant. Regional disparities already presented in the descriptive summary are confirmed in this
table, but urban residence is no longer statistically significant when other
variables are included. Similarly, number of relatives (children or siblings)
is not associated with MI score when other variables are included. We
have assumed that more relatives lead to more social interactions. The
Chinese fertility rate has been lower in the more economically developed
areas, resulting in fewer children and siblings in urban areas, but our
results suggest no strong effect on elderly cognition will follow.

MI is highly influenced by all SES factors. Compared with those who
are illiterate, people with some education have a better mental status,
which is consistent with the hypothesis that education is a determinant
factor of the heterogeneity in cognitive functions in old age (Leibovici et
al., 1996). The results also imply that higher education is related to higher
MI scores, as the size of coefficients become increasingly larger moving
from lower levels to higher ones. As expected, household expenditure is
positively associated with MI.

With a few exceptions community-level variables are not statistically
significant. Among the few that are significant, better mental intactness is
associated with shorter distance between community center and the most-
commonly used middle school and/or a library and a higher number of
bus lines. The share of female population exhibits a positive sign, even
though the female dummy is negatively associated with cognition. We

TABLE 12-6 OLS Analysis of Effects of SA on MI

Independent Variables	Dependent Variable: Mental Intactness (0–11)			
	(1)		(2)	
Social Activities (no participation omitted)				
Interacting with friends	0.093	(0.086)		
Playing Mahjong, chess, or cards	0.032	(0.107)		
Other social activities	0.153	(0.144)		
Any of the above activities			0.175**	(0.082)
Demographics				
Age (45+)	0.129***	(0.048)	0.128***	(0.047)
Age squared/100	−0.135***	(0.039)	−0.135***	(0.038)
Female	−0.508***	(0.089)	−0.499***	(0.087)
Urban	0.110	(0.115)	0.107	(0.115)
Zhejiang	0.732***	(0.145)	0.723***	(0.145)
No. of children	0.058*	(0.034)	0.059*	(0.034)
No. of siblings	−0.012	(0.021)	−0.012	(0.021)
SES				
Education (illiterate omitted)				
Sishu/home school and below	1.293***	(0.115)	1.297***	(0.115)
Elementary school	1.497***	(0.120)	1.498***	(0.120)
Middle school	1.808***	(0.137)	1.812***	(0.136)
High school and above	2.262***	(0.160)	2.273***	(0.158)
Log PCE	0.130**	(0.052)	0.128**	(0.051)
Community				
% of female	0.021***	(0.007)	0.021***	(0.007)
# of big surnames	−0.036	(0.038)	−0.036	(0.038)
# of kindergartens	0.069*	(0.038)	0.068*	(0.038)
Distance from kindergarten	0.004	(0.007)	0.004	(0.007)
# of primary schools	0.057	(0.121)	0.056	(0.121)
Distance from primary school	0.112*	(0.058)	0.112*	(0.058)
# of middle schools	−0.005	(0.137)	−0.000	(0.137)
Distance from middle school	−0.061***	(0.018)	−0.061***	(0.018)
# of senior high schools	−0.132	(0.249)	−0.131	(0.249)
Distance from senior high school	−0.001	(0.005)	−0.001	(0.005)
# of post offices	0.020	(0.153)	0.020	(0.152)
Distance from post office	0.002	(0.013)	0.003	(0.013)
# of libraries	0.095	(0.078)	0.093	(0.078)
Distance from the library	−0.012**	(0.005)	−0.012**	(0.005)
# of theatres	−0.179	(0.186)	−0.164	(0.186)
Distance from the theatre	−0.005	(0.004)	−0.004	(0.004)
# of nursing homes	0.046	(0.171)	0.037	(0.171)
Distance from nursing home	0.006*	(0.003)	0.007*	(0.003)
# of bus lines	0.023*	(0.012)	0.024**	(0.012)
Distance from bus line	0.009	(0.010)	0.009	(0.010)
Distance from train station	0.000	(0.001)	0.001	(0.001)
% of people having telephones	0.001	(0.002)	0.001	(0.002)
% of people having cellphones	0.000	(0.002)	0.000	(0.002)
Log public expenditure during the past year	−0.000	(0.009)	−0.000	(0.009)
Log per capita income	−0.015	(0.060)	−0.015	(0.060)
Whether the medical care is poor	−0.528	(0.346)	−0.527	(0.346)
Observations	1,873		1,873	
R-squared	0.397		0.397	

NOTE: Standard errors in parentheses.* denotes p < 0.1; ** p < 0.05; *** p < 0.01.
SOURCE: Data from CHARLS 2008 Pilot.

think that the female population share represents the level of economic and social conditions in local areas. As shown in Table 12-5, although the share of female population is normal overall (50.1%), the maximum share reaches 53.3% and the lowest 48.6%. The unbalanced gender ratio is due to two reasons. First, in areas of longer life expectancy, women outlive men to create a higher ratio of females in the population. Second, in less developed areas where sons are valued more than daughters, sex-selective abortion produced highly skewed gender ratio among the younger population (Ebenstein, 2010). In both cases, a higher ratios of females is associated with better life conditions, which may be positively correlated with community cognition levels. Other community-level variables may not be able to fully capture these regional disparities. With prefecture fixed effects (not shown), the significance of percentage female disappears, supporting the hypotheses here.[9]

Table 12-7 illustrates a parallel OLS association estimation in which EM is regressed on variables representing social activities and the same set of other control variables included in the MI model.[10] Both any social activity participation collectively and interacting with friends or playing card games are strongly statistically associated with EM. In addition, in the second model that includes the single measure of participation in any social activity it is strongly related to our measure of episodic memory.

Looking next at the control variables, once again memory increases with age at a decreasing rate. Memory level reaches its peak at 47 ($= (0.134 * 100)/(2 * 0.142)$) years of age, after which it starts declining. Unlike the disparity between men and women for mental intactness, there is generally no sex difference for EM and no statistically significant relationship with the number of relatives. All regional measures—urban and province—are also not significant, suggesting that the other covariates (mostly likely education and income) pick up the regional disparities displayed in the descriptive tables. Once again, education and log PCE are strongly related to our cognitive measure—in this case, episodic memory.

From the bottom panel, most community-level variables are statistically insignificant. Similar to the prior table, distance between community center and most-commonly used middle school is negatively correlated with episodic memory. Episodic memory is positively associated with the number of kindergartens in the community. These results indicate that availability and access to education resources may play important roles in improving people's mental health. Taking account of unobserved

---

[9]A prefecture is an administrative district that is between province and county or county-level city.

[10]As the two dependent variables have different missing values, observations of these two regressions are slightly different.

TABLE 12-7 OLS Analysis of Effects of SA on EM

Independent Variables	Dependent Variable: Episodic Memory (0–10)			
	(1)		(2)	
Social Activities (no participation omitted)				
Interacting with friends	0.222**	(0.088)		
Playing Mahjong, chess, or cards	0.459***	(0.110)		
Other social activities	0.186	(0.149)		
Any of the above activities			0.404***	(0.084)
Demographics				
Age (45+)	0.133***	(0.049)	0.134***	(0.049)
Age squared/100	−0.140***	(0.040)	−0.142***	(0.040)
Female	0.036	(0.091)	0.004	(0.090)
Urban	0.157	(0.118)	0.155	(0.118)
Zhejiang	−0.191	(0.147)	−0.196	(0.147)
No. of children	−0.028	(0.035)	−0.026	(0.035)
No. of siblings	0.000	(0.022)	−0.002	(0.022)
SES				
Education (illiterate omitted)				
Sishu/home school and below	0.610***	(0.118)	0.632***	(0.118)
Elementary school	0.866***	(0.123)	0.877***	(0.123)
Middle school	1.541***	(0.141)	1.562***	(0.140)
High school and above	1.508***	(0.165)	1.564***	(0.163)
Log PCE	0.160***	(0.053)	0.169***	(0.052)
Community				
% of female	0.012	(0.007)	0.013*	(0.007)
# of big surnames	0.085**	(0.039)	0.089**	(0.039)
# of kindergartens	0.067*	(0.039)	0.068*	(0.039)
Distance from kindergarten	−0.006	(0.007)	−0.006	(0.007)
# of primary schools	−0.008	(0.124)	−0.006	(0.124)
Distance from primary school	0.051	(0.060)	0.047	(0.060)
# of middle schools	−0.069	(0.142)	−0.035	(0.142)
Distance from middle school	−0.041**	(0.018)	−0.040**	(0.018)
# of senior high schools	−0.002	(0.260)	−0.021	(0.261)
Distance from senior high school	0.002	(0.005)	0.002	(0.005)
# of post offices	0.224	(0.155)	0.203	(0.155)
Distance from post office	−0.006	(0.013)	−0.007	(0.013)
# of libraries	0.146*	(0.081)	0.153*	(0.081)
Distance from the library	0.005	(0.006)	0.005	(0.006)
# of theatres	−0.126	(0.190)	−0.112	(0.190)
Distance from the theatre	−0.005	(0.005)	−0.006	(0.005)
# of nursing homes	−0.228	(0.176)	−0.248	(0.177)
Distance from nursing home	0.001	(0.004)	0.002	(0.004)
# of bus lines	0.004	(0.013)	0.004	(0.013)
Distance from bus line	0.006	(0.010)	0.006	(0.010)
Distance from train station	0.000	(0.001)	0.001	(0.001)
% of people having telephones	0.003	(0.002)	0.003	(0.002)
% of people having cellphones	−0.001	(0.002)	−0.001	(0.002)
Log public expenditure during the past year	−0.019**	(0.009)	−0.018**	(0.009)
Log per capita income	0.136**	(0.061)	0.142**	(0.061)
Whether the medical care is poor	0.041	(0.356)	0.041	(0.356)
Observations	1,901		1,901	
R-squared	0.279		0.276	

NOTE: Standard errors in parentheses.* denotes $p < 0.1$; ** $p < 0.05$; *** $p < 0.01$.
SOURCE: Data from CHARLS 2008 Pilot.

prefecture level variations in culture, climate, and geographic factors that may affect cognition, we also estimated prefecture fixed effects models. The results (not shown) are remarkably similar to those contained in Tables 12-6 and 12-7. The significance and magnitudes of coefficients on SA do not change much.

Summarizing our results, OLS association regressions with multiple SA measures provide evidence of a positive correlation between cognitive functioning and participation in social activities. Despite the salient association, closer scrutiny is needed because OLS regressions may be biased due to the endogeneity of people's participation decisions, an issue presented in the next section.

THE ASSOCIATION OF COMMUNITY FACILITIES AND COGNITIVE FUNCTION

OLS estimates of the association between social activities and cognitive functions do not have a causal interpretation as unobserved heterogeneity may introduce a correlation between social activities and cognitive function. Sources of this unobserved heterogeneity may include aspects of the environment, people's preferences, and personalities. While the natural environment is controllable to some extent by including community-level variables in the models, the other sources of individual heterogeneity are not easy to control. Although we include a rich set of individual and spatial variables in our model, they cannot be perfectly controlled for. Another possible source of bias is reverse causality—taking part in social activities requires some minimum cognitive skills or people with cognitive impairment deliberately seek social activities as therapy for slowing down the decline.

One option to get around this problem is to find instrumental variables. We have a set of instruments in mind, i.e., the availability of community facilities that accommodate social gatherings. For example, in 1995, the Chinese government started the Universal Exercise Plan (1995–2010) encouraging Chinese people to participate in physical activities. In the past decade, especially during pre-Olympic years, enforcement of the plan was strengthened. Accompanying this was a larger governmental investment in community recreational facilities/organizations and advocacy for participating in exercises. This development is different across community/village because of variation in the capacity for building facilities and the strength of local leaders. Because there is no evidence that this difference is directly related to cognition function, these variables can serve as candidates for IVs for social activities. However, probably because the number of communities in our sample is relatively small, these variables do not pass weak instrument tests. Thus, instead of directly tackling the causal relationship, we opt to estimate OLS reduced form equations to test whether these variables are associated with cognitive function.

The CHARLS community survey contains information on whether a village/community has certain facilities/organizations shown on a list. There are 15 items on the list: (1) a basketball court, (2) a swimming pool, (3) outside exercising facilities, (4) outdoor sports facilities, (5) rooms for card games and chess games, (6) rooms for playing ping-pong, (7) calligraphy and painting associations, (8) other entertainment facilities, (9) dancing teams or other exercise organizations, (10) organizations for helping the elderly and the frail, (11) employment services, (12) healthcare organizations, (13) activity centers for elderly, (14) elderly associations, and (15) nursing homes.

The first variable of community facility, "outdoor facilities," takes value 1 if the community has outdoor recreational facilities (1–4 on the list). Having outdoor facilities provide people with place(s) to gather. The second variable, "whether there are activity centers for the elderly" (item 13) is necessary for people to play Mahjong, chess, or cards, or participate in a club. The third variable is the dummy indicating whether the community has organizations that help the elderly and the handicapped (item 10). We also create a variable indicating whether the community has any of the three types of facilities. The items in the survey question not utilized include employment service, healthcare organizations, elderly associations, and nursing homes. Though important facilities and organizations, these items are omitted due to their possible direct impact on people's cognitive health (for instance, employment services teach people job skills and knowledge that improves cognition, and healthcare organizations enhance mental intactness and cure cognitive diseases such as dementia). As the purpose of examining the facilities is to explore the effect of social activities on cognition, we only keep those that are likely to affect cognition through affecting social activities. The detailed distributions of these facility variables by residency and province are reported in Appendix Table 12-A1.

Table 12-3 depicts the relationship between facility variables and their corresponding SAs, showing that the facility variables are highly associated with SA participation among the elderly, consistent with the mechanisms discussed above. Tables 12-8 and 12-9 give the OLS reduced form estimates of the associations of community facilities and the two types of cognitive functions, MI and EM, respectively. Similarly as before, we employ two models in each table. Model 1 includes the three types of facilities separately, while Model 2 only the aggregate facility measure "any of the above facilities." From Table 12-8, the facility measures do not significantly affect mental intactness, which is consistent with the results in the OLS association estimation in Table 12-6, where almost all social activity measures lack significance on the correlation with mental intactness.

Table 12-9 replaces MI as the dependent variable with EM. As seen from the first model, having activity centers for the elderly is significantly (at 1% level) associated with better episodic memory, while the other two types of facilities are not. These results are also consistent with the OLS association estimates in Table 12-6 where we see significant (at 1% level) correlation between playing Mahjong, chess, or cards. The likely explanation is that having activity centers for the elderly allowing for more involvement in playing Mahjong, chess, or cards, which further promotes episodic memory. Accordingly, from the second model, we see significant correlation between any of the facilities and episodic memory, which is most likely driven by the effect of having activity centers for the elderly.

In sum, we interpret our results as providing some support for the hypothesis that taking part in social activities could help slow down the cognitive decline of the elderly. The results are consistent with findings from Glei et al. (2005) that employed a similar definition and was based on data from Taiwan, where the tradition of living arrangement is most similar. This indicates that social participation plays an important role even in a society where family members are more likely to live together, regardless of level of economic development. Our results also imply that providing more activity facilities in the community could be helpful to the cognitive health of the elderly as facilities involve more people in social activities. We are cautious in our interpretation since we do not directly estimate the causal effects especially in light of the relatively small sizes in the CHARLS pilot, which was fielded in only two provinces. Most sample sizes in the HRS network of surveys exceed 10,000 households, and China is a very heterogeneous country, which makes larger samples even more important. The availability of the full CHARLS survey, especially its panel, in a few years with much higher samples will help provide additional tests of our hypothesis.

CONCLUSIONS

With data from the 2008 CHARLS pilot, this chapter explores the relation between SA and cognitive outcomes for Chinese elderly aged 45 and older, where cognition is composed of two dimensions—MI and EM. There are several key limitations to our analysis. Most important, we are only able to examine two Chinese provinces with moderate sample sizes and must rely for now on cross-sectional analysis. A larger sample size spanning the entire country would not only address the issue of representativeness, but also provide greater variation across communities—the

TABLE 12-8 OLS Reduced Form Analysis of Community Facilities on MI

Independent Variables	Dependent Variable: Mental Intactness (0–11)			
	(1)		(2)	
Community Facilities				
Outdoor facilities	0.042	(0.166)		
Activity centers for the elderly	0.028	(0.125)		
Organizations for helping the elderly and the handicapped	−0.069	(0.128)		
Any of the above			−0.046	(0.128)
Demographics				
Age (45+)	0.128***	(0.048)	0.129***	(0.048)
Age squared/100	−0.135***	(0.039)	−0.135***	(0.039)
Female	−0.499***	(0.087)	−0.499***	(0.087)
Urban	0.121	(0.117)	0.117	(0.115)
Zhejiang	0.736***	(0.166)	0.760***	(0.146)
No. of children	0.056	(0.035)	0.056	(0.035)
No. of siblings	−0.011	(0.021)	−0.011	(0.021)
SES				
Education (illiterate omitted)				
Sishu/home school and below	1.294***	(0.115)	1.296***	(0.115)
Elementary school	1.504***	(0.120)	1.506***	(0.120)
Middle school	1.827***	(0.137)	1.826***	(0.137)
High school and above	2.313***	(0.158)	2.311***	(0.158)
Log PCE	0.135***	(0.052)	0.139***	(0.051)
Community				
% of female	0.022***	(0.007)	0.022***	(0.007)
# of big surnames	−0.039	(0.039)	−0.038	(0.038)
# of kindergartens	0.075*	(0.041)	0.069*	(0.038)
Distance from kindergarten	0.004	(0.007)	0.004	(0.007)
# of primary schools	0.053	(0.123)	0.056	(0.121)
Distance from primary school	0.101*	(0.060)	0.113*	(0.060)
# of middle schools	0.016	(0.141)	0.001	(0.137)
Distance from middle school	−0.062***	(0.018)	−0.062***	(0.018)
# of senior high schools	−0.189	(0.277)	−0.133	(0.250)
Distance from senior high school	−0.001	(0.005)	−0.001	(0.005)
# of post offices	0.012	(0.160)	0.037	(0.155)
Distance from post office	0.003	(0.013)	0.002	(0.013)
# of libraries	0.092	(0.079)	0.089	(0.079)
Distance from the library	−0.012**	(0.006)	−0.012**	(0.005)
# of theatres	−0.165	(0.187)	−0.173	(0.186)
Distance from the theatre	−0.004	(0.004)	−0.005	(0.004)
# of nursing homes	0.032	(0.176)	0.049	(0.173)
Distance from nursing home	0.007*	(0.004)	0.007*	(0.003)
# of bus lines	0.025*	(0.013)	0.022*	(0.012)
Distance from bus line	0.007	(0.010)	0.008	(0.010)
Distance from train station	0.000	(0.001)	0.000	(0.001)
% of people having telephones	0.001	(0.002)	0.001	(0.002)
% of people having cellphones	0.000	(0.002)	0.000	(0.002)
Log public expenditure during the past year	0.000	(0.009)	−0.000	(0.009)
Log per capita income	−0.012	(0.067)	−0.010	(0.061)
Whether the medical care is poor	−0.552	(0.353)	−0.519	(0.346)
Observations	1,873		1,873	
R-squared	0.396		0.396	

NOTE: Standard errors in parentheses.* denotes $p < 0.1$; ** $p < 0.05$; *** $p < 0.01$.
SOURCE: Data from CHARLS 2008 Pilot.

TABLE 12-9 OLS Reduced Form Analysis of Effects of Community Facilities on EM

Independent Variables	Dependent Variable: Episodic Memory (0–10)			
	(1)		(2)	
Community Facilities				
Outdoor facilities	0.266	(0.171)		
Activity centers for the elderly	0.408***	(0.128)		
Organizations for helping the elderly and the handicapped	−0.022	(0.132)		
Any of the above			0.540***	(0.131)
Demographics				
Age (45+)	0.129***	(0.049)	0.130***	(0.049)
Age squared/100	−0.139***	(0.040)	−0.141***	(0.040)
Female	−0.010	(0.090)	−0.014	(0.090)
Urban	0.142	(0.120)	0.133	(0.119)
Zhejiang	−0.239	(0.168)	−0.231	(0.149)
No. of children	−0.019	(0.036)	−0.018	(0.036)
No. of siblings	0.001	(0.022)	0.002	(0.022)
SES				
Education (illiterate omitted)				
Sishu/home school and below	0.615***	(0.119)	0.614***	(0.119)
Elementary school	0.887***	(0.123)	0.878***	(0.123)
Middle school	1.570***	(0.141)	1.544***	(0.141)
High school and above	1.635***	(0.163)	1.631***	(0.162)
Log PCE	0.183***	(0.053)	0.184***	(0.052)
Community				
% of female	0.010	(0.007)	0.009	(0.007)
# of big surnames	0.068*	(0.040)	0.076*	(0.039)
# of kindergartens	0.091**	(0.042)	0.046	(0.039)
Distance from kindergarten	−0.005	(0.008)	−0.005	(0.008)
# of primary schools	0.037	(0.126)	0.028	(0.124)
Distance from primary school	0.017	(0.061)	−0.021	(0.062)
# of middle schools	0.045	(0.146)	−0.034	(0.142)
Distance from middle school	−0.037**	(0.019)	−0.033*	(0.019)
# of senior high schools	−0.359	(0.289)	−0.131	(0.262)
Distance from senior high school	0.002	(0.005)	0.006	(0.005)
# of post offices	0.051	(0.163)	0.088	(0.158)
Distance from post office	−0.002	(0.013)	−0.002	(0.013)
# of libraries	0.171**	(0.081)	0.191**	(0.082)
Distance from the library	0.005	(0.006)	0.006	(0.006)
# of theatres	−0.111	(0.192)	−0.178	(0.190)
Distance from the theatre	−0.006	(0.005)	−0.008*	(0.005)
# of nursing homes	−0.390**	(0.182)	−0.336*	(0.178)
Distance from nursing home	0.001	(0.004)	0.002	(0.004)
# of bus line	0.003	(0.013)	0.006	(0.013)
Distance from bus line	0.001	(0.010)	0.003	(0.010)
Distance from train station	0.001	(0.001)	0.001	(0.001)
% of people having telephones	0.002	(0.002)	0.002	(0.002)
% of people having cellphones	0.000	(0.002)	0.001	(0.002)
Log public expenditure during the past year	−0.017*	(0.009)	−0.016*	(0.009)
Log per capita income	0.099	(0.068)	0.101	(0.062)
Whether the medical care is poor	−0.071	(0.364)	−0.003	(0.357)
Observations	1,901		1,901	
R–squared	0.272		0.274	

NOTE: Standard errors in parentheses.* denotes p < 0.1; ** p < 0.05; *** p < 0.01.
SOURCE: Data from CHARLS 2008 Pilot.

analytical center of our analysis. Panel samples will aid in identification of causal pathways.

Our major findings are roughly half of Chinese aged 45 and older take part in social activities. Second, participation in social activities is highly dependent on respondents' socioeconomic status and community environment. Third, OLS association results show that playing Mahjong, chess, or card games and interacting with friends are significantly related to episodic memory, both individually and taken as a whole (any of the three activities); individually, they are not related to mental intactness, while taken as a whole they are. Fourth, having an activity center in the community is significantly related to higher episodic memory but has no relation to mental intactness. These results point to a possible causal relationship between social activities and cognitive function, especially in strengthening short-term memory. Our research suggests that an effective way to maintain cognitive abilities at advanced ages may be to improve community facilities, such as by providing Mahjong rooms or other entertainment facilities.

APPENDIX TABLE 12-A1 Distribution of Community Facilities

Instrumental Variables	All	Region		Province	
		Urban	Rural	Zhejiang	Gansu
Outdoor facilities	0.101	0.161	0.053	0.080	0.126
	(.301)	(.368)	(.223)	(.271)	(.332)
Activity centers for the elderly	0.496	0.698	0.335	0.753	0.187
	(.500)	(.459)	(.472)	(.431)	(.390)
Organizations for helping the elderly and the handicapped	0.307	0.528	0.130	0.335	0.272
	(.461)	(.500)	(.337)	(.472)	(.445)
For any SA: Any of the facilities above	0.591	0.824	0.405	0.814	0.322
	(.492)	(.381)	(.491)	(.389)	(.468)
Number of facilities	0.904	1.387	0.518	1.168	0.585
	(.901)	(.901)	(.690)	(.770)	(.943)
Observations	2,293	1,017	1,276	1,253	1,040

NOTE: Standard errors in parentheses.* denotes p < 0.1; ** p < 0.05; *** p < 0.01.
SOURCE: Data from CHARLS 2008 Pilot.

REFERENCES

Allaire, J.C., and M. Marsiske. (1999). Everyday cognition: Age and intellectual ability correlates. *Psychology and Aging* 14(4):627-644. Available: http://www.ncbi.nlm.nih.gov/pmc/articles/PMC2904910/.

China Center for Economic Research, Peking University. (2008). *China Health and Retirement Longitudinal Survey.* Available: http://charls.ccer.edu.cn/charls/data.asp.

Ebenstein, A. (2010). The "missing girls" of China and the unintended consequences of the one child policy. *Journal of Human Resources* 45:87-115.

Engelhardt, H., I. Buber, V. Skirbekk, and A. Prskawetz. (2010). Social involvement, behavioural risks and cognitive functioning among the aged. *Ageing and Society* 30. doi: 10.1017/S0144686X09990626. Available: http://www.share-austria.at/fileadmin/user_upload/articles/2010_Cognitivefunctioning.pdf.

Glei, D.A., D.A. Landau, N. Goldman, Y-L. Chuang, G. Rodríguez, and M. Weinstein. (2005). Participating in social activities helps preserve cognitive function. *International Journal of Epidemiology* 34(4):864-871. Available: http://www.ncbi.nlm.nih.gov/pubmed/15764689.

Hauser, R.M. (2009). Causes and consequences of cognitive functioning across the life course. *Educational Researcher* 39(2):95-109.

Hsu, H.C. (2007). Does social participation by the elderly reduce mortality and cognitive impairment? *Aging & Mental Health* 11(6):699-707.

Lei, X., Y. Hu, J.J. McArdle, J.P. Smith, and Y. Zhao. (2011). *Gender Differences in Cognition Among Older Adults in China.* Working Paper #WR-881. Available: http://www.rand.org/content/dam/rand/pubs/working_papers/2011/RAND_WR881.pdf.

Leibovici, D., K. Ritchie, B. Ledesert, and D. Touchon. (1996). Does education level determine the course of cognitive decline? *Age and Ageing* 25:392-397.

Levy, R. (1994). Aging-associated cognitive decline. *International Psychogeriatrics* 663-668. Available: http://journals.cambridge.org/action/displayAbstract?fromPage=online&aid=272198.

Löckenhoff, C.E., and L.L. Carstensen. (2004). Socio-emotional selectivity theory, aging, and health: The increasingly delicate balance between regulating emotions and making tough choices. *Journal of Personality* 72(6):1,395-1,424. Available: http://www.ncbi.nlm.nih.gov/pubmed/15509287.

McArdle, J.J., J.P. Smith, and R. Willis. (2011). Cognition and economic outcomes in the Health and Retirement Survey. Pp. 209-236 in *Explorations in the Economics of Aging,* D. Wise (Ed.). Chicago: University of Chicago Press.

Schaie, K.W. (1994). The course of adult intellectual development. *American Psychologist* 49:304-313.

Smith, J.P., Y. Shen, J. Strauss, Z. Yang, and Y. Zhao. (2012). The effects of childhood health on adult health and SES in China. *Economic Development and Cultural Change.*

Strauss, J., and D. Thomas, D. (2008). Health over the life course. In *Handbook of Development Economics, Volume 4,* T.P. Schultz and J. Strauss (Eds.). Amsterdam: North Holland Press.

Tilvis, R.S., M.H. Kähönen-Väre, J. Jolkkonen, J. Valvanne, K.H. Pitkala, and T.E. Strandberg. (2004). Predictors of cognitive decline and mortality of aged people over a 10-year period. *The Journals of Gerontology. Series A, Biological Sciences and Medical Sciences* 59(3): 268-274. Available: http://www.ncbi.nlm.nih.gov/pubmed/15031312.

Verhaegen, P., and T.A. Salthouse. (1997). Meta-analyses of age-cognition relations in adulthood. Estimates of linear and nonlinear age effects and structural models. *Psychological Bulletin* 122(3):231-249.

Wang, H.X., A. Karp, B. Winblad, and L. Fratiglioni. (2002). Decreased risk of dementia: A longitudinal study from the Kungsholmen Project. *American Journal of Epidemiology* 155(12):1,081-1,087.

Yip, W., S.V. Subramanian, A.D. Mitchell, T.S.L. Dominic, J. Wang, and I. Kawachi. (2007). Does social capital enhance health and well-being? Evidence from rural China. *Social Science & Medicine* 64:35-49.

Zhao, Y., J. Strauss, A. Park, Y. Shen, and Y. Sun. (2009). *Chinese Health and Retirement Longitudinal Study, Pilot, User's Guide.* Peking: Peking University, National School of Development.

Zunzunegui, M-V., B.E. Alvarado, T. Del Ser, and A. Otero. (2003). Social networks, social integration, and social engagement determine cognitive decline in community-dwelling Spanish older adults. *The Journals of Gerontology. Series B, Psychological Sciences and Social Sciences* 58(2):S93-S100. Available: http://www.ncbi.nlm.nih.gov/pubmed/12646598.

Health and Well-Being

13

Socioeconomic Success and Health in Later Life: Evidence from the Indonesia Family Life Survey[1]

Firman Witoelar, John Strauss, and *Bondan Sikoki*

Indonesia has been undergoing a health and nutrition transition over the past 20 years and more. Overall, health of the population has been improving, as indicated by a continuing rise in attained adult heights for men and women over the entire 20th century (heights of both men and women increased by about 1 cm per decade over this period, Strauss and Thomas, 1995; Strauss et al., 2004). In Indonesia, infectious diseases caused 72% of all deaths in 1980; by 1992, noninfectious conditions caused more than half of the country's deaths (Indonesian Public Health Association, 1993). As part of the reason for the increase in deaths from chronic conditions, body mass indices (BMIs) have been rising for middle-aged people and the elderly, as has been noted more generally in Asia (see, for example, Monteiro et al., 2004; Popkin, 1994; Strauss and Thomas, 2008; Strauss et al., 2004). In Indonesia, body mass among the aged population has been rising rapidly, especially for women, as has waist circumference. On the other hand, hemoglobin levels have also been rising, though from low levels, leading to improved health. Yet, other health measures have been fairly steady as shown in the Indonesia Family Life Survey (IFLS),

---

[1]An earlier version of this chapter was presented at the annual meetings of the Population Association of America, April 2009, Detroit, Michigan, and the World Congress of the International Union for the Scientific Study of Population, October 2009, Marrakesh, Morocco. We thank Paul Heaton, James P. Smith, and other participants of the RAND Labor and Population Workshop for their very helpful comments. All errors are ours. Witoelar gratefully acknowledges the financial support of the World Bank's Research Support Budget. The views expressed here do not necessarily reflect those of the World Bank and of its member countries.

including the prevalence of hypertension. In terms of measures of health outcomes, while some trends seem upwards, specifically the movement out of undernutrition and communicable diseases, there seems at the same time to have been a movement toward more risk factors that are likely to lead to future chronic problems, but not universally so. Related to this, other symptoms, such as low levels of HDL cholesterol, are very high, especially for men, and the extremely high rate of current male smoking does not yet show a downward trend (Witoelar, Strauss, and Sikoki, 2009).

The backdrop of these important health and nutrition transitions is a country where the formal social safety system is still in its infancy and policies and programs that are designed to address specific challenges brought about by an aging population are still lacking.[2,3] As in many developing countries in the region, elderly in Indonesia mostly rely on children and family networks for old-age support, either through co-residency or transfers (Cameron and Cobb-Clark, 2008). With the elderly population becoming more exposed to risk of chronic and noncommunicable diseases, the issues of elderly care are becoming increasingly important.[4] Understanding the socioeconomic status (SES) correlates of elderly health outcomes will help to improve knowledge that could be useful in designing health as well as social programs to improve the well-being of the elderly in Indonesia.

In this chapter, we document the health and nutrition transition that the elderly population in Indonesia has undergone in the 15 years between 1993 and 2008, using the four full waves of the Indonesia Family Life Survey (IFLS).[5] This period spans a period of rapid economic growth from 1993 to 1997, a major financial crisis starting at the end of 1997 going through 1998 and 1999, and a major economic expansion starting in 2000, continuing through early 2008. IFLS is uniquely suited to look at changes over time, both for age groups and for birth cohorts in Indonesia, as it is a panel survey covering most of the country. Indonesia, like other developing countries in Asia and Latin America, has been aging rapidly. In 1980, only 3.4% of the population was aged 65 and older; by 2010, it was projected to be 6.1%, and by 2040, 14.7% (Kinsella and He, 2009). The population aged 65 and older is projected to double between 2000 and 2020 and again by 2040. We examine the IFLS sample 45 years and older

---

[2]An important bill on social safety nets was passed in October 2004 (Law no 40/2004). It includes a number of provisions that are important for elderly such as pensions, old-age savings, and health coverage, but has yet to be implemented.

[3]See Abikusno (2009) for a review of past and recent laws and government policies related to elderly in Indonesia.

[4]Van Eeuwijk (2006) argues that the epidemiological health transition has necessitated a shift from a "cure" to "care" paradigm in healthcare delivery in urban areas in Indonesia.

[5]IFLS1 was fielded in 1993, IFLS2 in 1997, IFLS3 in 2000, and IFLS4 in 2007–2008.

in each of the four waves, pretending that we have a series of independent cross-sections. Age 45 is chosen because it corresponds to early retirement age in Indonesia and is the age cutoff used in the new Health and Retirement Study type surveys being done in Asia.[6]

We focus in this chapter on examining changes over time for a series of health outcomes and behaviors, mainly using biomarkers. The health outcomes that we focus on are body mass index (BMI), waist circumference (a measure of body fat, given BMI), blood hemoglobin, total and HDL cholesterol levels, hypertension, cognition measured by word recall, and an index of depression (the short CES-D).[7] This is a much broader set of health indicators than is usually analyzed, in large part because such a rich set of health data is not usually available in broad-purposed socioeconomic surveys.

In addition to looking at trends in IFLS, we examine the correlations between these health outcomes and behaviors, and a series of SES variables: own education and the log of household per-capita expenditure (*pce*). In all cases, we examine the data separately for men and women and include age, period, and cohort effects (normalized), as well as dummy variables for province and rural area, alone and interacted with year of survey.

We find that the nutrition transition has progressed strongly in Indonesia over the 15-year period 1993–2008. Large increases in overweight have occurred for both men and women aged 45 years and older. For women, a full 33% are now overweight and for men, 10 percentage points less. On the other side of the coin, underweight has dramatically decreased, although among the current older population, it is still a problem. Related to nutrition, blood hemoglobin has improved over this period, especially since 2000. However, levels of hemoglobin are still low by international standards. On the other hand, hypertension has been constant over the period since 1997, since IFLS has been measuring it.

We find strong, positive correlations between SES and good health outcomes in most cases except hypertension and cholesterol. We recognize that causality runs both ways. We allow for interactions between one SES variable—education—and age and find that education tends to suppress the negative impact of age on many health outcomes. For hypertension we have data not only on measured prevalence, but also on doctor

---

[6]These are the China Health and Retirement Longitudinal Study (CHARLS), Japanese Study of Aging and Retirement (JSTAR), Korean Longitudinal Study of Ageing (KLoSA), and Longitudinal Study of Aging in India (LASI).

[7]We also examine the degree to which older Indonesians have difficulties with Activities of Daily Living and Instrumental Activities of Daily Living (ADLs and IADLS, respectively) and their self-reported general health status, as well as two important inputs for elderly health: smoking and physical activity. The results are available in Witoelar, Strauss, and Sikoki (2009).

diagnosis. We find a very high level of underdiagnosis of hypertension, which is strongly, negatively associated with SES for women, but not associated for men. Even among those who have been diagnosed, a large proportion claim not to be taking medications. We speculate that for other chronic health conditions, the degree of underdiagnosis is likely to also be quite high, suggesting the need for major health campaigns directed both at the general population and very specifically at doctors and other health providers.

DATA AND METHODOLOGY

The Indonesia Family Life Survey is a general-purpose survey designed to provide data for studying many different behaviors and outcomes. The survey contains a wealth of information collected at the individual and household levels, including indicators of economic and noneconomic well-being. In particular for this chapter, IFLS collects a rich set of information on health outcomes, in particular on many biomarkers.

IFLS is an ongoing longitudinal survey. The first wave, IFLS1, was conducted in 1993–1994. The survey sample represented about 83% of the Indonesian population living in 13 of the country's 26 provinces.[8] IFLS2 followed up with the same sample four years later, in 1997. IFLS2 ended in December 1997, just as the financial crisis was beginning, so it serves as an immediate baseline. IFLS3 was fielded on the full sample in 2000, three years after the crisis, and IFLS4 in 2007–2008, some 10 years after. Thus, IFLS from 1993 to 2008 provides a period of still-strong economic growth, followed by a major economic crash and recovery.

In this chapter, for some purposes we treat each year as though it were an independent cross-section, in order to explore how prevalence of different measures have evolved cross-sectionally for a particular age group, those aged 45 and older. For the regressions, though, we test pooling across years and then pool with some interactions after we fail to reject that SES coefficients are the same over the four waves. We do not employ dynamic models in this chapter and so do not use the panel nature directly; we will deal with these topics in another chapter.

One potential worry in a study like this over a 15-year period is sample

---

[8]Public-use files from IFLS1 are documented in six volumes under the series title *The 1993 Indonesian Family Life Survey*, DRU-1195/1–6-NICHD/AID, The RAND Corporation, December 1995. IFLS2 public-use files are documented in seven volumes under the series *The Indonesia Family Life Survey*, DRU-2238/1-7-NIA/NICHD, RAND, 2000. IFLS3 public-use files are documented in six volumes under the series *The Third Wave of the Indonesia Family Life Survey (IFLS3)*, WR-144/1-NIA/NICHD. IFLS4 public-use files are documented in the six volumes under the series *The Fourth Wave of the Indonesia Family Life Survey (IFLS4)*, WR-675/1-NIA/NICHD.

attrition. However, the attrition in IFLS is quite low. In IFLS1, 7,224 households were interviewed, and detailed individual-level data were collected
from over 22,000 individuals. In IFLS2, 94.4% of IFLS1 households were
re-contacted (interviewed or died). In IFLS3, the re-contact rate was 95.3%
of IFLS1 dynasty households (any part of the original IFLS1 households).
In IFLS4, the recontact rate of original IFLS1 dynasties was 93.6% (of
course, the period between waves was seven years, not three). Among
IFLS1 dynasties, 90.3% were either interviewed in all four waves or died.
Of some 6,523 households, 6,329, or 87.6%, were actually interviewed in
all four waves.[9] These re-contact rates are as high as or higher than most
longitudinal surveys in the United States and Europe. For the regressions,
we do not weight, but for the descriptive tables we do weight, both for
the sampling procedures (which oversampled urban areas and some outer
provinces) and for attrition (see Strauss et al., 2009, for details of weight-
ing). The weights provide the inverse probability that a household and
individual were sampled and appeared in IFLS in each wave.

To look at the associations of SES and health outcomes under a multivariate context, we run a set of regressions. The specification, which is
used for all health outcomes analyzed in this chapter, is as follows. In
results not shown, we first test for pooling across waves, for those health
outcomes that we have data for multiple waves. We find that the age,
schooling, and *pce* coefficients are not significantly different across years
although the province/rural-urban dummies are (results are available
upon request). Consequently, we pool the data across rounds of the survey (IFLS1, 2, 3, and 4), but allow for interactions between year dummies
and the province/rural-urban dummies. These interactions will capture
community/time differences in prices, healthcare availability and quality,
and health conditions. The sample for each regression consists of adults
who are aged 45 and older at the time of the survey, and for whom the
physical measurements (or other measures) are available. Estimation for
males and females are done separately. We use ordinary least squares
for continuous dependent variables and linear probability (LP) model
for binary dependent variables. LP model estimates are consistent for
estimating average partial effects of the regressors, which is what we are
interested in. Robust standard errors of the regression coefficients are
computed, which also allow for clustering at the community level. By
using robust standard errors for the linear probability regressions, we
ensure that these standard error estimates are consistent.

Table 13-1 shows means and standard deviations from the IFLS4 data
for our covariates. We create dummy variables for age indicating whether
an individual is aged 55 and older, 65 and older, and 75 and older. In this

---

[9]See Thomas et al. (forthcoming) for a more detailed discussion of IFLS attrition rates.

TABLE 13-1 Descriptive Statistics of the Socioeconomic Variables, 2007

Variable	Male (N = 4,014)		Female (N = 4,629)	
	Mean	Std. Dev	Mean	Std. Dev
Age (yrs)	57.94	10.465	58.47	10.786
Age (dummy vars.):				
45–54	0.466	0.499	0.455	0.498
55–64	0.272	0.445	0.261	0.439
65–74	0.178	0.383	0.191	0.393
75+	0.084	0.277	0.093	0.291
Years of education (yrs)	6.046	4.661	4.015	4.273
School completion (dummy vars.)				
No schooling	0.150	0.357	0.337	0.473
Some primary school	0.281	0.450	0.290	0.454
Completed primary school	0.276	0.447	0.206	0.405
Completed junior high	0.293	0.455	0.167	0.373
Monthly *pce* (Rp)	562,568	834,740	590,319	1,064,606
Residence (dummy vars.)				
Rural	0.503	0.500	0.492	0.500
Province				
North Sumatra	0.055	0.229	0.061	0.239
West Sumatra	0.049	0.216	0.055	0.229
South Sumatra	0.047	0.211	0.045	0.208
Lampung	0.044	0.205	0.036	0.187
Jakarta	0.064	0.245	0.060	0.238
West Java	0.166	0.372	0.157	0.364
Central Java	0.138	0.345	0.145	0.352
Yogyakarta	0.072	0.259	0.074	0.261
East Java	0.155	0.362	0.162	0.369
Bali	0.054	0.226	0.054	0.226
West Nusa Tenggara	0.059	0.236	0.058	0.234
South Kalimantan	0.047	0.211	0.040	0.195
South Sulawesi	0.049	0.215	0.052	0.223

SOURCE: Data from IFLS4.

way, the coefficients on the dummy variables indicate the marginal change from the next lowest age group (not from the omitted group) of being in the reference group. Similarly, for education, the dummy coefficients show the marginal change over the next lowest education group: We use a dummy variable for having at least some primary education, completed primary school or more, and completed junior high school or more. For per capita expenditures (*pce*), we take logs and then use a linear spline with a knot at the median of log *pce*.[10] For health measures that we have

---

[10]The coefficient on the second log *pce* variable we report is the change in the coefficient from the slope to the left of the knot point.

data on from more than one wave, we include dummy variables if the observations are from 1997 and after (if 1993 observations are available), 2000 and after, or 2007, and, as stated, interaction of these period effects with province and province-rural dummies. For the few health variables that we only have data for 2007–2008, we just include the province and province-rural dummies. Also for measures that data exist for multiple waves, we use five-year birth cohort dummy variables.[11,12] It is, of course, not possible to separately identify age, cohort, and period effects without untestable assumptions made. In our case, we aggregate ages into 10-year intervals and birth cohorts into five-year groups.[13] Because we are pooling the four waves for each age group, we have several birth-year cohorts, helping identification.

Nevertheless, we are not so interested in the age, cohort, or year effects as we are in the SES coefficients. However, if we left out age and/or birth cohort variables, we would bias the education coefficients positively, as the estimated education impacts would then also capture cohort effects. This would arise because younger birth cohorts have more schooling and also faced better health conditions when they were babies and in the fetus, compared to older cohorts. There is an accumulation of evidence now that better health conditions when young are associated with better health in old age (for instance, Barker, 1994; Gluckman and Hanson, 2005; and Strauss and Thomas, 2008, for an economist's perspective).

We have to be careful not to interpret the SES coefficients from these regressions as causal (Strauss and Thomas, 1995, 1998, 2008). Causality runs in both directions between SES and health outcomes. However, we add one variable that can help some in this regard, an interaction between years of education and de-meaned age. Using de-meaned age is helpful for interpretation because then the coefficients on the education dummies show the differentials at the sample mean age. The interaction coefficient then shows how that differential changes with age differences compared to the mean age. What we are looking for is whether education mitigates the powerful negative influence of aging on our health outcomes. If it does, then this is more consistent with a causal interpreta-

---

[11]The birth-year cohort dummy variables included are as follows: –1928, 1929–1933, 1934–1938, 1939–1943, 1944–1948, 1949–1953, 1954–1958, with 1959–1963 omitted as the base.

[12]For health measures that we only have data from 2007, of course, we do not use either year or birth cohort dummies, but we still use the age dummies. For these cases, the age dummies must be interpreted with even more caution, since it is not possible to disentangle age from birth cohort from time effects.

[13]The year dummy variables are aged 55 and older, 65 and older, 75 and older, with 45 and older omitted as the base.

tion of our education coefficients.[14,15] Studies of child height have shown that mother's education has its largest impact on heights when the child is less than three years (Barrera, 1990; Thomas, Strauss, and Henriques, 1990, 1991). This is thought to be the period during which children are most vulnerable to infection from dirty water and ill-prepared food, so that mother's schooling might well have its biggest impact during that period. Among the mechanisms for this enhanced impact is thought to be an allocative efficiency effect of mother's schooling, knowing, or being better at acquiring information regarding what inputs are better and safer for children, such as boiling water. A similar argument might be applied to our measures of health, which are largely general; at older ages, people are more susceptible to problems, hence one's own schooling may have a larger allocative impact at these ages (though possibly from affecting health inputs and behaviors from years earlier).

RESULTS

Physical Measurement:
Anthropometry, Hemoglobin Level, and Hypertension BMI

We first look at a number of biomarkers: BMI, waist circumference, blood hemoglobin levels, and hypertension.[16] BMI, which is weight (in kg)

---

[14]While this interaction coefficient could also represent a nonlinear effect of schooling, the fact that we enter schooling with level dummies protects us in part against this potential confounding effect.

[15]Another empirical strategy we could have taken would be to include household fixed effects. That would have captured all factors at the household level, but still would not have addressed the issue of unobserved individual factors. Household fixed effects would have required there to be multiple men aged 45 and older within the same household and likewise for adult women. We examined the cell sizes for our samples, using as our definition of household, the "dynastic" 1993 households (that is combining all households that split from a given 1993 household into one household). We found that an average dynastic household contained 1.1 adult male or adult female members aged 45 and older. In the case of CES-D, for example, we had 3,900 individual men in our sample and 3,683 dynasties. That means we only had 217 individuals from multiple member households, and it is this group that would be used to estimate the SES coefficients. We judged that this was too small a group from which to reliably get estimates. This case is typical. For health outcomes that we measure over time, like BMI, we have numerous persons for whom we have multiple measures over waves. We thus could have used individual fixed effects in that case, but that should be part of a dynamic analysis, which is a different research exercise than this chapter.

[16]Heights were measured using a lightweight SECA aluminum height board, the SECA 214 portable stadiometer. Weights were measured using a portable digital scale, the CAMRY EB6171. Hemoglobin was measured using a small, hand-held meter, the Hemocue Hb301 analyzer. A finger prick was made using a lancet and a drop of blood inserted into the Hemocue microcuvette. Blood pressure was taken with a digital meter, the Omron HEM 712c meter. Total and HDL cholesterol were measured using a CardiochekPA meter. This meter measures over the range 100–400 for total cholesterol and 15–100 for HDL.

divided by height (in m) squared, provides a convenient summary of height and weight of adults. We use World Health Organization (WHO) standards whereby adults whose BMI is under 18.5 are considered undernourished and those whose BMI is 25 or greater are considered overweight. Extreme values of BMI are associated with elevated hypertension, diabetes, and other causes of mortality.

Figures 13-1a and 13-1b plot the cumulative distribution functions (CDF) of BMI for adult males and females aged 45 and older using data from IFLS1, 2, 3, and 4. The CDFs are shifted down for each year after 1993 for both men and women. The shift for 2007 from 2000 is especially large. The fact that the CDFs do not cross means that each successive year first order stochastically dominates the last. In the case of BMI, unlike income, stochastic dominance across the entire distribution does not have a clear welfare implication. On the one hand, undernourishment is unambiguously dropping, but on the other hand, overweight is unambiguously increasing. Table 13-2 shows the percentages of adults aged 45 and older who are undernourished and overweight in 2007. The percentage of adult males who are undernourished was around 17.5 in 2007. This number continues the decline from 28.3 in 1993 to 23.5 in 2000 (see Witoelar, Strauss, and Sikoki, 2009).[17] The numbers are similar for women, with around 17.4% who were undernourished in 2007, compared to 29.7% in 1993. But what is more interesting has to do with the proportion of those overweight. In 2007, around 31% of elderly women have BMI 25 or over, more than double the fraction of 1993. Among elderly men in 2007, 17% are overweight, compared to 8.5% in 1993. Among the different age groups, it is the 45–54 age group who have both the lowest fraction of undernourished and the largest fraction of overweight.

The increase over the years and the substantial degree of overweight suggests that overnutrition and health conditions associated with it have become increasingly important in Indonesia. At the same time, undernutrition has not entirely disappeared, though its magnitude among the aged has sharply dropped.

Holding BMI constant, greater waist circumference increases the risks of various cardiovascular diseases. For people who are overweight or obese, the risk of future mortality is higher if their waist circumference is greater than 120 cm for men or 88 cm for women. The CDF of waist circumference for both men and women shifted to the right between 2000 and 2007 (see Witoelar, Strauss, and Sikoki, 2009). Around 30% of women aged 45 and older in 2007 had waist circumferences that are greater than 88 cm compared to around 20% in 2000. This CDF does not control for BMI changes, so a lot of the increase in waist circumference may simply be

---

[17]Percentages of adults 45+ who are undernourished and overweight in all four survey waves of the IFLS are presented in Witoelar, Strauss, and Sikoki (2009).

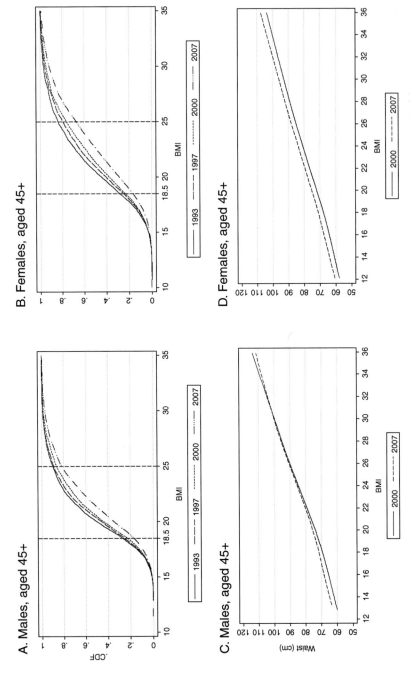

FIGURE 13-1 CDF of body mass index and waist circumference by body mass index, adults aged 45 and older.
SOURCE: Data from IFLS, Waves 1-4.

TABLE 13-2 Under/Overnutrition, Low Hemoglobin Level, High Total Cholesterol, and Low HDL Level Among 45+ in 2007

	Male		Female	
	%	# obs.	%	# obs.
45–54 years				
% undernourished	9.46	1,870	9.39	2,106
% overweight	22.65	1,870	40.18	2,106
% low blood hemoglobin	17.72	1,869	28.08	2,091
% high total cholesterol	12.49	1,832	20.02	2,054
% low HDL	70.59	1,832	40.81	2,054
55–64 years				
% undernourished	18.22	1,096	16.64	1,211
% overweight	17.26	1,096	30.57	1,211
% low blood hemoglobin	26.01	1,093	32.82	1,212
% high total cholesterol	12.66	1,071	26.00	1,204
% low HDL	64.79	1,071	36.25	1,204
65–74 years				
% undernourished	27.95	713	29.57	878
% overweight	8.59	713	18.82	878
% low blood hemoglobin	40.86	728	40.25	886
% high total cholesterol	9.48	716	23.07	884
% low HDL	59.49	715	41.31	883
75+ years				
% undernourished	38.05	338	33.60	438
% overweight	6.31	338	13.96	438
% low blood hemoglobin	52.24	350	50.06	461
% high total cholesterol	8.60	339	21.63	448
% low HDL	65.22	339	34.47	448
All adults 45+				
% undernourished	17.54	4,017	17.40	4,633
% overweight	17.31	4,017	31.14	4,633
% low blood hemoglobin	27.12	4,040	33.81	4,650
% high total cholesterol	11.66	3,958	22.33	4,590
% low HDL	66.55	3,957	39.09	4,589
Mean BMI	21.75	4,017	22.90	4,633
Mean blood hemoglobin	13.99	4,040	12.42	4,650
Mean total cholesterol	178.16	3,958	198.46	4,590
Mean HDL	34.94	3,957	44.97	4,589

SOURCE: Data from IFLS4. Undernourished = BMI < 18.5, overweight = BMI ≥ 25, low blood hemoglobin = < 13.0 mg/dL (male) or < 12.0 mg/dL (female), high total cholesterol = (≥ 240 mg/dL, low HDL = < 40 mg/dL).

due to an increase in BMI, but not all. Figures 13-1c and 13-1d plot waist circumference against BMI for men and women in 2000 and 2007. For men at higher BMI levels, there is not much change in waist circumference, so that the upward shift in waist circumference for men between 2000 and 2007 is largely a result of increasing BMI. Not so for women, however, who have a shift up in mean waist circumference by BMI. In 2007 being over 188 cm in waist size is associated with a BMI of 26, instead of 28, which was the case in 2000.

Table 13-3 shows the regression results for BMI. Men who completed junior high or more are likely to have higher BMI than those with less schooling. For women, BMI seems to increase with education; this is true for those with some primary education compared to no schooling at all and for those with completed primary or more compared to some primary. However, having completed junior high or more does not have any additional effect (the marginal coefficient is slightly negative, but not significant). Thus the BMI-education gradient flattens out for women with junior high school (nine years) or more schooling, very similar to the effect found by Strauss and Thomas (2008). Education variables are jointly significant for both men and women. *Pce* variables turn out to be statistically significant and positive, similar to findings in previous studies that have found BMI is positively correlated with income. For both men and women, the results show that BMI decreases at old ages. In results not shown, BMIs are also lower for successively older birth cohorts.

One important result from this table is that the effect of education (as well as its interaction with age in the case of men) and *pce* are still significant even after we control for province and province-urban interactions, as well as province-urban-year interactions. The province-urban-year interactions are themselves also jointly statistically significant. This is an important finding that suggests that there is a degree of inequality of health outcomes among the elderly population even after we control for some regional characteristics, a theme that we will see again in some other health biomarkers.

The negative interaction coefficient on the age-schooling interaction for men can be interpreted as meaning that better educated men lose more BMI as they age compared to the less educated. This effect is small in magnitude, however. For a man 10 years older than the mean, 58, and with 10 years of schooling, BMI falls an additional .15. Note that for women, the interaction is close to zero and not significant, consistent with the flattening out of the BMI education gradient for women compared to men.

TABLE 13-3 Multivariate Regressions: BMI and Hemoglobin Levels

	BMI				Hemoglobin			
	Male		Female		Male		Female	
	Coeff.	t-stat	Coeff.	t-stat	Coeff.	t-stat	Coeff.	t-stat
Age Group (dummy variables)								
55 and older	-0.0004	[-0.004]	0.1806	[1.523]	-0.2742***	[-2.738]	-0.0463	[-0.836]
65 and older	-0.3004***	[-2.651]	-0.0401	[-0.291]	-0.2447***	[-2.623]	-0.1418*	[-1.730]
75 and older	-0.4224***	[-2.938]	-0.6853***	[-4.152]	-0.3392***	[-2.814]	-0.2890***	[-3.544]
Years of Education (dummy variables)								
At least some primary	0.2194**	[2.342]	0.7537***	[5.202]	0.1072	[1.455]	0.1051**	[2.158]
Completed primary school or more	0.3443***	[3.548]	0.6045***	[4.330]	0.0140	[0.221]	0.1454***	[2.912]
Completed junior high or more	1.0519***	[8.106]	0.0804	[0.423]	0.2614***	[4.372]	0.0194	[0.218]
Education × Age Interaction								
Years of education × age[a]	-0.0015*	[-1.754]	-0.0011	[-0.841]	0.0001	[0.140]	0.0019***	[2.935]
Per Capita Expenditures (splines)[b]								
0 - median pce	0.6904***	[7.730]	0.8015***	[6.983]	0.2712***	[4.409]	0.1244**	[2.425]
>= median pce	0.0996	[0.669]	0.0409	[0.245]	-0.0606	[-0.701]	-0.0591	[-0.803]
Year Dummy Variables								
1997 and after	-0.4722*	[-1.963]	-0.0677	[-0.220]	0.2680**	[2.196]	0.1544	[0.945]
2000 and after	-0.1163	[-0.543]	-0.4053	[-1.570]	-0.4854***	[-3.000]	0.0375	[0.243]
2007	-0.2097	[-0.630]	-0.2841	[-0.987]				
Constant	14.4015***	[14.600]	15.5432***	[12.079]	10.9429***	[15.749]	10.6710***	[18.213]
Observations	12,836		14,735		10,305		11,853	
R-squared	0.226		0.222		0.123		0.057	
Cohort Dummy Variables	Yes		Yes		Yes		Yes	
Province × Rural Dummy	Yes		Yes		Yes		Yes	
Variables + Province × Rural × Year Interactions								

continued

TABLE 13-3 Continued

	BMI				Hemoglobin			
	Male		Female		Male		Female	
	Coeff.	t-stat	Coeff.	t-stat	Coeff.	t-stat	Coeff.	t-stat
F-tests for joint significance:	F-stat	p(values)	F-stat	p(values)	F-stat	p(values)	F-stat	p(values)
Age group dummy variables	5.869	0.001	8.284	0.000	3.948	0.008	5.057	0.002
Education variables	47.550	0.000	27.479	0.000	10.818	0.000	6.651	0.000
Educ. years + educ. age interactions	41.392	0.000	21.542	0.000	8.220	0.000	6.635	0.000
Per capita expenditures	82.506	0.000	78.482	0.000	30.996	0.000	6.474	0.002
Cohort dummy variables	5.143	0.000	11.298	0.000	2.067	0.046	1.649	0.120
Year dummy variables	1.963	0.119	1.292	0.277	5.154	0.006	0.639	0.528
Province × rural dummy variables	4.626	0.000	6.787	0.000	4.182	0.000	4.208	0.000
Year × prov × rural variables interactions	2.233	0.000	2.815	0.000	4.687	0.000	2.728	0.000

NOTES: The dependent variable for BMI regressions is the BMI; for hemoglobin, the hemoglobin level (g/dL). Blood hemoglobin level was not collected in 1993. t-statistics (in brackets) are based on standard errors that are robust to clustering at the community level. * denotes significant at 10%; ** significant at 5%; *** significant at 1%. The omitted group for age dummy variable is 45 and older, for education, "no schooling," and for province, Jakarta. Birth-year cohort dummy variables included are as follows: −1928, 1929–1933, 1934–1938, 1939–1943, 1944–1948, 1949–1953, 1954–1958, with 1959–1963 omitted.

[a]The interaction term is between years of education and the de-meaned age. Means of age in the BMI sample are 58.2 (male), 58.5 (female); in the hemoglobin sample: 58.3 (male), 58.8 (female).

[b]Knot point is at the median *pce*, coefficient represent change in the slope.

SOURCE: Data from IFLS, Waves 1–4.

Hemoglobin

Levels of hemoglobin in blood are of interest because low levels indicate problems of anemia, which can have various negative consequences. Iron deficiency is associated, for instance, with lower endurance for physical activity.[18] For some types of employment, this deficiency may affect productivity significantly (see Thomas et al., 2008).

Figure 13-2 displays the CDF of blood hemoglobin levels for elderly for 1997, 2000, and 2007 (blood hemoglobin level was not collected in 1993).[19] The vertical lines at 13.0 dL for males and 12.0 g/dL for females in Figure 13-2 show the thresholds that are used in previous studies.[20] The figure shows the shift to the right from previous rounds for both men and women, indicating higher levels of blood hemoglobin levels in the population, and lower proportion of elderly who are below the thresholds. Indeed the proportion of elderly men with blood hemoglobin levels lower than the threshold of 13.0 g/dL has declined from 40.6 in 1997 to 27.12 in 2007. For women, the proportion below the threshold of 12.0 g/dL has declined from 41.9 to 33.8. Given what we know about what blood hemoglobin levels can tell us, this change shows an improvement in one dimension of health in Indonesia over the years. Even so, the 2007 levels are still high compared to what is found in industrial countries, consistent with much evidence that low hemoglobin levels exist in low-income countries (Tolentino and Friedman, 2007).

The regressions presented in Table 13-3 show that older age has a strong impact on lowering blood hemoglobin levels for both and women. There are no significant cohort effects for women, though there are for men, with older cohorts having lower hemoglobin levels. For men, having completed junior high school or more education is associated with higher levels of hemoglobin compared to those with less schooling. For women, having some primary schooling has a strong positive correlation and completed primary schooling even more so. The relationship flattens out with junior high school or more. Log *pce* has a strongly positive correlation with hemoglobin at low levels of income. The age-education interaction is strongly significant and positive for women, meaning that the negative association with age for women is weakened for those with more schooling. For a woman having completed primary school, with 6 years of schooling and 15 years older than mean age, the marginal impact of being over 75 is cut in half, a large impact.

---

[18]Hemoglobin levels may also be low if a person has an infection or for other reasons.

[19]A validation study reported by Crimmins et al. (2011) shows that the Hemocue meter performs well compared to a gold standard of hemoglobin measured from venous blood.

[20]Studies have also shown that the relationship between hemoglobin level and work capacity is nonlinear; higher level above the thresholds have no impact on work capacity; see for, instance, Thomas et al. (2008).

A. Males, aged 45+

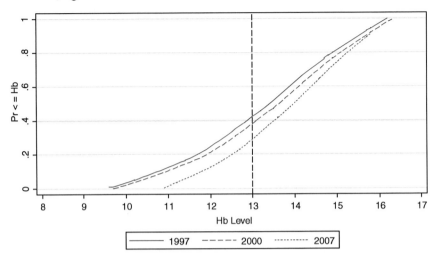

B. Females, aged 45+

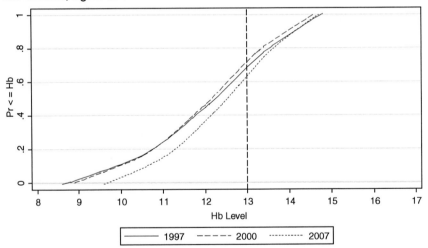

FIGURE 13-2 CDF of hemoglobin levels, adult aged 45 and older, 1997, 2000, and 2007.
SOURCE: Data from IFLS, Waves 2-4.

Cholesterol

Lipids, in particular high total cholesterol and low HDL, were measured, non-fasting, in IFLS4. Lipids are strongly correlated in the medical literature with cardiovascular risk (e.g., Kannel, Castelli, and Gordon, 1979). It is thus of considerable interest to explore their levels in a low-income country like Indonesia, and, as well, their associations with SES variables.[21] Table 13-2 shows the 2007 sample means and fractions above the threshold for total cholesterol and below for HDL, using standard WHO thresholds. For total cholesterol, high levels are not large, only 12% for men, but higher for women at 22%.[22] However, the situation for low HDL is completely different. Levels below the threshold of 40 are large, especially for men, 67%, and 39% for women. Small fractions of high total cholesterol but large fractions of low HDL is a pattern that is being found in several low-income countries where it has been looked at (e.g., Crimmins et al., 2011; Gurven et al., 2009), including the Tsimane study of primitive Amazon Indians in Bolivia and the CHARLS study in China (Crimmins et al., 2011). Figure 13-3 plots the fraction above and below the thresholds of total and HDL cholesterol against age. One can see that there is little relationship for total cholesterol, with a small increasing tendency to have high total cholesterol for women until the mid-50s, when the curve flattens. For HDL there is some decline in the incidence of low levels with age.

Table 13-4 reports the regressions. There is very little SES correlation with either the probability of having high total cholesterol or low HDL. There are *pce* correlations for men for total and for women for HDL. For men, having higher per capita household expenditure is associated with a higher chance of being above the threshold for total cholesterol, then the *pce* curve flattens out above the median. For women for HDL, having a higher *pce* is associated with a lower chance at being below the HDL threshold, but then flattens out above the median level of *pce*. For men's HDL, however, we do not see any association with *pce*. There are also quite strong community effects that are found, though from the dummies we cannot say what exactly they represent; perhaps impacts of local food prices, through diets, but it could be through other mechanisms as well.

---

[21]Crimmins et al. (2011) report a validation study of the Cardiochek PA meter against venous blood for both total and HDL cholesterol. The results look quite similar. It is the case, however, that the distributions for Cardiochek PA samples are censored at the measurement bounds of the meter (see footnote 16). However, we define our dependent variables as the fraction above or below thresholds ($\geq$ = 240 for total and <40 for HDL). These thresholds are within the measurement bounds of the meter, so this censoring should not matter for this chapter.

[22]This same gender differential is found in the CHARLS data for China, see Crimmins et al. (2011).

A. High total cholesterol

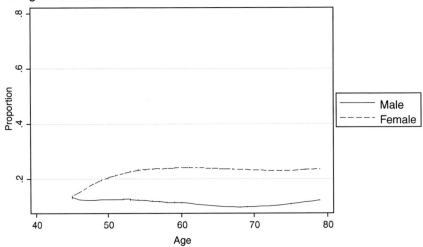

B. Low HDL

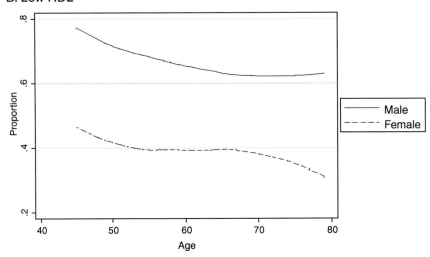

FIGURE 13-3 Proportion with high total cholesterol and low HDL, adults aged 45 and older, 2007.
SOURCE: Data from IFLS4.

TABLE 13-4 Multivariate Regressions: High Total Cholesterol and Low HDL Levels, Aged 45 and Older in 2007

	High Total Cholesterol				Low HDL			
	Male		Female		Male		Female	
	Coeff.	t-stat	Coeff.	t-stat	Coeff.	t-stat	Coeff.	t-stat
Age Group (dummy variables)								
55 and older	0.0112	[0.378]	-0.0082	[-0.229]	0.0375	[0.920]	0.0132	[0.326]
65 and older	-0.0175	[-0.643]	-0.0019	[-0.050]	0.0431	[0.751]	0.0275	[0.636]
75 and older	-0.0022	[-0.047]	-0.0209	[-0.390]	0.0110	[0.162]	0.0459	[0.794]
Years of Education (dummy variables)								
At least some primary	-0.0048	[-0.367]	0.0347*	[1.853]	0.0285	[1.186]	-0.0188	[-0.857]
Completed primary school or more	0.0159	[1.286]	-0.0006	[-0.032]	-0.0320*	[-1.700]	0.0238	[1.153]
Completed junior high or more	0.0223	[1.421]	0.0230	[0.997]	0.0320	[1.520]	-0.0022	[-0.084]
Education × Age Interaction								
Years of education × age^a	-0.0001	[-0.574]	-0.0001	[-0.337]	0.0001	[0.309]	-0.0001	[-0.568]
Per Capita Expenditures (splines)^b								
0 - median *pce*	0.0438***	[3.202]	0.0218	[1.161]	-0.0285	[-1.104]	-0.0874***	[-3.677]
>= median *pce*	-0.0372	[-1.552]	-0.0072	[-0.250]	0.0344	[0.954]	0.1188***	[3.467]
Constant	-0.4599***	[-2.699]	-0.1567	[-0.657]	1.1763***	[3.571]	1.5265***	[5.018]
Observations	3,960		4,591		3,958		4,589	
R-squared	0.069		0.074		0.047		0.068	
Cohort Dummy Variables	Yes		Yes		Yes		Yes	
Province × Rural	Yes		Yes		Yes		Yes	

continued

TABLE 13-4 Continued

	High Total Cholesterol				Low HDL			
	Male		Female		Male		Female	
F-tests for Joint Significance:	Coeff. F-stat	t-stat p(values)	Coeff. F-stat	t-stat p(values)	Coeff. F-stat	t-stat p(values)	Coeff. F-stat	t-stat p(values)
Age group dummy variables	0.185	0.907	0.063	0.979	0.521	0.668	0.357	0.784
Education variables	1.838	0.139	2.289	0.078	1.437	0.231	0.526	0.664
Educ. vars + educ. age interactions	1.572	0.180	1.868	0.115	1.096	0.358	0.571	0.684
Per capita expenditures	6.692	0.001	1.736	0.177	0.610	0.544	6.908	0.001
Cohort dummy variables	1.649	0.120	1.649	0.120	1.649	0.120	1.649	0.120
Year dummy variables	0.639	0.528	0.639	0.528	0.639	0.528	0.639	0.528
Province × rural dummy variables	6.756	0.000	8.508	0.000	4.386	0.000	8.971	0.000

NOTES: The dependent variable for high total cholesterol is 1 if individual has total cholesterol level ≥ 240 mg/dL, 0 otherwise. The dependent variable for low HDL level is 1 if individual has HDL level < 40 mg/dL, 0 otherwise. Blood cholesterol levels were only measured in 2007. t-statistics (in brackets) are based on standard errors that are robust to clustering at the community level. * denotes significant at 10%; ** significant at 5%; *** significant at 1%. The omitted group for age dummy variable is 45 and older, for education, "no schooling," and for province, Jakarta. Birth-year cohort dummy variables included are as follows: −1928, 1929–1933, 1934–1938, 1939–1943, 1944–1948, 1949–1953, 1954–1958, with 1959–1963 omitted.

[a]The interaction term is between years of education and the de-meaned age. Means of age in the sample are 58.0 (male) and 58.6 (female).
[b]Knot point is at the median *pce*, coefficient represent change in the slope.
SOURCE: Data from IFLS4.

Hypertension

Along with BMI and waist circumference, blood pressure is a useful indicator of risk of coronary heart diseases. Blood pressure measures are available from IFLS2, 3, and 4.[23] Figure 13-4 plots the proportion of those who are hypertensive (those whose systolic is greater than or equal to 140 or diastolic is greater than or equal to 90) against age. For both men and women, there is a strong positive relationship between age and being hypertensive.

Looking at the levels of measured hypertension over the years in Table 13-5 Panel A, there seems to be little change. Among men aged 45 and older, around 44% had hypertension in 2007, the same percentage as in 1997. Similarly among women, 53% were hypertensive, and the number does not change much over the years. However, it is important to note that the percentage of those with hypertension is substantial, so clearly hypertension is a major health issue for the elderly.

A major public health issue, given the nutrition and health transitions that Indonesians are undergoing, is whether the health system, which is set up to focus on young children and mothers and infectious diseases, can adequately care for chronic disease among the elderly. Are the elderly being diagnosed and treated? In IFLS4 2007, the respondents were asked whether or not they had ever been diagnosed with hypertension by a modern medical provider. We take the union of those who answer yes and those whom we measured to have hypertension (of course, there is an overlap) to arrive at a sum of persons who have hypertension.[24] We then tabulate the fraction of those who have hypertension who say they have been diagnosed, in Table 13-5 Panel B and show the bivariate relationship with level of education. Almost 75% of men and 62% of women are undiagnosed according to Table 13-5 Panel B. [25] By education level there is a drop in undiagnosed hypertension with higher education for both men and women; for women, the drop occurs for those with any schooling. Panel C shows among those who are report being diagnosed, what fraction are not taking medications for hypertension, and by level of schooling. A very high percentage of those diagnosed are not taking

---

[23]In IFLS2 1997 and IFLS3 2000, blood pressure was measured only once. In IFLS4 2007, blood pressure was measured three times. For 2007, we use the average of the three measures for our analysis.

[24]This is the usual way in HRS-type data to calculate levels of hypertension (for example, see Gurven et al., 2009; Strauss et al., 2010).

[25]In China, the same analysis has been done with the CHARLS pilot data (see Strauss et al., 2010). There the underdiagnosis rate is 45%. The fraction of those who are diagnosed who take medications is much higher, 75–80%. For Mexico the situation for hypertension is the same (Parker et al., 2010). Clearly, the health system in Indonesia has a major problem of healthcare for the elderly.

A. Males, aged 45+

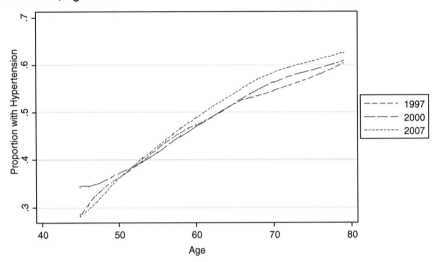

B. Females, aged 45+

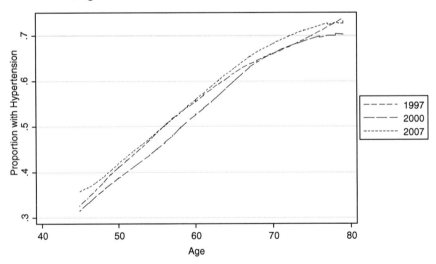

FIGURE 13-4 Proportion with hypertension by age, 1997, 2000, and 2007.
SOURCE: Data from IFLS, Waves 2–4.

TABLE 13-5 Hypertension, Underdiagnosis, and Medication Take Up, Age 45+

PANEL A. Incidence of hypertension, diagnosis, and medication take up						
	Men			Women		
	1997	2000	2007	1997	2000	2007
Observations	2856	3,477	4,044	3,307	3,631	4,674
% measured as hypertensive	43.8	44.2	44.2	52.6	49.6	52.7
% not measured, but diagnosed as hypertensive[a]			6.5			11.6
Total hypertensive (%)[b]	43.8	44.4	50.7	52.6	50	63.3

PANEL B. Underdiagnosis of hypertension by completed education, adults 45+[c]		
Education	2007	2007
no schooling	79.0	69.5
primary schooling	74.4	58.2
junior high	73.2	52.1
senior high +	68.0	62.1
all adults 45+	73.6	62.1

PANEL C. Hypertensive and not taking medication, by completed education, aged 45+[d]		
Education	2007	2007
no schooling	91.5	92.6
primary schooling	89.1	89.3
junior high	73.6	79.4
senior high +	77.9	86.8
all adults 45+	85.0	89.2

[a]Diagnosed" if answered "Yes" to the question "*Has a doctor/nurse/paramedic ever told you that you have hypertension?*" The question was only asked in 2007. Percentages of those diagnosed with hypertension are out of individuals aged 45+.

[b]Percentages are out of individuals 45+.

[c]Percentages are out of individuals 45+ who are measured and/or diagnosed to be hypertensive.

[d]Percentages are out of individuals 45+ who are diagnosed to be hypertensive.

SOURCE: Data from IFLS Waves 2–4.

medications and the percentage is higher for women, 89%, than for men, 85%. Education level gradients exist, particularly for men.

The multivariate regressions presented in Table 13-6 confirm what we saw in Figure 13-4 that the probability of having hypertension increases with age, although the increase with birth cohort is even larger. For men, education levels are jointly significant, with higher levels of schooling

TABLE 13-6 Hypertension and Underdiagnosis of Hypertension: Linear Probability Models

	Hypertension				Underdiagnosis of hypertension			
	Male		Female		Male		Female	
	Coeff.	t-stat	Coeff.	t-stat	Coeff.	t-stat	Coeff.	t-stat
Age Group (dummy variables)								
55 and older	0.0478**	[2.434]	0.0390**	[2.143]	−0.0290	[−0.910]	0.0310	[1.152]
65 and older	0.0257	[1.230]	0.0558***	[3.115]	−0.0351	[−1.111]	0.0200	[0.692]
75 and older	0.0695***	[2.634]	0.0300	[1.372]	−0.0259	[−0.684]	−0.0289	[−0.892]
Years of Education (dummy variables)								
At least some primary	−0.0067	[−0.385]	0.0105	[0.680]	−0.0144	[−0.396]	−0.1249***	[−4.704]
Completed primary school or more	0.0255*	[1.658]	−0.0018	[−0.113]	−0.0213	[−0.736]	0.0287	[1.030]
Completed junior high or more	0.0333**	[2.172]	−0.0060	[−0.286]	−0.0358	[−1.075]	0.0298	[0.872]
Education × Age Interaction								
Years of education × age^a	−0.0001	[−0.984]	0.0004***	[2.984]	−0.0003	[−1.334]	−0.0003	[−1.250]
Per Capita Expenditures (splines)^b								
0 - median pce	0.0172	[1.095]	0.0371**	[2.540]	−0.0507	[−1.342]	−0.0998***	[−3.244]
>= median pce	0.0022	[0.096]	−0.0285	[−1.397]	0.0263	[0.484]	0.0753*	[1.652]
Year Dummy Variables								
2000 and after	0.0580	[1.610]	0.0385	[1.068]				
2007	0.1166***	[2.674]	0.0608	[1.401]				
Constant	−0.0267	[−0.147]	−0.1018	[−0.610]	1.3425***	[2.802]	1.7300***	[4.411]
Observations	10,376		11,994		1,966		2,745	
R-squared	0.064		0.088		0.045		0.072	
Cohort Dummy Variables	Yes		Yes		No		No	
Province × Rural Dummy Variables +	Yes		Yes		Province × rural		Province × rural	
Province × Rural × Year Interactions								

F-tests for Joint Significance:

Age group dummy variables	3.447	0.017	3.630	0.013	1.163	0.323	0.988	0.398
Education variables	4.206	0.006	0.171	0.916	1.280	0.281	7.586	0.000
Educ. years + educ. age interactions	3.953	0.004	2.913	0.021	1.253	0.288	7.305	0.000
Per capita expenditures	2.569	0.078	4.424	0.012	1.891	0.152	8.253	0.000
Cohort dummy variables	7.374	0.000	4.417	0.000				
Year dummy variables	4.791	0.009	1.990	0.138				
Province x rural dummy variables	1.769	0.019	3.293	0.000	2.653	0.000	6.955	0.000
Year x prov x rural variables interactions	1.979	0.000	2.682	0.000				

NOTES: The dependent variable for the hypertension regressions is whether the individual is hypertensive = 1, 0 otherwise; and for the under-diagnosis of hypertension, the dependent variable is 1 if the individual has ever been diagnosed with hypertension, 0 otherwise, conditional of being hypertensive. Blood pressure measurement was not collected in 1993, and question about diagnosis was only asked in 2007. t-statistics (in brackets) are based on standard errors that are robust to clustering at the community level. * denotes significant at 10%; ** significant at 5%; *** significant at 1%. The omitted group for age dummy variable is 45 and older, for education, "no schooling," and for province, Jakarta. Birth-year cohort dummy variables included are as follows: –1928, 1929–1933, 1934–1938, 1939–1943, 1944–1948, 1949–1953, 1954–1958, with 1959–1963 omitted.

[a] The interaction term is between years of education and the de-meaned age. Means of age in the hypertension sample are: 58.3 (male), 58.9 (fe-male); in the underdiagnosis sample: 60.3 (male), 60.8 (female).

[b] Knot point is at the median *pce*, coefficient represent change in the slope.

SOURCE: Data from IFLS, Waves 2–4.

associated with a great likelihood of being hypertensive. *Pce* on the other hand is not significantly related to hypertension for men. For women, it is *pce* and not education levels that is significantly related to hypertension, with higher *pce* being associated with higher chances of having hypertension. For underdiagnosis of hypertension, the regression results suggest that among women with hypertension, having some primary education reduces the probability of being underdiagnosed compared to those with no schooling, although having higher levels of schooling show no additional effects. The education variables are jointly significant for both women and men. On the other hand, *pce* is significant at under 1% for women. The higher per capita expenditure, the lower is underdiagnosis, so underdiagnosis is larger for lower income and uneducated people, particularly women.

Cognition: Word Recall

Cognition has been found to be an important issue among the elderly (see McArdle, Fisher, and Kadlec, 2007). We use immediate and delayed word recall as one of the cognitive measures, namely the episodic memory measure. In IFLS4, like the U.S. Health and Retirement Study (HRS), respondents are read a list of 10 simple nouns, and they are immediately asked to repeat as many as they can, in any order. After answering unrelated questions on morbidity, maybe 10 minutes later, the respondents are then asked again to repeat as many words as they can. We use the average number of correctly immediate and delayed recalled words as our memory measure (McArdle, Smith, and Willis, 2009).

On average, elderly men are able to recall 2.9 words, and elderly women are able to recall 3.2 words. Figure 13-5a shows a strong negative binary relationship between the number of words recalled and age. Note that in the top panel, the line for men is higher than that of women. This is partly due to the fact that at any given age, men on average are better educated than women. Along the same lines, part of the reason that the lines coincide is that for any given years of education, men are typically older than women. The multivariate analysis, presented in Table 13-7, sheds more light on these associations.

The regressions show a strong negative relationship between age and memory for men and women. A strong, positive relationship between education and memory is also evident, with a negative coefficient on the age-schooling interaction term for men, suggesting that education reinforces the negative effects of aging on memory in this case. The *pce* variables are jointly significant, positively correlated with word recall, with the effect at low levels of *pce* for men and at high levels for women.

A. Words recalled and age

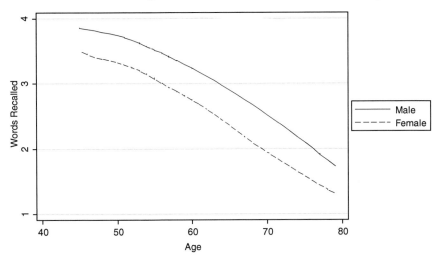

B. CES-D score and age

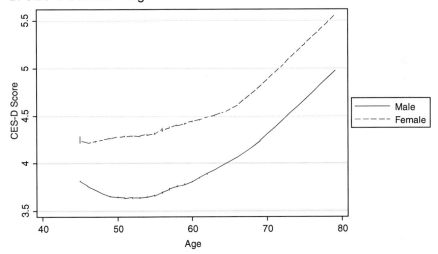

FIGURE 13-5 Words recalled and CES-D 10 (2007), adults aged 45 and older.
SOURCE: Data from IFLS4.

TABLE 13-7 Multivariate Regressions: Number of Words Recalled and the CES-D 10 Score

	Word Recall				CES-D 10			
	Male		Female		Male		Female	
	Coeff.	t-stat	Coeff.	t-stat	Coeff.	t-stat	Coeff.	t-stat
Age Group (dummy variables)								
55 and older	-0.2597***	[-3.530]	-0.2800***	[-4.455]	0.1468	[1.105]	0.0425	[0.292]
65 and older	-0.4163***	[-4.962]	-0.4913***	[-6.805]	0.5017***	[2.997]	0.2468	[1.452]
75 and older	-0.6090***	[-5.560]	-0.3392***	[-3.262]	0.5974**	[2.387]	0.7027***	[3.020]
Years of Education (dummy variables)								
At least some primary	0.4525***	[4.724]	0.5753***	[8.541]	-0.3082*	[-1.743]	-0.3000**	[-2.165]
Completed primary school or more	0.5900***	[7.949]	0.7014***	[9.822]	-0.1542	[-1.152]	-0.3948***	[-2.758]
Completed junior high or more	0.5740***	[7.873]	0.5622***	[6.850]	-0.5087***	[-3.529]	-0.6314***	[-3.623]
Education × Age Interaction								
Years of education × age[a]	-0.0019***	[-3.338]	-0.0008	[-1.203]	-0.0015	[-1.373]	-0.0005	[-0.356]
Per Capita Expenditures (splines)[b]								
0 - median *pce*	0.2001**	[2.536]	0.0360	[0.495]	-0.2731	[-1.589]	-0.2583	[-1.371]
>= median *pce*	0.0135	[0.119]	0.2082**	[1.992]	-0.0684	[-0.269]	0.0423	[0.162]
Constant	0.1745	[0.175]	2.1664**	[2.361]	8.3122***	[3.822]	8.2205***	[3.421]
Observations	3,748		4,063		3,900		4,399	
R-squared	0.283		0.315		0.066		0.068	
Province × Rural	Yes		Yes		Yes		Yes	
F-tests for Joint Significance:								
Age group dummy variables	43.322	0.000	50.164	0.000	7.318	0.000	6.522	0.000
Education variables	104.477	0.000	169.400	0.000	11.726	0.000	21.114	0.000
Educ. years + educ. age interactions	83.455	0.000	137.819	0.000	9.220	0.000	15.859	0.000
Per capita expenditures	13.403	0.000	10.295	0.000	7.236	0.001	2.950	0.053
Province × rural dummy variables	5.347	0.000	5.761	0.000	5.998	0.000	9.180	0.000

NOTES: The dependent variable for the word recall regression is the average number of the words recalled from the immediate and delayed recalls. Word recall question module was only administered in 2007. The dependent variable for the CES-D regression is the CES-D10 score. The score is computed in the way suggested by the Stanford group that created the CES-D, using numbers from 0 for rarely to 3 for most of the time, for negative questions such as "do you feel sad." For positive questions, such as "do you feel happy," the scoring is reversed from 0 for most of the time to 3 for rarely (see text). CESD-10 module was only asked in 2007. t-statistics (in brackets) are based on standard errors that are robust to clustering at the community level. * denotes significant at 10%; ** significant at 5%; *** significant at 1%. The omitted group for age dummy variable is 45 and older, for education, "no schooling," and for province, Jakarta.

[a]The interaction term is between years of education and the de-meaned age. Means of age in the word recall sample are 56.9 (male), 56.7 (female); and in the CES-D sample: 57.3 (male), 57.4 (female).

[b]Knot point is at the median *pce*, coefficient represent change in the slope.

SOURCE: Data from IFLS4.

CES-D 10 Score

As a measure of mental health, the respondents were administered a self-reported depression scale from the short version of the CES-D scale, one of the major international scales of depression used in general populations. Higher scores on the CES-D scale indicate a higher likelihood of having major depression.[26] Some recent studies have failed to find a relationship between depression and education or income (see Das et al., 2007, for example); however, other studies have found such correlations. (Patel and Kleinman, 2003, surveyed several studies that do find negative correlations between depression and SES.) For Indonesia, Friedman and Thomas (2008) find that the economic crisis fueled depression indicators, especially for the more vulnerable population.[27]

Figure 13-5b displays the relationships between CES-D scores and age. For both elderly men and elderly women, CES-D scores increase with age and are higher for women. The mean CES-D scores among people aged 45 and older are 3.3 for men and 3.8 for women.

The regressions using CES-D as dependent variable (Table 13-7) show that even in a multivariate setting, age has a strong positive correlation with CES-D scores. The education variables are jointly statistically significant for both men and women, with the more schooling, the lower the CES-D scores. The age-schooling interactions are not significant. The *pce* variables, while not individually significant, are jointly significant (at 10% or lower) and show a negative association between *pce* and CES-D scores.[28]

CONCLUSIONS

Indonesia has undergone major changes in multiple dimensions since the Indonesia Family Life Survey was first fielded in 1993. Among these changes has been moving along the health and nutrition transition. IFLS is very well suited to examine those changes.

Overall there have been significant changes in health outcomes among elderly Indonesians over the 15-year period of IFLS. Much of the change

---

[26]The answers for CES-D are on a four-scale metric, from rarely, to some days (1–2 days), to occasionally (3–4 days), to most of the time (5–7 days). We score these answers in the way suggested by the Stanford group that created the CES-D, using numbers from 0 for rarely to 3 for most of the time, for negative questions such as "do you feel sad." For positive questions, such as "do you feel happy," the scoring is reversed from 0 for most of the time to 3 for rarely.

[27]They also use IFLS data, from 1993 and 2000. Unfortunately the depression scale that IFLS had been using was not as widely used as the CES-D scale, so we switched scales in 2007 to be more comparable to other international surveys, especially the HRS-type surveys. This means that in this chapter, we can only use the CES-D scale for one year, 2007.

[28]Similar results are again found in the CHARLS data for China (see Strauss et al., 2011).

can be seen as improvements, such as the movement out of undernutrition and communicable disease as well as the increasing levels of hemoglobin, which, however, are still at low levels compared to high-income countries. On the other hand, other changes, such as the increase in overweight and waist circumference, especially among women, and continuing high levels of hypertension and high levels of low HDL cholesterol seem to be inadequately addressed by the health system. These conditions indicate that the elderly population in Indonesia is increasingly exposed to higher risk factors that are correlated with chronic problems such as cardiovascular diseases and diabetes.

This is quite interesting because this period has seen major gyrations in economic activity, including strong growth from 1993 to 1996, a major economic collapse from late 1997 to 1998, and a strong recovery from 2000 to 2007. The financial crisis may have slowed the nutrition transition, and some of our evidence is consistent with that conjecture.

The relationship between health and SES at different stages in the life cycle is always difficult to disentangle. IFLS enables us to provide some important findings that contribute to our understanding of the relationships. In this chapter we examine correlations between SES and many health outcomes and behaviors for the elderly. Past work has usually been limited to just a small number of health outcomes and has not usually examined the elderly. To the extent that controlling for time, community, and their interactions account for differences in prices, healthcare availability, and quality in the communities over time, the significant correlations that still exist between SES and many of the health outcomes indicate a substantial degree of inequality of health among the elderly population. We find positive correlations between SES and most of the good health outcomes and that education tends to suppress the negative impacts of age on some health outcomes.

Of some importance, we find a very large rate of underdiagnosis for hypertension, the one chronic disease of the elderly for which we have data. These rates are differential by SES for women, with lower SES women having a greater chance of being undiagnosed. This is very likely true for other chronic conditions that we could not calculate. This lack of diagnosis indicates that the Indonesian health system, like most others in low-income countries, is still not set up to adequately care for chronic conditions of the elderly.

REFERENCES

Abikusno, N. (2009). Evaluation and implementation of ageing-related policies in Indonesia. In *Older Persons in Southeast Asia: An Emerging Asset*, E.N. Arifin and A. Ananta (Eds.). Singapore: ISEAS.

Barker, D. (1994). *Mothers, Babies, and Health in Later Life*. London: BMJ Publishing.

Barrera, A. (1990). The role of mother's schooling and its interaction with public health programs in child health production. *Journal of Development Economics 32(1)*:69-92.

Cameron, L.A., and D. Cobb-Clark (2008). Do co-residency and financial transfers from the children reduce the need for elderly parents to works in developing countries? *Journal of Population Economics 21*:1,007-1,033.

Crimmins, E., J. Hu, P. Hu, W. Huang, J. Kim, Y. Shi, J. Strauss, L. Zhang, and Y. Zhao. (2011). *CHARLS Pilot: Blood-based Biomarker Documentation*. Peking University, China Center for Economic Research.

Das, J., Q.-T. Do, J. Friedman, D. McKenzie, and K. Scott. (2007). Mental health and poverty in developing countries. *Social Science and Medicine 65(3)*:467-480.

Friedman, J., and D. Thomas (2008). Psychological health, before, during and after an economic crisis: Results from Indonesia 1993-2000. *World Bank Economic Review 23(1)*:57-76.

Gluckman, P., and M. Hanson (2005). *The Fetal Matrix: Evolution, Development and Disease*. Cambridge: Cambridge University Press.

Gurven, M., H. Kaplan, J. Winking, D.E. Rodriguez, S. Vasunilashorn, J.-K. Kim, C. Finch, and E. Crimmins. (2009). Inflammation and infection do not promote arterial aging and cardiovascular disease risk factors among lean horticulturalists. *PLoS One 4(8)*:e6590. doi:10.1371/journal.pone.0006590.

Indonesia Family Life Survey, Wave 1. (1994). Available: http://www.rand.org/labor/FLS/IFLS.html.

Indonesia Family Life Survey, Wave 2. (1997). Available: http://www.rand.org/labor/FLS/IFLS.html.

Indonesia Family Life Survey, Wave 3. (2000). Available: http://www.rand.org/labor/FLS/IFLS/ifls3.html.

Indonesia Family Life Survey, Wave 4. (2008). Available: http://www.rand.org/labor/FLS/IFLS/ifls4.html.

Indonesian Public Health Association. (1993). *Analysis of the Health Transition in Indonesia: Implications for Health Policy*. Jakarta: Indonesian Public Health Association.

Kannel, W.B., W.P. Castelli, and T. Gordon. (1979). Cholesterol in the prediction of atherosclerotic disease. New perspectives based on the Framingham study. *Annals of Internal Medicine 90(1)*:85-91.

Kinsella, K., and W. He (2009). *An Aging World: 2008*. U.S. Census Bureau, International Population Reports, PS95/09-1. Washington, DC: U.S. Government Printing Office.

McArdle, J., G. Fisher, and K. Kadlec. (2007). Latent variable analysis of age trends in tests of cognitive ability in the Health and Retirement Survey, 1992-2004. *Psychology and Aging 22(3)*:525-545.

McArdle, J., J.P. Smith, and R. Willis. (2009). Cognition and Economic Outcomes in the Health and Retirement Survey, manuscript, RAND Corporation, Santa Monica, CA.

Monteiro, C., E. Moura, W. Conde, and B. Popkin (2004). Socioeconomic status and obesity in adult populations of developing countries. *Bulletin of the World Health Organization 82(12)*:940-946.

Parker, S., G. Teruel, and L. Rubalcava. (2010). Perceptions and Knowledge of Underlying Health Conditions in Mexico. Paper presented at the Population Association of America Annual Meetings, Dallas, Texas.

Patel, V., and A. Kleinman. (2003). Poverty and common mental disorders in developing countries. *Bulletin of the World Health Organization 81(8)*:609-615.

Popkin, B. (1994). The nutrition transition in low-income countries: An emerging crisis. *Nutrition Reviews 52(9)*:285-298.

Strauss, J., and D. Thomas (1995). Human resources: Empirical modeling of household and family decisions. In *Handbook of Development Economics, Volume 3A*, J.R. Behrman and T.N. Srinivasan (Eds.). Amsterdam: North Holland Press.

Strauss, J., and D. Thomas (1998). Health, nutrition and economic development. *Journal of Economic Literature 36(3)*:766-817.

Strauss, J., and D. Thomas. (2008). Health over the life course. In *Handbook of Development Economics, Volume 4*, T.P. Schultz and J. Strauss (Eds.). Amsterdam: North Holland Press.

Strauss, J., K. Beegle, A. Dwiyanto, Y. Herawati, D. Pattinasarany, E. Satriawan, B. Sikoki, Sukamdi, and F. Witoelar. (2004). *Indonesian Living Standards Before and After the Financial Crisis*. Singapore: Institute for Southeast Asian Studies.

Strauss, J., F. Witoelar, B. Sikoki, and A.M. Wattie. (2009). *User's Guide for the Indonesia Family Life Survey, Wave 4: Volume 2*. Working Paper WR-675/2-NIA/NICHD, Labor and Population Program. Santa Monica, CA: RAND Corporation.

Strauss, J., X. Lei, A. Park, Y. Shen, J.P. Smith, Z. Yang, and Y. Zhao. (2010). Health outcomes and socio-economic status among the elderly in China: Evidence from the CHARLS Pilot. *Journal of Population Ageing 3(3)*:111-142.

Thomas, D., J. Strauss, and M.-H. Henriques. (1990). Child survival, height for age and household characteristics in Brazil. *Journal of Development Economics 33(2)*:197-234.

Thomas, D., J. Strauss, and M.-H. Henriques. (1991). How does mother's education affect child height? *Journal of Human Resources 26(2)*:183-211.

Thomas, D., E. Frankenberg, J. Friedman, J.-P. Habicht, M. Hakimi, N. Ingwersen, Jaswadi, N. Jones, C. McKelvey, G. Pelto, B. Sikoki, T. Seeman, J.P. Smith, C. Sumantri, W. Suriastini, and S. Wilopo. (2008). Causal effect of health on social and economic prosperity: Experimental evidence, manuscript, Department of Economics, Duke University.

Tolentino, K., and J.F. Friedman. (2007). An update on anemia in less developed countries. *American Journal of Tropical Medicine and Hygiene 77(1)*:44-51.

van Eeuwijk, P. (2006). Old age vulnerability, ill-health and care support in urban areas of Indonesia. *Ageing and Society 26(1)*:61-80.

Witoelar, F., J. Strauss, and B. Sikoki. (2009). *Socioeconomic Success and Health in Later Life: Evidence from the Indonesia Family Life Survey*. RAND Labor and Population Working Paper No. WR-704. Santa Monica, CA: RAND Corporation.

14

Healthcare and Insurance Among the Elderly in China: Evidence from the CHARLS Pilot[1]

John Strauss, Hao Hong, Xiaoyan Lei, Lin Li,
Albert Park, Li Yang, and Yaohui Zhao

W e are concerned in this chapter with measuring health insurance in China: who has it, which types, what are the key parameters of the insurance, and who uses inpatient and outpatient facilities, by using new data from the China Health and Retirement Longitudinal Study (CHARLS) pilot. These are important issues in China now, with many changes instituted recently related to the programs' availability and generosity.

In very recent years, there has been a large set of reforms begun regarding health insurance and healthcare, and a growing literature has analyzed these reforms (see, for instance, a recent issue of *Health Economics* devoted to this topic, Wagstaff et al., 2009). The older rural system, the Rural Cooperative Medical System, collapsed with the advent of the newer Household Responsibility System (Brown and Theoharides, 2009; Wagstaff et al., 2009). Because of this massive change, health insurance was virtually nonexistent in rural areas after the economic reforms and before 2003.

In general, urban health insurance coverage was directly tied to

[1]Comments from two referees, the editors, Gordon Liu, Richard Suzman, and David Weir are greatly appreciated. An earlier version was presented at the 2nd International Conference on Health and Retirement in China, July 2009, Beijing. The research was supported by the National Institute on Aging (Grant Number R21AG031372), Natural Science Foundation of China (Grant Numbers 70773002 and 70910107022), the World Bank (Contract 7145915), and the Fogarty International Center (Grant Number R03TW008358). The content is solely the responsibility of the authors and does not necessarily represent the official views of any of the funders.

formal employment status, with coverage of other family members not provided. Previous government and state-owned enterprise insurance programs have been subsumed by the Basic Medical Insurance program in urban areas, which is funded by employer and employee contributions (6–10% and 2% of wages, respectively) split between individual medical savings accounts and socially pooled accounts. Growing informalization of the urban labor market caused by the closing of many State Owned Enterprises starting in the late 1980s led to falling health insurance coverage rates in urban areas. In 2005, only 47% of those living in cities and 33% of those living in towns were covered by health insurance (World Bank, 2009). The problem of low health insurance coverage was exacerbated by rising healthcare costs (which were then not covered) caused in part because doctors had a strong incentive to overprescribe treatments and medicines to generate income (World Bank, 2009).

Recent reforms have aimed to increase health insurance coverage of the population. In urban areas, coverage has been extended to the non-employed (e.g., students, children, elderly, those unemployed or out of the labor force) by a new voluntary Urban Resident Basic Medical Insurance Scheme, which was introduced in September 2007 in 79 cities. It enrolled 43 million people by year-end 2007, with plans to expand to 229 cities in 2008 (Lin, Liu, and Chen, 2009; World Bank, 2009).

The New Cooperative Medical Scheme (NCMS), a new rural health insurance program, was established on a pilot basis in 2003 and expanded nationally over time. When the program began, the health insurance coverage rate in rural China was about 20%, but by the end of 2007, the NCMS had grown to reach 2,451 counties (86% of all counties nation-wide) (World Bank, 2009). The program is underwritten by both the central and provincial governments, but the county-unit governments have the responsibility for setting parameters of the program, such as user fees and premiums and reimbursement rates. Many counties have fixed the fees at 10 Yuan per person per year, supplemented with a local government contribution of at least 20 Yuan per person, plus a central government contribution also typically of 20 Yuan per person (Brown and Theoharides, 2009).[2] However, a number of concerns have also been

---

[2]For the premiums, the central government contributes a certain amount and also has a minimum requirement of how much the local government should pay. The amount has increased over time: From 2003–2004, the central government paid 10 Yuan/person/ year and required the local government to pay at least 10; in 2005–2007, these numbers were 20; in 2008–2009, they were raised to 40, and in 2010, to 60. The actual contributions of the local governments differ depending on their economic capability, but they must satisfy the minimum requirement. The minimum individual contribution was 10 Yuan in 2003–2007; it was raised to 20 in 2008, and then to 30, in 2010. It was waived for very poor households such as those receiving Wubao, a welfare program.

raised about the new program, including large differences across counties in coverage (which hospitals permit coverage and for what) and percentage of reimbursement. Discussion has ensued about low and unreliable reimbursement procedures and lack of coverage of outpatient expenses (Brown and Theoharides, 2009; World Bank, 2009; Yi et al., 2009). Yi et al. (2009) found lower reimbursement rates for higher medical costs in the five provinces their study covers, which means that major medical bills are not well covered. In April 2009, the Chinese government announced a plan to spend 850 billion Yuan over the next three years to improve the healthcare system, with a goal of covering 90% of the population with basic health insurance by 2011.

Regional variations in the implementation and timing of pension, health insurance, and social assistance programs provide opportunities to study the impact of policies and programs. China is in a critical phase of designing and reforming its social insurance programs, and CHARLS will be able to track whether programs are reaching the elderly and evaluate how such programs are affecting the behavior and welfare of the elderly. In this chapter we take a first look at the CHARLS pilot data from Zhejiang and Gansu provinces, fielded in the summer of 2008.

We find that the overwhelming majority of our respondents over age 45 report having health insurance of some kind, particularly the new rural insurance scheme. Premiums that are paid by individuals are low in rural areas and higher in urban areas, which reflect the higher degree of government subsidization in rural areas. Most importantly, the schemes as they have been instituted so far cover mostly inpatient use, not outpatient. Reimbursement rates for inpatient services range from 30-40% in rural and urban areas, respectively. These new schemes are not covering catastrophic illnesses, at least not on average, and have no major medical insurance component. Incomes are very highly correlated with inpatient service use, and having insurance is also positively correlated with inpatient use for men.

In the rest of this chapter, we briefly discuss some data issues and the results, starting with the insurance results and then utilization. Finally, we offer some conclusions.

DATA

We use the CHARLS pilot data, which is described in Zhao et al. (2009). CHARLS was designed after the Health and Retirement Study in the United States as a broad-purposed social science and health survey of the elderly in Zhejiang and Gansu provinces. These provinces were chosen because they represented the extremes of living standards in China at the time: Zhejiang being among the richest and fastest-growing provinces and Gansu being the poorest. The pilot survey was conducted in July–September 2008. The CHARLS pilot sample is representative of people aged 45 and older, and their spouses, living in households in Gansu and Zhejiang provinces.

The CHARLS pilot sample was drawn in four stages. In each province, all county-level units were stratified by whether they were urban districts (*qu*) or rural counties (*xian*), and by region within each classification. Both urban districts and rural counties can contain both urban and rural communities, but the concentration of urban and rural populations is quite different in the two. With a goal of sampling 16 county-level units per province, the number of counties to be sampled in each stratum was determined based on population size. Before the pilot survey, the Beijing CHARLS office first obtained a list of county units and their populations in each of the provinces from official statistics. Counties were randomly selected within each stratum with probabilities proportionate to size as measured by population.

After the county units were chosen, the National Bureau of Statistics helped us to sample villages and communities within county units using recently updated village-level population data. As primary sampling units (PSUs), our sample used administrative villages (*cun*) in rural areas and neighborhoods (*shequ*), which comprise one or more former resident committees (*juweihui*), in urban areas. We selected three PSUs within each county-level unit, using PPS (probabilities proportional to size) sampling. As noted above, rural counties contain both rural villages and urban neighborhoods, and it is also possible for urban districts to contain rural administrative villages.

In each PSU, we selected a sample of dwellings from our frame, which was constructed based on maps prepared by advance teams with the support of local informants. For rural villages, in many cases the lead persons on the advance teams were able to use maps drafted for the agricultural census in 2006 as a starting point, which they updated in consultation with local leaders. For urban communities, existing building maps were frequently used as the basis for the frame. All buildings in each PSU were numbered, and dwellings within each building were listed and coded using standardized methods. The advanced team verified that all buildings in the PSU had been properly identified and that dwelling units within multidwelling buildings had been correctly coded before choosing the sample of households.

Once the sampling frame for a PSU was completed and entered into the lead person's computer, the team used CAPI (computer-assisted personal interviewing) to sample the households automatically. The number of households sampled was greater than the targeted sample size of 16 households per PSU in anticipation of nonresponse and sampled households not having any members aged 45 and older. The number of households sampled was 36 in urban PSUs and 30 in rural PSUs. We interviewed all age-eligible sample households in each PSU that were willing to participate in the survey, ultimately interviewing 1,570 households containing 2,685 respondents aged 45 and older and their spouses.

We use data on all respondents aged 45 and older.[3] Tables and figures are weighted using individual sample weights.[4] All figures are nonparametric and drawn using LOWESS. Regressions are run unweighted since the sample selection is independent of our dependent variables. All analyses are disaggregated by gender. Health outcomes have long been known to differ by gender, and they do for the elderly in China (see, for instance, Strauss et al., 2010). Hence, it is natural to explore whether health insurance coverage and healthcare utilization also differ by gender.

RESULTS

Insurance Coverage

In the five years before 2008, a major change began in terms of the availability of health insurance to the Chinese population. We can see this in Table 14-1, which shows the fraction of the men and women separately who claim they have some health insurance (public or private). Overall, 91% of our sample over 45 has some insurance. By age, the fraction with insurance stays fairly constant, with a slight drop among those over 75 years. There are no major differences between men and women. Among those who do not have insurance, a small percentage, 15% of men and 13% of women, lost their insurance recently,[5] but most never had any after the collapse of the old system. Five years prior to 2008, very few people would have had insurance coverage, especially in rural areas.

We examine the different types of publicly provided insurance separately in Table 14-2, for men and women respectively. Three new public insurance programs had come into existence in the five years prior to 2008.[6] The NCMS is designed for rural areas and is the most prevalent of the three. Two insurance schemes dominate urban areas: the Urban Employee Medical Insurance and the Urban Resident Basic Medical

---

[3]Spouses who are under 45 years old are dropped from this analysis.

[4]Here we use the sample weights allowing for household nonresponse; see Zhao et al. (2009) for details.

[5]In the CHARLS pilot, we asked respondents who did not have health insurance if they had lost any coverage.

[6]Although there are other types of insurance in China, such as government medical insurance and private health insurance, these three types of insurance are the most common, so we only focused on them.

TABLE 14-1 Insurance Coverage, by Age and Gender

	Men		Women		All	
	%	N	%	N	%	N
45–54	90.3	447	92.0	493	91.1	940
	(2.5)		(1.9)		(1.9)	
55–64	94.3	423	93.4	404	93.8	827
	(1.6)		(1.9)		(1.6)	
65–74	90.9	279	90.1	229	90.5	508
	(2.5)		(2.1)		(1.7)	
75+	86.1	119	81.3	112	83.5	231
	(4.2)		(4.8)		(3.3)	
Total (45+)	91.1	1,268	90.5	1,238	90.8	2,506
	(1.5)		(1.5)		(1.3)	

NOTE: Standard errors in parentheses.
SOURCE: Authors' calculations using CHARLS pilot data.

Insurance, with the former being more prevalent in our sample. The employee insurance is given mainly through employers, while the resident insurance is a public program provided through the community. As seen in Table 14-2, the rural insurance scheme is targeted to people with a rural hukou,[7] not necessarily those living only in rural areas.[8] While in rural areas there is little spillover from the rural to the urban insurance schemes, in urban areas many residents have the rural insurance because they are farmers and still have rural hukou. For example, Table 14-2 Panel B shows that 48.7% of men in urban areas have NCMS insurance, while only 7.4% have it for those with an urban hukou. Almost no difference exists for men in having some insurance by rural or urban area, or by rural or urban hukou. For women, Table 14-2 Panel C shows that having a rural hukou makes it a little more likely that they will have some coverage. Women with an urban hukou are much more likely to have the Urban Resident Basic Medical Insurance, and men almost only have the Urban Employee Medical Insurance.

If we define a migrant as a person whose hukou is in a different county than where he or she currently resides, migrants are severely

---

[7]Hukou is a form of registration, attached to an area and agricultural or nonagricultural. People may live in urban areas with an agricultural, or rural, hukou, because many formerly rural areas have become urban. Migrants typically have their hukou in their place of origin. Not having a hukou for one's place of residence results in some loss of public benefits.

[8]The rural definition we use in this chapter is the State Bureau of Statistics (SBS) definition. Some of the SBS urban communities are in fact rural in nature, and many of their populations are farmers with rural hukou.

TABLE 14-2 Coverage of Different Insurance Types

PANEL A Both Men and Women

	Urban Employee Medical Insurance	Urban Resident Basic Medical Insurance	New Cooperative Scheme Medical Insurance	Other Insurances	Without Insurance	N
Urban Hukou	53.7 (5.9)	16.2 (3.0)	9.9 (2.8)	18.1 (4.8)	10.3 (2.3)	497
Rural Hukou	0.9 (0.3)	0.3 (0.2)	88.6 (1.5)	2.7 (0.7)	8.9 (1.4)	2,010
Urban Area	24.7 (5.1)	7.7 (1.5)	51.6 (6.3)	10.8 (2.8)	10.3 (2.2)	1,106
Rural Area	1.4 (0.3)	0.2 (0.2)	89.3 (1.6)	1.8 (0.5)	8.2 (1.5)	1,401
Total	12.4 (2.8)	3.7 (0.8)	71.5 (3.6)	6.1 (1.5)	9.2 (1.3)	2,507

PANEL B Men

	Urban Employee Medical Insurance	Urban Resident Basic Medical Insurance	New Cooperative Scheme Medical Insurance	Other Insurances	Without Insurance	N
Urban Hukou	63.0 (5.8)	11.4 (2.6)	7.4 (2.3)	18.3 (3.5)	7.9 (2.2)	268
Rural Hukou	1.1 (0.4)	0.4 (0.3)	87.4 (1.8)	3.5 (1.2)	9.2 (1.6)	1,001
Urban Area	30.2 (6.1)	5.7 (1.4)	48.7 (6.1)	11.6 (2.4)	9.2 (2.5)	541
Rural Area	2.2 (0.6)	0.4 (0.4)	87.0 (1.9)	2.8 (0.8)	8.8 (1.7)	728

	Urban Employee Medical Insurance	Urban Resident Basic Medical Insurance	New Cooperative Scheme Medical Insurance	Other Insurances	Without Insurance	N
Total	14.9	2.8	69.7	6.8	8.9	1,269
	(3.1)	(0.7)	(3.5)	(1.3)	(1.5)	

PANEL C Women

	Urban Employee Medical Insurance	Urban Resident Basic Medical Insurance	New Cooperative Scheme Medical Insurance	Other Insurances	Without Insurance	N
Urban Hukou	43.5	21.5	12.6	18.0	12.9	229
	(7.2)	(5.0)	(4.3)	(7.3)	(3.3)	
Rural Hukou	0.6	0.1	89.9	1.9	8.5	1,009
	(0.3)	(0.1)	(1.7)	(0.6)	(1.6)	
Urban Area	19.4	9.5	54.4	10.1	11.3	565
	(4.8)	(2.3)	(7.0)	(4.1)	(2.5)	
Rural Area	0.4	0.0	91.9	0.8	7.6	673
	(0.2)	(0.0)	(1.8)	(0.5)	(1.9)	
Total	9.8	4.7	73.4	5.4	9.5	1,238
	(2.7)	(1.2)	(4.2)	(2.2)	(1.5)	

NOTE: Standard errors in parentheses.
SOURCE: Authors' calculations using CHARLS pilot data.

disadvantaged. One-third of migrants, both male and female, have no insurance whatever, up from the 9% in the general population.[9] Clearly, migrants are a vulnerable population in this regard. If a migrant has insurance, it is most likely the rural NCMS insurance. This makes sense because their hukou are in most cases rural places, even though they may live in an urban area.[10]

It is of some interest to examine whether the insured are in better or worse health than the non-insured. No causality can be attached to these correlations in this chapter. We have many available measures of health to use; here, we use a self-reported measure of general health on a scale of excellent, very good, good, fair, or poor. While self-reported general health measures have biases (see Strauss and Thomas, 1998, for example), they also have signal, since they predict future mortality well (Banks et al., 2009). As shown in Table 14-3, there are no significant differences in insurance coverage among those in poor health versus those not in poor health. This is of interest for several reasons, among which it appears that adverse selection is not a major problem in our sample, at least not for all programs taken together. Lin et al. (2009), however, do find adverse selection in their analysis of the Urban Resident Basic Medical Insurance, but they do not focus exclusively on the older population.

Table 14-4 provides regression results for having any insurance for men and women, respectively. We start in column 1 with a model that includes major socioeconomic status (SES) variables: a set of dummy variables for age group (under 55 years the left-out group), for education levels completed (no schooling the left out group), and a linear spline in log of per capita expenditure (*pce*).[11] *Pce* is preferred to income because income is measured with much more error than *pce* (see Lee, 2009, for instance) and because *pce* is a better measure of long-run resources because it is smoothed in the face of annual income shocks. The knot point for the spline is at the median of log *pce*. We also include dummies for province interacted with rural area of residence. In column 2, we add a set of variables that are arguably endogenous: a dummy for migrant status (not a migrant being left out), and dummies for being widowed and being divorced or never married (the two are both very small in number and cannot be statistically distinguished in our data). Column 3 replaces

---

[9]Note that the cell sizes are extremely small, especially for women.

[10]Note that if we define migrant as having a rural hukou but living in an urban area, the insurance coverage of this population is nearly identical to nonmigrants. In part, this is a function of these people not really being migrants but just being farmers and living in urban areas that are arguably rural.

[11]A linear spline allows different slopes to the left and right of the knot point with the two lines being joined at the knot point. The first coefficient reported is the slope to the left of the knot point, and the second coefficient is the change in the slope from the left-hand portion.

TABLE 14-3 Coverage of Insurance for Men and Women, by Self-reported Health

	Men				Women			
	With insurance (%)	Without insurance (%)	N	P-value	With insurance (%)	Without insurance (%)	N	P-value
Poor health	89.7 (3.1)	10.3 (3.1)	241		92.5 (1.8)	7.5 (1.8)	341	
Nonpoor health	91.1 (1.7)	8.9 (1.7)	872		90.2 (1.7)	9.8 (1.7)	781	
All	90.9 (1.6)	9.1 (1.6)	1,113	0.658	90.8 (1.5)	9.2 (1.5)	1,122	0.221

NOTE: Standard errors in parentheses. P-values are from tests of equality of insurance coverage between people having poor health and nonpoor health, separately for men and women.
SOURCE: Authors' calculations using CHARLS pilot data.

TABLE 14-4 Regression for Having Any Insurance, Men and Women

	Men			Women		
	(1)	(2)	(3)	(1)	(2)	(3)
Aged 55–64	0.031*	0.027	0.017	0.019	0.019	0.016
	(0.018)	(0.019)	(0.016)	(0.022)	(0.024)	(0.021)
Aged 65–74	0.037	0.044*	0.025	-0.018	-0.013	-0.016
	(0.023)	(0.026)	(0.026)	(0.024)	(0.025)	(0.024)
Aged 75 and older	-0.002	-0.006	-0.008	-0.124***	-0.081*	-0.113**
	(0.035)	(0.043)	(0.042)	(0.047)	(0.047)	(0.049)
Can read and write	0.026	0.032	0.032	0.057**	0.058**	0.047**
	(0.022)	(0.022)	(0.021)	(0.025)	(0.027)	(0.021)
Finished primary	0.021	0.032	0.033	0.025	0.023	0.002
	(0.024)	(0.025)	(0.022)	(0.032)	(0.033)	(0.031)
Junior high and above	0.034	0.044*	0.030	0.087***	0.096***	0.067**
	(0.022)	(0.024)	(0.023)	(0.030)	(0.031)	(0.026)
logPCE (< median)	0.034*	0.021	0.010	0.001	0.003	0.002
	(0.017)	(0.017)	(0.013)	(0.012)	(0.012)	(0.013)
logPCE (> median, marginal)	0.001	0.019	0.012	0.013	0.014	0.008
	(0.027)	(0.027)	(0.022)	(0.030)	(0.035)	(0.029)
Migrant		-0.262***	-0.197**		-0.302**	-0.188
		(0.076)	(0.079)		(0.118)	(0.144)
Widowed		-0.105***	-0.128***		-0.053	-0.044
		(0.038)	(0.037)		(0.032)	(0.033)
Divorced or never married		0.088***	0.081***		-0.075	-0.140
		(0.019)	(0.016)		(0.141)	(0.147)

	(1)	(2)	(3)	(4)	(5)	(6)
Having poor health		0.011	0.017		0.022	0.026*
		(0.020)	(0.022)		(0.016)	(0.015)
Rural Zhejiang	0.007	0.005		0.043	0.045	
	(0.032)	(0.033)		(0.039)	(0.041)	
Urban Gansu	−0.021	−0.021		−0.093	−0.091	
	(0.047)	(0.051)		(0.057)	(0.055)	
Rural Gansu	0.079***	0.076**		0.070*	0.072	
	(0.026)	(0.030)		(0.042)	(0.046)	
Community FE	NO	NO	YES	NO	NO	YES
F-test for all age dummies	2.02	1.66	0.66	3.06**	1.82	2.70**
(p-value)	(0.117)	(0.181)	(0.576)	(0.032)	(0.149)	(0.050)
F-test for all education dummies	0.88	1.19	1.04	3.56**	3.98**	3.30**
(p-value)	(0.453)	(0.320)	(0.379)	(0.017)	(0.010)	(0.024)
F-test for all logPCE splines	5.17***	2.91*	1.61	0.16	0.27	0.15
(p-value)	(0.007)	(0.060)	(0.206)	(0.855)	(0.761)	(0.857)
F-test for all marital status dummies		17.73***	19.60***		1.53	1.33
(p-value)		(0.000)	(0.000)		(0.223)	(0.268)
F-test for all location dummies	4.23***	3.44**	1.98***	3.23**	3.57**	1.84***
(p-value)	(0.008)	(0.020)	(0.000)	(0.026)	(0.017)	(0.001)
Observations	1,262	1,107	1,107	1,233	1,118	1,118

NOTE: Robust standard errors in parentheses, all clustered at community level. * denotes $p < .1$; ** $p < .05$; *** $p < .01$. logPCE (> median, marginal) represents the change in the slope from the interval for logPCE below the median.
SOURCE: Authors' calculations using CHARLS pilot data.

province-rural dummies with community fixed effects.[12] The idea here is that each community has factors that will affect insurance and healthcare utilization that are not captured by the provincial dummies interacted with rural or urban. These factors will include healthcare prices, inherent healthiness of the area, public health infrastructure, and other factors. F-tests for all combinations of dummy variables are reported as well.

Regressions are all ordinary least squares (OLS). For binary dependent variables, this represents linear probability (LP) models. LP models consistently estimate average treatment effects, which is what we are interested in. Furthermore, all of our standard errors are calculated for robustness to heteroskedasticity and allow clustering at the community level. The robustness makes our standard error estimates consistent when we are estimating LP models (Wooldridge, 2002).

For men, age dummies are weakly significant (at the 10% level), except when we add community fixed effects, and show that men aged 55–64 are about 3% more likely to have insurance than younger men. For women, the age dummies are highly significant (at the .001 level), and older women over 75 years are 10–14% less likely to be insured, a large impact.

For men, education does not seem to have significant effects on possessing any insurance, but for women, it raises the likelihood of having insurance. On the other hand, for men, higher *pce* is associated with a higher probability of having some insurance, but not for women.

Reporting poor general health is not correlated with having insurance for men. It is weakly (at the 10% level) positively correlated for women, with some evidence of adverse selection for women.

Being a migrant male is associated with a 22% decline in the likelihood of being insured, a very large difference; the difference for women is similar in magnitude and significance. The NCMS generally does not reimburse migrants for their medical expenses incurred in urban areas where the migrants are working, so the incentive for them to participate in the NCMS is low. The two major urban insurance schemes also do not cover migrants. In May 2006, a separate medical insurance pooling fund was set up to cover expenses for migrants, but the effectiveness of this program has not been evaluated to date.

Being widowed also is associated with a large (10%) decline in the odds of being insured for men, though a much less large difference for women and not significant in most cases.

Men and women who live in rural Gansu have a somewhat higher chance of having health insurance, once individual and household SES

---

[12]Since the binary dependent variables cannot be all 1 or 0 for a given community, some communities had to be aggregated.

factors are controlled. This is interesting, and one might have expected the reverse. However, even the unconditional probabilities of having insurance are a bit higher in rural areas of Zhejiang and Gansu. When we add the community dummies in column 3, they are jointly significant at the .001 level for both men and women.[13] Now the migrant dummy loses magnitude and significance for women and its magnitude drops by 30% for men. Apparently, important, unmeasured factors exist at the community level that affect access to insurance for those who do not get it.

In results not shown, we repeat the regressions for respondents who have a rural hukou and are thus eligible in principle to join the NCMS.[14] Most of the results for the rural insurance are similar to the main results: Older women, migrants, and male widowers are substantially less likely to be insured with this scheme. However, the associations of education and *pce* with belonging to the NCMS are generally not significant, except for women for being able to read and write, but not for those with more schooling.

Healthcare Utilization

About 16.5% of men and 21% of women aged 45 and older said they used outpatient services at least once over the past month (see Table 14-5).[15] Most of those who went used a hospital or a village or private clinic. Township hospitals and healthcare posts were also important destinations, especially in rural areas. Table 14-5 shows that inpatient use over the past year was less frequent, 6.7% for men and 6% for women. Virtually all of the inpatient use was at hospitals, general hospitals being the most important destination by far, followed equally by specialized hospitals, Chinese medicine hospitals, and township hospitals.

Regressions for outpatient utilization (see Table 14-6) show that for men, being older and more educated have positive associations with use,

---

[13]With community fixed effects, testing the joint significance of the community dummies is not straightforward. Because there are in our case few observations per cluster, we cannot cluster the standard errors after estimation using community fixed effects and use an F-test to test for the joint significance of clusters (Wooldridge, personal communication). To test the community dummies, we re-estimate the model with community dummies and just robust standard errors, without clustering, and do the F-test.

[14]We consider sample sizes for people with urban hukou and thus eligible for the urban insurance schemes too small to analyze with regressions. Lin et al. (2009) find that income has a U-shaped association with having the Urban Resident Basic Medical Insurance, with low- and high-income persons more likely to have it.

[15]While these outpatient rates may seem high, they correspond closely to other populations. In the Indonesia Family Life Survey, wave 4, for instance, 15% of men and 21% of women over 45 years used an outpatient service over the same one-month period. The inpatient usage rates in Indonesia are lower, only 4.7% of men and 3.5% of women aged 45 and older.

TABLE 14-5 Percentage of People Who Used Medical Service in the Past Month, by Age and Gender

	Outpatient						Inpatient					
	Men		Women		All		Men		Women		All	
	%	N	%	N	%	N	%	N	%	N	%	N
45–54	11.7	395	20.0	459	15.6	854	2.9	395	4.5	459	3.7	854
	(2.0)		(2.4)		(1.4)		(0.8)		(1.0)		(0.7)	
55–64	23.6	374	23.6	367	23.6	741	9.3	374	5.1	367	7.1	741
	(4.0)		(3.8)		(3.1)		(1.9)		(1.4)		(1.2)	
65–74	15.4	249	16.7	204	16.0	453	10.3	249	7.3	204	8.9	453
	(2.5)		(2.6)		(1.9)		(2.6)		(2.6)		(1.9)	
75+	17.4	92	25.6	94	22.1	186	6.5	92	9.5	94	8.2	186
	(4.9)		(6.5)		(4.3)		(2.8)		(4.1)		(2.7)	
Total (45+)	16.5	1,110	21.2	1,124	18.9	2,234	6.7	1,110	5.9	1,124	6.3	2,234
	(1.7)		(2.1)		(1.5)		(0.9)		(0.9)		(0.7)	

NOTE: Standard errors in parentheses.
SOURCE: Authors' calculations using CHARLS pilot data.

TABLE 14-6 Regression for Using Medical Service for Outpatients

	Men		Women	
	(1)	(2)	(1)	(2)
Aged 55–64	0.082***	0.073**	0.009	–0.009
	(0.030)	(0.030)	(0.029)	(0.030)
Aged 65–74	0.072**	0.060	0.010	–0.014
	(0.033)	(0.037)	(0.036)	(0.037)
Aged 75 and older	0.084*	0.097**	0.111*	0.099
	(0.044)	(0.047)	(0.058)	(0.060)
Can read and write	0.078**	0.081**	–0.017	–0.025
	(0.030)	(0.034)	(0.034)	(0.038)
Finished primary	0.036	0.035	0.026	–0.001
	(0.033)	(0.038)	(0.047)	(0.055)
Junior high and above	0.067*	0.073*	0.012	–0.023
	(0.036)	(0.038)	(0.045)	(0.045)
logPCE (< median)	0.016	0.022	0.022*	0.019
	(0.014)	(0.014)	(0.013)	(0.012)
logPCE (> median, marginal)	0.024	0.005	0.058*	0.047
	(0.027)	(0.029)	(0.035)	(0.034)
Having any insurance	0.040	0.021	0.004	–0.004
	(0.035)	(0.037)	(0.043)	(0.051)
Rural Zhejiang	0.001		0.010	
	(0.030)		(0.034)	
Urban Gansu	0.019		0.078	
	(0.033)		(0.048)	
Rural Gansu	0.061		0.119***	
	(0.037)		(0.041)	
Community FE	NO	YES	NO	YES
F-test for all age dummies	3.00**	2.46*	1.23	1.15
(p-value)	(0.035)	(0.068)	(0.304)	(0.334)
F-test for all education dummies	2.37*	2.30*	0.25	0.20
(p-value)	(0.076)	(0.083)	(0.861)	(0.893)
F-test for all logPCE splines	2.09	1.59	6.65***	4.50**
(p-value)	(0.129)	(0.210)	(0.002)	(0.014)
F-test for all location dummies	1.08	1.12	3.58**	1.84***
(p-value)	(0.360)	(0.231)	(0.017)	(0.000)
Observations	1,104	1,104	1,118	1,118

NOTE: Robust standard errors in parentheses, all clustered at community level. * denotes $p < .1$; ** $p < .05$; *** $p < .01$. logPCE (> median, marginal) represents the change in the slope from the interval for logPCE below the median.
SOURCE: Authors' calculations using CHARLS pilot data.

while for women, having higher *pce* is positively related to outpatient service use, as is living in rural Gansu, controlling for SES. The community dummies are highly significant for women, though not for men. Again, unmeasured factors at the community level are important for women seeking outpatient care.

For inpatient care (see Table 14-7), income (*pce*) is highly significant and positively related to care for both men and women. Other factors being equal, being in Gansu, rural or urban, is associated with more inpatient care use for women and living in urban Gansu for men. It is, of course, of prime interest to examine how having insurance is associated with outpatient and inpatient care. The problem is that having insurance is endogenous, and there is no good way with these data to identify a structural relationship. Still, looking at the correlations is of interest. Insurance is positively and significantly correlated with inpatient use by men, though it is not significant for women and it is not significantly related to outpatient use. A man with insurance is 4.5% more likely to seek inpatient care than a man without any insurance. These results are consistent with the results of Gao, Raven, and Tang (2007) and Wagstaff and Lindelow (2008), who also found a positive correlation of insurance with inpatient use.

Health Insurance Parameters and Reimbursement

Having health insurance does not tell anything about the nature of that insurance. The CHARLS pilot collected data about some of the characteristics of the insurance, in particular about the premiums paid, as well as, for those who had insurance and who went for inpatient or outpatient services, what fraction of their total costs they anticipated would be reimbursed. For the Urban Resident Basic Medical Insurance, not enough respondents reported their premiums so our sample is too small to report. For the Urban Employee Medical Insurance and the NCMS insurance, we report mean premiums in Table 14-8.

The mean reported premium for the NCMS is about 20 RMB per year. The mean premium is lower in rural Gansu, only 13 RMB, and higher in rural Zhejiang, about 28 RMB. These are remarkably low premiums even compared to low rural incomes in Gansu of 5,000 RMB *pce*. Even in Zhejiang, both rural and urban, about 20% say they did not pay any premiums for their NCMS insurance. For the Urban Employee Medical Insurance scheme, premiums are much higher, around 300 RMB per year in urban Gansu, about the same for women in urban Zhejiang, but much higher, 600 RMB per year, for men in urban Zhejiang. Even these levels, however, are not large relative to annual *pce* of between 7,500 RMB and 10,000 RMB per year in Gansu and Zhejiang. We have to be a bit careful because our

TABLE 14-7 Regression for Using Inpatient Medical Service

	Men		Women	
	(1)	(2)	(1)	(2)
Aged 55–64	0.051***	0.058***	0.001	0.005
	(0.018)	(0.018)	(0.019)	(0.019)
Aged 65–74	0.078***	0.087***	0.013	0.013
	(0.028)	(0.029)	(0.020)	(0.020)
Aged 75 and older	0.043	0.053	0.054	0.057*
	(0.030)	(0.033)	(0.034)	(0.034)
Can read and write	0.019	0.019	−0.023	−0.024
	(0.023)	(0.024)	(0.016)	(0.017)
Finished primary	−0.020	−0.021	0.007	0.009
	(0.020)	(0.021)	(0.024)	(0.025)
Junior high and above	−0.017	−0.013	−0.026	−0.025
	(0.022)	(0.022)	(0.024)	(0.023)
logPCE (< median)	0.014*	0.016**	0.004	0.007
	(0.008)	(0.008)	(0.005)	(0.006)
logPCE (> median, marginal)	0.038	0.032	0.062***	0.060**
	(0.025)	(0.024)	(0.021)	(0.023)
Having any insurance	0.046**	0.053*	0.024	0.020
	(0.021)	(0.028)	(0.023)	(0.024)
Rural Zhejiang	0.012		0.007	
	(0.021)		(0.016)	
Urban Gansu	0.098***		0.049**	
	(0.036)		(0.020)	
Rural Gansu	0.019		0.046**	
	(0.018)		(0.022)	
Community FE	NO	YES	NO	YES
F-test for all age dummies	3.68**	4.62***	0.98	0.99
(p-value)	(0.015)	(0.005)	(0.407)	(0.400)
F-test for all education dummies	1.20	1.17	0.99	1.10
(p-value)	(0.313)	(0.325)	(0.403)	(0.353)
F-test for all logPCE splines	5.21***	5.78***	6.06***	5.88***
(p-value)	(0.007)	(0.004)	(0.003)	(0.004)
F-test for all location dummies	2.46*	1.09	2.72**	0.71
(p-value)	(0.068)	(0.337)	(0.049)	(0.890)
Observations	1,104	1,104	1,118	1,118

NOTE: Robust standard errors in parentheses, all clustered at community level. * denotes $p < .1$; ** $p < .05$; *** $p < .01$. logPCE (> median, marginal) represents the change in the slope from the interval for logPCE below the median.
SOURCE: Authors' calculations using CHARLS pilot data.

TABLE 14-8 Mean of Premium of Different Medical Insurances

		Urban Employee Medical Insurance		New Cooperative Medical Scheme Insurance	
		Men	Women	Men	Women
Gansu Urban	Mean	289.0	337.4	18.1	18.7
		(116.4)	(114.6)	(6.0)	(6.5)
	= 0	6%	0%	1%	0%
	N	41	20	67	86
Gansu Rural	Mean			13.0	12.9
				(0.7)	(0.7)
	= 0			0%	0%
	N			368	340
Zhejiang Urban	Mean	608.1	324.3	18.2	24.1
		(173.3)	(158.9)	(3.6)	(6.2)
	= 0	12%	11%	18%	17%
	N	70	52	211	220
Zhejiang Rural	Mean			28.2	26.8
				(4.7)	(4.6)
	= 0			20%	22%
	N			267	273
Total	Mean	495.4	318.3	20.3	21.8
		(127.4)	(123.4)	(2.1)	(2.6)
	= 0	5%	3%	10%	10%
	N	122	76	913	919

NOTE: Standard errors in parentheses. "= 0" represents the number of people whose premium is zero.
SOURCE: Authors' calculations using CHARLS pilot data.

cell sizes are not large, but it is quite interesting that for this insurance plan, unlike the rural plan, premiums are lower for women, particularly in urban Zhejiang. We do not know why as yet. The other point to note from Table 14-8 is that in urban Zhejiang, a little more than 10% get their Urban Employee Medical Insurance without any premium.

Another important parameter of the new insurance schemes is the reimbursement rate. Reimbursements depend on the plan and on the parameters, which are set at the county or district level.[16] They vary greatly across county-units and depend on many factors, such as total medical expenditures, which type of facility the respondent went to and whether that type of facility is covered by the particular insurance

---

[16]In the national baseline survey conducted in 2011, a special policy module was administered at the county or district level to collect detailed plan information. Since there are 150 county-units in the national baseline, these can be analyzed at the county-unit level. In the pilot survey data we use in this chapter, that is not possible

policy, and the specific treatment received. The NCMS has four models to reimburse patients for in- and outpatient services (Lei and Lin, 2009). The most frequent model, used in two-thirds of the rural counties, uses a medical savings account. Each household has its own medical savings account, with household members depositing their contributions into this account and then spending money from it. Only household members are entitled to the funds in the account, which is used mainly for outpatient services. There is a deductible and a reimbursement cap for using a medical savings account.

Traditionally, the reimbursements for the NCMS have put more emphasis on inpatient than outpatient services. However, a more recent, general trend includes outpatient services and physical check-ups in patient reimbursements (Du and Zhang, 2007). In addition, some counties provide insurance coverage for an annual physical examination. Overall, there has been an increasing trend in the amount of coverage per capita and an increase in the range of services offered (Du and Zhang, 2007).

We calculated individual reimbursement rates by first asking the respondent if they went for outpatient service in the past month or inpatient service in the past year. If the answer was yes, then we got details about the last visit, including the total costs of the service, including medicines. We then asked how much he or she expected to pay, not just what he or she had paid to date.[17] One could reasonably worry how well respondents can answer these cost questions, but they were thoroughly pretested, and it is our judgment that these answers are reliable. For the cost repayment estimates, we aggregated men and women to maximize our cell sizes, which are small. We also used only those respondents who reported that they have insurance, as otherwise this question does not make sense.[18]

The reimbursement rates for inpatient service are 40% and 30% in urban and rural areas, respectively (not, however, significantly different at standard levels), similar between Gansu and Zhejiang (see Table 14-9). By hukou status, the reimbursement rates are 58% for urban hukou holders and 28% for rural hukou holders (these are significantly different at the .01 level). By hukou, there were some important differences across provinces; the rates for rural hukou holders were higher in Gansu (35% versus

---

[17]Respondents who reported a visit were asked about their last visit "What was the total cost of medical treatment?" and "How much will you eventually pay out of pocket for the total costs of the visit?" This was followed by equivalent questions about medications from this visit.

[18]The number of respondents who reported going for inpatient care and who do not have insurance is too small to separately and reliably report their expenditures. For outpatient care, sample size for those without insurance is very small, just 34, but in general their total costs are somewhat lower than for those with insurance.

362

TABLE 14-9 Inpatient Cost for People with Insurance

PANEL A by Urban/Rural and Province

	Urban				Rural				
	Total cost mean	Share of out-of-pocket cost (%)	Reimbursement rate (%)	N	Total cost mean	Share of out-of-pocket cost (%)	Reimbursement rate (%)	N	P-value
Gansu	3,329.3 (658.5)	57.6 (5.9)	42.4 (5.9)	33	3,631.6 (732.4)	67.9 (5.7)	32.1 (5.7)	37	0.210
Zhejiang	14,591.7 (4,844.3)	61.2 (9.7)	38.8 (9.7)	34	9,449.0 (1,316.4)	70.2 (6.0)	29.8 (6.0)	25	0.431
Total	10,562.9 (3,223.4)	59.9 (6.5)	40.1 (6.5)	67	6,981.1 (995.8)	69.3 (4.2)	30.7 (4.2)	62	0.226

PANEL B by Hukou and Province

	Urban Hukou				Rural Hukou				
	Total cost mean	Share of out-of-pocket cost (%)	Reimbursement rate (%)	N	Total cost mean	Share of out-of-pocket cost (%)	Reimbursement rate (%)	N	P-value
Gansu	4,080.7 (974.1)	54.4 (7.3)	45.6 (7.3)	17	3,284.6 (592.2)	65.2 (4.8)	34.8 (4.8)	53	0.211
Zhejiang	18,165.4 (9,372.0)	35.6 (12.4)	64.4 (12.4)	14	10,086.0 (1,430.0)	76.9 (3.9)	23.1 (3.9)	45	0.003
Total	13,247.0 (6,131.9)	42.1 (8.9)	57.9 (8.9)	31	7,351.6 (1,012.1)	72.4 (3.2)	27.6 (3.2)	98	0.002

NOTE: Standard errors in parentheses. P-values are from tests of equality of reimbursement rates between rural and urban residents or rural and urban Hukou, separately or jointly for Gansu and Zhejiang provinces.
SOURCE: Authors' calculations using CHARLS pilot data.

23%), while the rates among urban hukou holders were much higher in Zhejiang (64% compared to 46%). Furthermore, the standard error of the reimbursement rate was much higher for urban hukou in Zhejiang than for Gansu (12.4 versus 7.3).[19] This is important because the county-level units are allowed to set the parameters for the health insurance, and apparently there is a wider variance of experience related to reimbursement rates in urban Zhejiang than in urban Gansu. Also since Zhejiang is far richer than Gansu, there is more scope for higher reimbursement rates should the county-unit choose.

We checked the variation in reimbursement rates between and within counties, using an analysis of variance (ANOVA), and find that counties account for 24% of the variation for inpatient rates in Gansu and 56% for Zhejiang. Our finding that more variation exists between counties in Zhejiang than in Gansu makes sense given that there seems to be more experimentation in insurance policy parameters among counties in Zhejiang than in Gansu, in part perhaps because of its greater wealth.[20] When we disaggregate plans and run an ANOVA for inpatient respondents with the NCMS, we find 41% of the variation in Zhejiang is between counties versus 30% in Gansu. We do find important variation between counties, which we expect since counties have control over setting parameters of the programs, but even more variation within counties. Reasons for this variation include not only that we are aggregating over different insurance schemes (because of sample size consideration), but also because even for a given program, reimbursement depends on factors such as the particular reason (illness) for going to a health facility, the type of facility visited, and the total cost. These factors vary by individual and are apparently important.[21]

Yi et al. (2009) report that in the five provinces in which they did their study (which did not include either Gansu or Zhejiang), as total costs of inpatient treatment increased, reimbursement rates fell for the NCMS, often to quite low levels, around 10%. If total costs are taken as a proxy of severity of the health problem, then this strongly suggests that the major new rural health insurance scheme is not covering catastrophic illnesses well and is certainly not adequately covering catastrophic health expenditures.

The CHARLS pilot data show a very interesting, and somewhat different, story. We start in Figure 14-1 by nonparametrically plotting reimbursement rates for inpatient services against total inpatient costs,

---

[19]This is not due to outliers; even the interquartile range is much larger in Zhejiang.

[20]If there is little systematic variation between counties in Gansu in reimbursement rates, that will result in a lower R^2 when regressing reimbursement rates on county dummies.

[21]Of course, measurement error will also contribute to within-county variation.

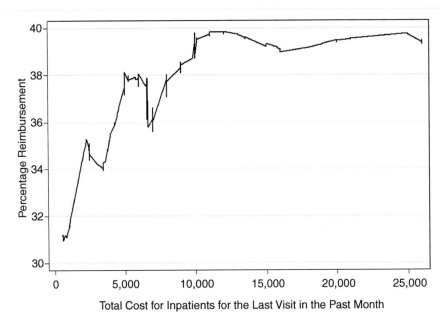

FIGURE 14-1 Reimbursement rates for inpatients with any insurance for the last visit in the past month, by total cost.
SOURCE: CHARLS pilot data.

using data on respondents with any insurance who reported inpatient utilization over the past year.[22] It is clear that reimbursement rates rise, not fall, as total costs rise. Reimbursement rates rise from 31% to a plateau of 40% at a total cost of 10,000 Yuan, which is right at the 75th percentile for the total cost distribution. Mean *pce* for our households is approximately 8,000 Yuan, and the median is 5,800, so an expense of 10,000 is quite large compared to mean *pce*. For costs above 10,000 Yuan, though, reimbursement rates stay flat at 40%. If the system were effective in covering catastrophic health expenditures, then the reimbursement rates should continue to rise; they do not.

So the glass seems to be half full. There is nontrivial coverage for inpatient expenses that does rise some as total costs rise, at least up to a point. Furthermore, when this situation is compared to the period before

---

[22]Our sample size is only 129. These are respondents who went for inpatient service (and so we have cost data for them) and who have insurance (so we have reimbursement data). Some caution needs to be taken because of the limited sample size. When we plot the figure for those who have NCMS insurance, some 96 observations, the curve slopes gently upwards at high levels of total cost, but has a peak of more than 30%.

2003, this represents a large improvement. Finally, we note that further reform and experimentation is ongoing, so this is not the final story.

For outpatient reimbursement, the story is quite different. The new health insurance schemes, particularly the rural scheme, were initially designed to help with inpatient service, so many county-units are apparently choosing not to reimburse for outpatient service (see Table 14-10 Panel A). The mean rural reimbursement rate is only 8.5%, being slightly higher in Zhejiang. The urban rates are considerably higher, a mean of 30%, but more than double in Zhejiang (36%) than in Gansu (14%). The urban reimbursement rates are significantly higher than the rural ones in Zhejiang and aggregating both provinces. Again, the standard error is much higher in urban Zhejiang than in urban Gansu, suggesting more experimentation in urban Zhejiang.[23]

If we split the sample by rural and urban hukou, the differences in reimbursement rates become starker (see Table 14-10 Panel B). Now, urban hukou holders face 63% reimbursement in Zhejiang and 17% in Gansu, which is still double the reimbursement rates for rural hukou holders in Gansu. Urban-rural hukou differences are significantly different at .01.

If we look only at reimbursement rates for people holding rural insurance through the NCMS (results not shown), we see a similar pattern to the rural population. Rates of reimbursement are about 10% for urban residents and 8% for rural, and the provincial differences are quite small. Clearly, this insurance scheme was not designed to cover outpatient service, just inpatient. However, it remains to be seen in the future whether these same patterns hold. It may be that over time, reimbursement rates may rise for outpatient service, as they have for the urban plans in Zhejiang.

Table 14-11 reports regressions on the cost share paid, separately by men and women, for outpatient service.[24] The sample is those persons who used outpatient services in the last one month and who have insurance that could be used to get reimbursement. The SES variables, education, and *pce* are insignificant in all cases. Age is important for men, but not women. Older men have lower out-of-pocket costs as a percentage of the total. The regional dummies are significant, with lower repayment rates in urban Zhejiang, as we saw in the previous tables. The community dummies are also significant.[25] This is interesting because, as discussed

---

[23]Some 35% of the variation in outpatient reimbursement rates in Zhejiang is between counties, but only 7% for Gansu. A high fraction of rural outpatients in Gansu have a zero reimbursement rate, which partly accounts for the low between-county variation.

[24]We considered the sample sizes for inpatient service too small to get meaningful results.

[25]The significance of the community dummies does not come from differences across provinces. Even using data from only Zhejiang or only Gansu, the community dummies are jointly significant.

TABLE 14-10 Outpatient Cost for People with Insurance

PANEL A Outpatient Cost for People with Insurance, by Urban/Rural and Province

	Urban				Rural				
	Total cost mean	Share of out-of-pocket cost (%)	Reimbursement rate (%)	N	Total cost mean	Share of out-of-pocket cost (%)	Reimbursement rate (%)	N	P-value
Gansu	229.4 (73.1)	85.6 (4.7)	14.4 (4.7)	58	180.8 (36.9)	92.5 (2.3)	7.5 (2.3)	131	0.186
Zhejiang	318.0 (59.1)	63.6 (9.8)	36.4 (9.8)	96	614.6 (178.1)	90.5 (1.7)	9.5 (1.7)	76	0.009
Total	293.4 (46.0)	70.1 (7.5)	29.9 (7.5)	154	413.0 (99.6)	91.5 (1.5)	8.5 (1.5)	207	0.006

PANEL B Outpatient Cost for People with Insurance, by Hukou and Province

	Urban Hukou				Rural Hukou				
	Total cost mean	Share of out-of-pocket cost (%)	Reimbursement rate (%)	N	Total cost mean	Share of out-of-pocket cost (%)	Reimbursement rate (%)	N	P-value
Gansu	192.0 (28.1)	82.6 (8.6)	17.4 (8.6)	41	201.6 (44.9)	92.3 (2.4)	7.7 (2.4)	148	0.301
Zhejiang	250.6 (67.0)	37.3 (9.7)	62.7 (9.7)	41	526.5 (114.5)	89.6 (1.9)	10.4 (1.9)	131	0.000
Total	231.4 (46.3)	53.6 (10.1)	46.4 (10.1)	82	400.5 (73.7)	90.7 (1.5)	9.3 (1.5)	279	0.000

NOTE: Standard errors in parentheses. P-values are from tests of equality of reimbursement rates between rural and urban residents or rural and urban Hukou, separately or jointly for Gansu and Zhejiang provinces.
SOURCE: Authors' calculations using CHARLS pilot data.

TABLE 14-11 Regression for the Share of Out-of-Pocket Cost in the Total Cost of the Past Visit for Outpatient Medical Service in the Past Month

	Men			Women		
	(1)	(2)	(3)	(1)	(2)	(3)
Aged 55–64	−0.083	−0.085*	−0.047	−0.039	−0.031	−0.027
	(0.050)	(0.050)	(0.053)	(0.046)	(0.047)	(0.040)
Aged 65–74	−0.225***	−0.232***	−0.206***	−0.109*	−0.102*	−0.131**
	(0.071)	(0.070)	(0.068)	(0.061)	(0.059)	(0.065)
Aged 75 and older	−0.362***	−0.380***	−0.298**	−0.053	−0.025	−0.040
	(0.112)	(0.111)	(0.119)	(0.084)	(0.090)	(0.084)
Can read and write	−0.042	−0.039	−0.045	0.055	0.061	0.048
	(0.083)	(0.084)	(0.085)	(0.045)	(0.046)	(0.053)
Finished primary	−0.066	−0.055	−0.040	−0.099	−0.094	−0.091
	(0.088)	(0.086)	(0.089)	(0.091)	(0.092)	(0.081)
Junior high and above	−0.116	−0.108	−0.048	−0.092	−0.087	−0.082
	(0.084)	(0.084)	(0.085)	(0.073)	(0.074)	(0.075)
logPCE (< median)	−0.018	−0.014	−0.017	0.007	0.008	0.005
	(0.044)	(0.047)	(0.043)	(0.018)	(0.018)	(0.018)
logPCE (> median, marginal)	0.037	0.030	0.036	−0.057	−0.056	−0.051
	(0.096)	(0.097)	(0.098)	(0.063)	(0.064)	(0.063)
Widowed		0.064	0.063		−0.026	−0.018
		(0.077)	(0.080)		(0.053)	(0.062)
Divorced or never married		0.018	−0.014		0.206***	0.040
		(0.105)	(0.096)		(0.069)	(0.088)

continued

TABLE 14-11 Continued

	Men			Women		
	(1)	(2)	(3)	(1)	(2)	(3)
Rural Zhejiang	0.232** (0.091)	0.233** (0.090)		0.137** (0.064)	0.143** (0.066)	
Urban Gansu	0.320*** (0.102)	0.316*** (0.102)		0.166** (0.081)	0.172** (0.083)	
Rural Gansu	0.237** (0.093)	0.230** (0.091)		0.123* (0.069)	0.133* (0.073)	
Community FE	NO	NO	YES	NO	NO	YES
F-test for all age dummies (p-value)	4.99*** (0.003)	5.39*** (0.002)	4.00** (0.011)	1.07 (0.368)	1.01 (0.395)	1.37 (0.257)
F-test for all education dummies (p-value)	0.71 (0.548)	0.65 (0.588)	0.12 (0.949)	1.13 (0.342)	1.15 (0.334)	0.86 (0.467)
F-test for all logPCE splines (p-value)	0.09 (0.918)	0.05 (0.952)	0.08 (0.923)	0.41 (0.667)	0.38 (0.688)	0.33 (0.722)
F-test for all marital status dummies (p-value)		0.34 (0.713)	0.34 (0.714)		4.55** (0.014)	0.18 (0.834)
F-test for all location dummies (p-value)	3.23** (0.027)	3.25** (0.027)	5.09*** (0.000)	1.59 (0.198)	1.62 (0.191)	2.79*** (0.003)
Observations	162	162	162	226	226	226

NOTE: Robust standard errors in parentheses, all clustered at community level. * denotes $p < .1$; ** $p < .05$; *** $p < .01$. logPCE (> median, marginal) represents the change in the slope from the interval for logPCE below the median.
SOURCE: Authors' calculations using CHARLS pilot data.

in Brown and Theoharides (2009), most of the choice regarding insurance parameters is set at the county-level. Thus, there is great scope for experimentation, which is evidently ongoing.

CONCLUSIONS

There was a major spread of health insurance in both urban and especially rural areas of China in the five years prior to the CHARLS pilot in 2008. In the CHARLS pilot data, some 90% of our sample report having some type of insurance, with the NCMS insurance the most prevalent. Reported premiums actually paid are low in rural areas, averaging 20 Yuan per year per person, though a good deal higher in urban areas. Thus, the degree of public subsidy is high. At the moment, in Zhejiang and Gansu, these schemes cover mainly inpatient care, and the reimbursement rates top out at 64% for respondents in Zhejiang having an urban hukou. For those with rural hukou, reimbursement rates are much lower, ranging from 23 to 35% in Zhejiang and Gansu. Reimbursement rates rise with total visit costs for all plans in the aggregate, and for the NCMS in particular. The rise in reimbursement rates with total costs stops when rates reach 40% at 10,000 Yuan in total costs, aggregating over all insurance types. For the NCMS, reimbursement rates top out at just over 30% for costs of 20,000 Yuan. In either case, people with high medical costs are still having to pay a large part of costs and are thus at risk of losing significant assets or not being able to pay. Outpatient service is just beginning to be covered by insurance in Zhejiang province, especially in urban areas and among those holding urban hukou, but not much yet in Gansu province.

Simple descriptive regressions show that respondents with lower incomes as measured by per capita expenditure (*pce*) have a lower chance of being insured, as do migrants, older women, and male widowers. Education has little significant correlation with being insured. There is a lot of variation across communities in coverage and reimbursement rates, as reported in earlier studies.

For inpatient use, having higher *pce* matters positively for both men and women, and it is also positively correlated with utilization for outpatient services for women. On the other hand, education is not correlated with utilization, conditional on *pce*. Unobserved community effects also are strongly correlated with utilization. Finally, although we cannot call it a causal relationship, having health insurance is positively correlated with inpatient use for men.

REFERENCES

Banks, J., A. Muriel, and J.P. Smith. (2009). Disease Prevalence, Incidence and Determinants of Mortality in the United States and England. Department of Economics, University College, London.

Brown, P., and C. Theoharides. (2009). Health seeking behavior and hospital choice in China's New Cooperative Medical System. *Health Economics 18(0)*:S47-S64.

China Health and Retirement Longitudinal Survey. (2008). China Center for Economic Research, Peking University. Available: http://charls.ccer.edu.cn/charls/data.asp.

Du, L., and W. Zhang (2007). *The Development on China's Health, No. 3*. Beijing: Social Science Academic Press.

Gao, J., J. Raven, and S. Tang. (2007). Hospitalization among the elderly in urban China. *Health Policy 84(2-3)*:210-219.

Lee, N. (2009). Measurement Error and Its Impact on Estimates of Income and Consumption Dynamics, mimeo, Department of Economics, Chinese University of Hong Kong.

Lei, X., and W. Lin. (2009). The New Cooperative Medical Scheme in rural China: Does more coverage mean more service and better health? *Health Economics 18*:S25-S46.

Lin, W., G. Liu, and G. Chen. (2009). The Urban Resident Basic Medical Insurance: A landmark reform toward universal coverage in China. *Health Economics 18(0)*:S83-S96.

Strauss, J., and D. Thomas. (1998). Health, nutrition and economic development. *Journal of Economic Literature 36(3)*:766-817.

Strauss, J., X. Lei, A. Park, Y. Shen, J.P. Smith, Z. Yang, and Y. Zhao. (2010). Health outcomes and socio-economic status among the elderly in China: Evidence from the China Health and Retirement Longitudinal Study, Pilot. *Journal of Population Ageing 3(3)*:111-142.

Wagstaff, A., and M. Lindelow. (2008). Can insurance increase financial risk?: The curious case of health insurance in China. *Journal of Health Economics 27(4)*:990-1,005.

Wagstaff, A., W. Yip, M. Lindelow, and W. Hsiao. (2009). China's health system and its reform: A review of recent studies. *Health Economics 18(0)*:S7-S23.

Wooldridge, J. (2002). *Econometric Analysis of Cross Section and Panel Data*. Cambridge, MA: MIT Press.

World Bank. (2009). *From Poor Areas to Poor People: China's Evolving Poverty Reduction Agenda*. Washington, DC: World Bank.

Yi, H., L. Zhang, K. Singer, S. Rozelle, and S. Atlas. (2009). Health insurance and catastrophic illness: A report on the New Cooperative Medical Scheme in rural China. *Health Economics 18(0)*:S119-S127.

Zhao, Y., J. Strauss, A. Park, Y. Shen, and Y. Sun. (2009). *China Health and Retirement Longitudinal Study Pilot User's Guide*. China Center for Economic Research, Peking University.

15

Health of the Elderly in India: Challenges of Access and Affordability

Subhojit Dey, Devaki Nambiar, J. K. Lakshmi,
Kabir Sheikh, and *K. Srinath Reddy*

India, the world's second most populous country, has experienced a dramatic demographic transition in the past 50 years, entailing almost a tripling of the population over the age of 60 years (i.e., the elderly) (Government of India, 2011). This pattern is poised to continue. It is projected that the proportion of Indians aged 60 and older will rise from 7.5% in 2010 to 11.1% in 2025 (United Nations Department of Economic and Social Affairs [UNDESA], 2008). This is a small percentage point increase, but a remarkable figure in absolute terms. According to UNDESA data on projected age structure of the population (2008), India had more than 91.6 million elderly in 2010 with an annual addition of 2.5 million elderly between 2005 and 2010. The number of elderly in India is projected to reach 158.7 million in 2025 (United Nations Department of Economic and Social Affairs, 2008), and is expected, by 2050, to surpass the population of children below 14 years (Raju, 2006).

Summary figures mask the unevenness and complexities of the demographic transition within India across Indian states with different levels of economic development, cultural norms, and political contexts. Projected estimates of population structure in 2025 for North India retain a "pyramidal" shape, while for south India, the share of the elderly population is expected to expand considerably. Linear growth in the population of the elderly is expected in the next 100 years, with steeper gradients of increase in central and east India and leveling off of absolute numbers of elderly in the north, south, west, and northeast (Aliyar and Rajan, 2008).

A few important characteristics of the elderly population in India are noteworthy. Of the 7.5% of the population who are elderly, two-thirds live in villages and nearly half are of poor socioeconomic status (SES) (Lena et al., 2009). Half of the Indian elderly are dependents, often due to widowhood, divorce, or separation, and a majority of the elderly are women (70%) (Rajan, 2001). Of the minority (2.4%) of the elderly living alone, more are women (3.49%) than men (1.42%) (Rajan and Kumar, 2003). Thus, the majority of elderly reside in rural areas, belong to low SES, and are dependent upon their families.

While the southern states (Andhra Pradesh, Karnataka, Kerala, and Tamil Nadu) may be considered the biggest drivers of aging in India, other Indian states (notably Haryana, Himachal Pradesh, Maharashtra, Orissa, and Punjab) are also experiencing an elderly population boom, largely in rural areas (Alam and Karan, 2010). Large-scale studies of the health behaviors of this growing elderly Indian population are scarce. However, information gathered from numerous surveys and regional and local studies point to the high prevalence of several risky behaviors, such as tobacco and alcohol use (Goswami et al., 2005; Gupta et al., 2005; Mutharayappa and Bhat, 2008), and physical inactivity (Rastogi et al., 2004; Vaz and Bharathi, 2004). With these stressors, predictably, aggregate data comparing the 52nd (1995–1996) and 60th Rounds (2004) of the National Sample Survey (NSS) suggest a general increase in the reports of ailments and utilization of healthcare services among the elderly (Alam and Karan, 2010; Rao, 2006). Access to services, however, is uneven across the country.

An analysis of morbidity patterns by age clearly indicates that the elderly experience a greater burden of ailments (which the National Sample Survey Organisation defines as illness, sickness, injury, and poisoning) compared to other age groups (see National Sample Survey Organisation, 2006, Fig. 1), across genders and residential locations. The elderly most frequently suffer from cardiovascular illness, circulatory diseases, and cancers, while the non-elderly face a higher risk of mortality from infectious and parasitic diseases (Alam, 2000; Kosuke and Samir, 2004; Shrestha, 2000). In developed countries advancing through demographic transition, there have been emerging epidemics of chronic non-communicable diseases (NCDs), most of which are lifestyle-based diseases and disabilities (Gruenberg, 1977; Waite, 2004). In contrast, India's accelerated demographic transition has not been accompanied by a corresponding epidemiological transition from communicable diseases to NCDs (Agarwal and Arokiasamy, 2010). As indicated in Figure 15-1, the Indian elderly are more likely to suffer from chronic than acute illness. There is a rise in NCDs, particularly cardiovascular, metabolic, and degenerative disorders, as well as communicable diseases (Ingle and Nath, 2008). While cardiovascular disease is the leading cause of death among the elderly

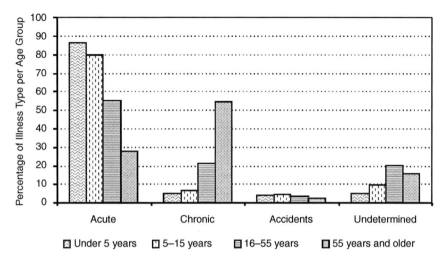

FIGURE 15-1 Burden of illness type among Indians.
SOURCE: Dror, Putten-Rademaker, and Koren (2008).

(Jha et al., 2006), multiple chronic diseases afflict them: chronic bronchitis, anemia, high blood pressure, chest pain, kidney problems, digestive disorders, vision problems, diabetes, rheumatism, and depression (Angra et al., 1997; Kumari, 2001; Raju, 2000; Roy, 1994; Shah and Prabhakar, 1997). Concurrently, the prevalence of morbidity among the elderly due to re-emerging infectious diseases is quite high, with considerable variations across genders, areas of residence, and socioeconomic status (Goldman, Korenman, and Weinstein, 1995; Gupta and Sankar, 2002; Kumar, 2003; Mini, 2008; National Sample Survey Organisation [NSSO], 1996; Radha et al., 1999; Rajan, Misra, and Sharma, 1999; Sudha et al., 2006). It is projected that NCD-related disability will increase and contribute to a higher proportion of overall national disability, in step with the greying of the population (Kowal et al., 2010). However, a very significant shortcoming of most of the above studies is the use of self-reported data, which, in the absence of autopsies and physician examinations of patients, represents enormous lacunae in data on the conditions affecting the elderly. More detailed studies are needed, other than surveys, to extract information on the epidemiology of health conditions experienced by the elderly.

This mixed disease burden among the Indian elderly places unique demands on the country's public healthcare system. In developing our conceptual model of elderly health in India, we began with a perusal of the larger health scenario in India, finding that "health care, far from helping people rise out of poverty, has become an important cause of household impoverishment and debt, the average national health indicators, though showing improvements in recent decade, hide vast regional and social disparities." Although some privileged individuals enjoy excellent health outcomes, others experience "the worst imaginable conditions" (Patel et al., 2011, p. 4). Among the elderly, we observed a number of barriers: from pathological progression (Lynch, Brown, and Taylor, 2009) to family nuclearization and dependency (Gupta and Sankar, 2002; Rajan and Prasad, 2008), from reductions in earning potential (Selvaraj, Karan, and Madheswaran, 2010) to the salience of pre-existing inequities on the axes of gender, caste, and religion (Chatterjee and Sheoran, 2007; Goel et al., 2003; Goldman, Korenman, and Weinstein, 1995; Gupta and Sankar, 2002; Kumar, 2003; Mini, 2008; National Sample Survey Organisation [NSSO], 1996; Radha et al., 1999; Rajan, Misra, and Sharma, 1999; Sudha et al., 2006). Across the board, we found that the elderly population (and subpopulations that form it) does not receive care commensurate to the conditions it suffers (access) and, second, that even where the care is physically accessible, costs of accessing this care hinder uptake (affordability).

The aim of this chapter, therefore, is to characterize and describe specific challenges in the domains of access and affordability, and the likely determinants of such challenges that must be addressed in the design and implementation of future health policymaking in India. Throughout, we aim to reveal areas where data gaps remain. A semi-structured literature review and secondary research methodology based upon Pope and colleagues (2000) was developed by the study authors with the collaborative assistance of two research assistants. All researchers undertook a literature review, drawing upon key informant experts in health systems research, government policy clearinghouses, and a review of scholarly journal articles, books, and program documentation comprising nongovernmental organization and government reports, presentations, and documents. All resources, including studies, reports, and policy briefs, were consolidated and summarized in league tables and discussed by the co-authors to determine key findings and themes under the headings of access and affordability. We discuss our findings in eponymous sections, following which we outline future policy directions under a universal health coverage framework that are pertinent to elderly health.

ACCESS: A CONTINUING CONCERN

Social Determinants of Access

A closer look at the literature on access to healthcare reveals variation across an age gradient. Older Indians have reported higher rates of outpatient and inpatient visits (Alam and Karan, 2010). The age gradient in elderly health access is overlaid by social determinants of health. For one, there is a feminization of the elderly population; according to the 2001 census, the gender ratio among the Indian elderly aged 60 years and older is 1,028 females for 1,000 males (Rajan and Aliyar, 2008). It is expected that by 2016, 51% of India's elderly will be women (in rural areas, this proportion will be much higher) (Kumari, 2001; Rao, 2006). More women report poor health status as compared to males, and yet a far greater proportion of men are hospitalized as compared to females (87 versus 67 per 1,000 aged persons) (Rajan and Sreerupa, 2008).

Unmet health needs are more pronounced among the 33.1% of the elderly in India who in 2001 were reported to have lost their spouses (Rajan and Aliyar, 2008), of whom a larger relative proportion is female (50% of female elderly are widows versus only 15% of male elderly who are widowers). Studies have shown that widows are disproportionately vulnerable to disability, illness, and poor healthcare utilization (Sreerupa, 2006) due to a number of mobility, employment, property, and financial constraints (Dreze, 1990).

In addition to gender and marital status, religion, caste, education, economic independence, and sanitation have bearing on elderly health. Count modeling of data from the 52nd Round of the NSS indicates that the number of diseases suffered by an elderly person, calculated independently for rural (Poisson Model) and urban populations (Negative Binomial Model), include age, gender, literacy, availability of drinking water and a toilet facility, and household monthly consumption expenditure (Alam, 2006). Another study of Uttar Pradesh (UP) and Maharashtra found that the *older* elderly (70 years and older) were significantly less likely to seek treatment compared to the 60–69 age category, while Muslims were between 62% and 49% more likely to seek treatment in UP and Maharashtra, respectively, compared to Hindus (Agrawal and Arokiasamy, 2009). This study found that elderly in scheduled tribe/scheduled caste (SC/ST) categories were 54% less likely and other backward classes (OBC) 35% less likely to seek treatment for existing ailments in Maharashtra compared to other castes. Finally, high school graduates were twice as likely in UP and four times as likely in Maharashtra to seek treatment compared to the illiterate group. However, in the above-mentioned study, a majority of the elderly suffered from multiple morbidity conditions, which makes interpreting the presented results difficult. The absence of rigorously designed studies that assess the types and severity of various disease conditions in the elderly further highlights this fact. Rajan (2006), using data from the same survey, concluded that 9.5% of rural inhabitants and 4.2% of urban inhabitants report lack of access to day-to-day requirements of medicine, close to double that of clothing and food.

Although broader trends of economic dependence are changing, kinship systems and social support still have strong bearing on access to healthcare among the elderly (see discussion below). A strong link can be established between ownership of property and kin-based caregiving arrangements. Traditional arrangements structured shared domicile of the elderly in their ancestral homes along with younger generations, who would later inherit this property (Rajan, 2006). While strong cultural emphasis was and continues to be placed upon respect for the elderly (Sivamurthy and Wadakannavar, 2001), kin conflict and such other broader considerations as caste order have historically hampered access to health (Cohen, 1998). Propertyless elders have a relatively higher likelihood of residence in old-age homes, living alone, and being looked after by relations other than their children when widowed (Kodoth and Rajan, 2008). More recently, arrangements of "living apart but together" are increasingly common, where joint family co-residence is discontinued but strong social support is immediately available, particularly in times of health crises (Sokolovsky, 2001). Given this variable provision of support, "discourses of neglect" may emerge, where in their everyday lives, the needs and problems of the elderly are invisible to those who offer them support in times of acute ill health (Sokolovsky, 2001). Moreover, research in India has shown that it is not the quantity but rather the quality of particular ties that relate to health. In some cases, having a continuous engagement or strong tie with a neighbor or child may have a more health-protective impact than having many (weak) ties to a host of family and community members (Sudha et al., 2006).

While systematic studies are rare, there have been increasing reports of material exploitation, financial deprivation, property grabbing, abandonment, verbal humiliation, and emotional and psychological torment in India, all of which compromise the mental and physical health of the elderly (Shankardass, 2009). In 2007, the Maintenance and Welfare of Parents and Senior Citizens Bill raised the profile of such practices, issuing penalties for abuse and neglect of elders exacted by members of their extended/joint family. At the same time, Delhi saw a tripling of police reports of elderly seeking protection in an 18-month period, and Mumbai's police helpline for seniors was receiving more than 80 calls daily (Datta, 2007). Reports of murder, rape, burglary, and violence inflicted upon the elderly remain and are more commonly reported in Indian metropolitan areas. (It is unclear whether they are more common, due to possible under-reporting or publication bias.)

The stigma of aging, as well as the health and social conditions the elderly commonly face (such as dementia, depression, incontinence, or widowhood), is another social barrier to access of health, manifest in the Indian case in unique ways (World Health Organization [WHO],

2002). Patel and Prince's qualitative study (2001) on the cultural perceptions of mental health needs among the aged in Goa, India, revealed
that despite being frequently observed in the elderly population, certain
mental health deficits were not acknowledged as health needs. Conditions
like dementia are viewed as normal aging and depression construed as
the result of neglect by family. Such cases were therefore not considered
the purview of health professionals and were more frequently acknowledged and addressed by community health workers. Access to mental
health services in the medical sector are limited, and, thus, most care
and support was provided ad hoc, informally, and in the family. Consequently, "dependency anxiety" was a common phenomenon among the
elderly, i.e., elderly felt the need to curtail their dependence upon the family and felt anxious about informing them about their health problems
(Patel and Prince, 2001). The stigma of widowhood has been examined
at length and leads to profound social ostracism that impinges not only
on access to healthcare, but also a broader range of fundamental human
rights, such as the right to shelter, food, property, and information (Chen,
1998; Dreze, 1990).

Physical Determinants of Access

A key physical barrier to access is that many elderly require home-
based care, a need arising from illness-related confinement following an
age gradient. Elderly confinement to the home is consistent in both rural
and urban areas (Aliyar and Rajan, 2008). Sample survey data suggest
that as many as 64 per 1,000 population in rural areas and 67 per 1,000
population in urban areas are confined to the home. For those aged 80
and older, as many as one in five are confined. Reduced mobility hinders
health-seeking.

While health-seeking is hindered, health needs tend to increase
through the life course and across geographies. According to NSSO data,
28.3% of the aged in rural areas and 36.8% in urban areas suffer from
one disease or another (Kumari, 2001). The greater reported morbidity
in urban areas is misleading. Census data reveal higher proportions of
people aged 60 and older in rural areas (7.7% of the population in 2001) as
compared to urban areas (6.7%), meaning that in absolute terms, the need
for elderly care is slightly higher in rural areas. Moreover, higher rates
of morbidity and hospitalization in urban areas are to be expected given
that most geriatric services are in urban areas and at the tertiary level
(Ingle and Nath, 2008). In contrast, the lack of infrastructure and health
service reach in rural areas is worrisome since of the 72% of the elderly
population that is not working, 69% is rural (Kumari, 2001). Moreover,
longitudinal data suggest the greatest deterioration in health status has

been of females living in urban areas (Husain and Ghosh, 2010). There is an acute need for expanding access to geriatric care beyond the tertiary level, in rural areas, and in service of the female elderly.

Even in cases where services are available, uptake is low because of lack of health promotion and community outreach. Goel and colleagues (2003) undertook a survey of 354 elderly rural inhabitants in Meerut, Uttar Pradesh, of whom only 53% were even aware of the geriatric welfare services available in their area and only 4% reported ever using them. Even in south India, where healthcare utilization is generally higher, evidence suggests similar trends. Another observational study of 213 elderly in Udupi, Karnataka, found that only 35.7% were aware of geriatric welfare services and 14.6% had used them (Lena et al., 2009).[1]

AFFORDABILITY: A COMPLEX CONUNDRUM

Affordability Through Income, Employment, and Assets

India has no population-wide mechanisms of social security. Given this scenario, Indians have to work as long as possible in order to support themselves (Mathew and Rajan, 2008). Employer insurance and pension schemes are available only to as low as 9% of rural males and 41.9% of urban males who are in the formal sector; among females, the figures are lower still (3.9% rural, 38.5% urban) (Rajan and Aiyar, 2008). The rest of the workforce comprises casual and self-employed workers who are not entitled to formal retirement benefits and, in order to afford healthcare in their early years, face the paradoxical challenges of remaining both healthy and employed in old age. Those in the formal sector may experience a halving of their incomes, which, in the face of rising inflation, leaves smaller proportions of income that may be allocated to health (Mathew and Rajan, 2008). As a result, a considerable proportion of the elderly are employed. An analysis of the Worker Population Ratios (WPRs) depicts that 56.79% of elderly males and 16.32% of elderly females were engaged in employment (proportions are higher in rural

---

[1]A corollary to confinement and multiple and chronic morbidity profile typical of the elderly is that multidrug use and polypharmaceutical use is common, heightening the propensity for inappropriate drug prescription and health-harming sequelae. A study of the elderly in Gujarat found that almost one-quarter in a sample of more than 400 patients received at least one inappropriate drug prescription according to Beer's 2003 criteria, most commonly for upper respiratory tract infection (URTI), abdominal pain, and congestive cardiac failure (Zaveri, Mansury, and Patel, 2010). Harugeri and colleagues (2010) found in a tertiary care facility that almost one-quarter of elderly patients engaged in potentially inappropriate medication use and, further, that the drug profile among the elderly is more varied than gold standard (Beer's) criteria used to assess medication use.

areas) (Mathew and Rajan, 2008). Among the elderly participating in the workforce, a majority (nearly 95%) is either self-employed or involved in casual labor with a maximum number of elderly being self-employed (79%) (Mathew and Rajan, 2008). Such employment arrangements may offer limited remuneration and require the elderly to keep working: NSS data suggest that almost one-fourth of males and one-sixth of females are employed even in the 80–84 age group (Mathew and Rajan, 2008).

In view of increasing the financial security of the elderly, higher tax exemption has been provided for the elderly, and the exemption age has also been reduced from 65 to 60 in the 2011 budget. Also, a new category called "very senior citizen" for elderly above 80 years of age has been introduced for greater tax exemption (Highlights of Union Budget 2011–2012, 2011). Notwithstanding these most recent developments, the overall pattern of employment in old age has required the pursuit of financial security up to later periods in life. The declining health and energy of the elderly discourages employers from hiring them in the regular workforce, forcing the elderly to opt for self-employment and casual labor, particularly in rural areas, where employment opportunities are generally low (Mathew and Rajan, 2008).

In the absence of state-level measures of providing social security, security in old age may be assured through movable or immovable property assets. In India, which is largely patriarchal, the ownership of land, house, or property is mostly owned and devolved among men with exceptions on the southwest coast and in the northeast (where matrilineal societies have existed) (Agarwal, 1994). Thus, ownership of property and assets is strongly affected by prevailing social norms related to gender and socioeconomic status (Agarwal, 1994; Agnes, 1999; Chen, 1998; Dreze, 1990). In the case of women, the basis of property rights not only is generally weak but also seems to be eroding. Ownership rights vary for women depending on their status as daughters or widows (Agarwal, 1994; Chen, 2000; Dreze, 1990). NSS data show that more than twice the number of male elderly own property or assets compared to female elderly in both urban and rural areas, a difference that is moderated by socioeconomic status (i.e., lower strata have greater gender disparities in property ownership) (Kodoth and Rajan, 2008). Transfer of property to children results in propertylessness, a phenomenon more common among rural elderly men and urban widowed women with sons. Lack of property means lack of assets or a safety net to rely on as health costs escalate through old age (Agnes, 1999).

Paying for Healthcare

Apart from individual-level socioeconomic issues that adversely affect affordability, a number of systemic factors underpin the reduced ability of people, particularly the elderly, to pay for healthcare. Although all forms of healthcare payments are available in India, 83% of healthcare expenses are private out-of-pocket (OOP) expenditures (Duggal, 2007). India's relatively unaccountable and inefficient public system of healthcare has led to the evolution of a highly varied, unregulated, and mostly expensive private sector that provides most healthcare, rendering Indians increasingly vulnerable to catastrophic health expenditures and poverty (Pal, 2010).

According to 2005 estimates, per capita expenditure on health is 125 Indian Rupees (INR), of which per capita OOP expenditure is 100 INR. The largest proportion of this OOP expenditure is spent on outpatient expenditures (74 INR), which overlaps to a great extent with the purchase of drugs (72 INR) (IIPS, 2007). The elderly, due to increased morbidity from chronic diseases, have long-term healthcare needs and a large likelihood of having health expenditures in general and OOP expenditures in particular. The need for healthcare increases with age. Those above 65 years spend on average 1.5 times on healthcare compared to those in the 60–64 year age category (Mahal, Berman, and Indicus Analytics, 2002). The elderly have little recourse as insurance does not cover outpatient or drug purchase. Moreover, insurance plans only cover inpatient hospital expenses (Shahrawat and Rao, 2011), and, thus, even insured elderly have a higher chance of falling into poverty, given that catastrophic expenditure occurs due to outpatient and drug expenses. In fact, the probability of catastrophic OOP expenses in households with elderly is much higher as compared to households without elderly members (Pal, 2010). Evidence suggests that if OOP payments for either medicines or outpatient care were removed, only 0.5% of people would fall into poverty due to health spending (Shahrawat and Rao, 2011).

Financial protection for health spending in India is largely in the form of savings and insurance. However, insurance in India is limited not only by its low coverage of conditions, but also by low coverage of populations. The National Family Health Survey of 2004–2005 indicates that only 10% of households in India had at least one member of the family covered by any form of health insurance (IIPS, 2007). Overall, the insurance market in India remains limited and fragmented in its presence. Benefits are accessed by only a few privileged sections of the population, such as those in the formal and civil service sectors like defense, civil services, and the railways, even after retirement long into old age (Acharya and Ranson, 2005; Ellis, Alam, and Gupta, 2000; Ranson, Sinha, and Chatterjee, 2006; Shiva Kumar et al., 2011). Lack of employment and income affect elderly utilization of medical insurance, as these populations are often incapable of paying regular insurance premiums. Finally, insurance companies often explicitly exclude the elderly due to age limits or eligibility restrictions for those with pre-existing conditions. This results in heightening the estrangement of the aged from a healthcare system and policy environment that has historically lagged in supporting the financially weak.

UNIVERSAL HEALTH COVERAGE: STRATEGIC DIRECTIONS AND DATA NEEDS

A pathway to national health reform has been envisioned by the Planning Commission in the lead-up to the 12th Five-Year Plan for India. In October 2010, a High-Level Expert Group (HLEG) was convened by the Planning Commission to recommend changes in health financing, drug procurement, community participation in health, health management, and physical and financial norms for health and human resources. Situating elderly health in a broader framework of universal access and affordability of Universal Health Coverage (UHC) has potential to transform the structural conditions that hamper the well-being of the aged. We summarize some of the ways in which UHC may serve these functions, throughout indicating the evidence gaps that will be required for these functions to be met.

Key UHC reforms pertinent to access include the provision of additional human resources at the Sub-Health Centre level (per 5,000 population), as well as the introduction of an additional Community Health Worker (like an Accredited Social Health Activist) in rural and low-income urban areas. These reforms would ensure that in addition to existing priorities of maternal and child health, emerging priorities in NCD control, as well as action on social and physical barriers to access, can be addressed locally (i.e., in tandem with Village Health and Sanitation Committees and their urban equivalent). Future research may help determine the scope of care at the Sub-Health Centre level and the range of promotive services provided at the village/community in order to cater to the needs of India's elderly.

It has been proposed by the HLEG, moreover, that an essential package of care (comprising primary-, secondary-, and tertiary-level services) be cashless at point of service through the use of a National Health Entitlement Card (which would also serve as an identifier for Electronic Medical Records, carrying patient histories and care-seeking profiles). This provision will be particularly useful for the elderly poor, and will require innovation and an expansive exercise in data collection and compilation on both the user and provider sides. To this end, methodological contributions from ongoing cohort studies such as the Longitudinal Study on Aging in India (LASI) and parallel efforts internationally will be highly valuable.

A number of regulatory mechanisms under the aegis of a newly proposed National Health Regulatory and Development Authority will ensure health system support, accreditation, and continuous health systems evaluation. This process may benefit, again, from the growing base of research on elderly users of the health system, who may have a longer duration of interactions with the system as well as great variation in terms of need and burden, influenced by varying social determinants. Health systems evaluation will additionally have to reflect age-specific morbidity and mortality patterns, as well as that of intersectional elderly groups (the widowed elderly, aged of religious minority status, and others).

Ensuring the functioning of entitlements to health under the UHC is an increase in overall health spending from 1.2% of gross domestic product to 3% by 2022, funded through general taxation. It is anticipated that this will, in turn, reduce private OOP spending to 33% of total spending in the same period, thereby increasing the affordability of health among the most vulnerable. The phasing of this reduction, with its anticipated and unanticipated consequences for the elderly, will have to be carefully mapped and characterized in future research studies.

The creation of state essential drugs and medical device lists—for both allopathic and traditional medicine systems—is also proposed to ensure that price inflation is curbed for critical products. Data on which critical products are already used, and in what combinations, is a critical area of research as populations age and the need grows ever more urgent to balance cost containment against monitoring and control of drug resistance in India. Here, too, the burden of both (over)medication and resistance may be disproportionately faced by the elderly. Patterns and priorities will have to be determined based on routine and careful examination of the evidence among the Indian elderly.

CONCLUSION

The growth of the elderly population in the coming decades will bring with it unprecedented burdens of morbidity and mortality across the country. As we have outlined, key challenges to access to health for the Indian elderly include social barriers shaped by gender and other axes of social inequality (religion, caste, socioeconomic status, stigma). Physical barriers include reduced mobility, declining social engagement, and the limited reach of the health system. Health affordability constraints include limitations in income, employment, and assets, as well as the limitations of financial protection offered for health expenditures in the Indian health system.

Among the most significant findings that emerged in developing this review was the incompleteness of data on the burdens of access and affordability among elderly populations in India. A major reason for this is that routine health data collection in India is not designed to reflect or characterize pathological progression: a process wherein, by virtue of being alive longer than others, the elderly are more likely to experience a pathology, leading to impairment, functional limitations, and ultimately disability (Lynch, Brown, and Taylor 2009). Many routine data collection procedures (National Sample Surveys, Census data, or death certificates) in India do not capture pathological progression nor do they disaggregate morbidity and disability outcomes among the elderly (as discussed at some length by Alam and Karan, 2010).

Recommendations under the UHC framework have prioritized primary and secondary prevention and health promotion, with the goal of creating enabling environments for healthy lifestyles, early detection, and routine screening among the aged and avoiding institutionalization. In order to ensure these needs are met, a concomitant program of dedicated research is required on how various UHC elements affect and may cater more appropriately to the growing demographic of Indian elderly.

REFERENCES

Acharya, A., and K. Ranson. (2005). Health care financing for the poor: Community-based health insurance schemes in Gujarat. *Economic and Political Weekly 40*:4,141-4,150.

Agarwal, B. (1994). Gender and command over property: A critical gap in economic analysis and policy in South Asia. *World Development 10*:1,455-1,478.

Agarwal, G., and P. Arokiasamy. (2010). Morbidity prevalence and health care utilization among older adults in India. *Journal of Applied Gerontology 29(2)*:155-179.

Agnes, F. (1999). Law and women of age. A short note. *Economic and Political Weekly 30*:51-54.

Alam, M. (2000). Ageing in India: A country profile. *Bold 10(3)*:5-22.

Alam, M. (2006). *Ageing in India: Socio-economic and Health Dimensions.* New Delhi: Academic Foundation.

Alam, M., and A. Karan. (2010). *Elderly Health in India: Dimensions, Differentials, and Over Time Changes.* Building Knowledge Base on Ageing in India: A series of Programmatic and Research Studies. New Delhi: United Nations Population Fund.

Aliyar, S., and S.I. Rajan. (2008). *Population Projections for India, 2001-2101.* Thiruvananthapuram: Centre for Development Studies.

Angra, S.K., G.V.S. Murthy, S.K. Gupta, and V. Angra. (1997). Cataract related blindness in India and its social implications. *Indian Journal of Medical Research 106*:312-324.

Chatterjee, C., and G. Sheoran. (2007). *Vulnerable Groups in India.* Mumbai: The Centre for Enquiry into Health and Allied Themes.

Chen, C. (1998). *Widows in India: Social Neglect and Public Action.* New Delhi: Sage.

Cohen, L. (1998). *No Aging in India.* Berkeley: University of California Press.

Datta, D. (2007). Home alone. *India Today,* July 16. Available: http://www.indiatoday.com/itoday/20070716/cover.html.

Dreze, J. (1990). *Widows in Rural India.* London: Development Economics Research Programme.

Dror, D.M., O. Putten-Rademaker, and R. Koren. (2008). Cost of illness: Evidence for a study of five resource-poor locations in India. *Indian Journal of Medical Research 127*:347-361.

Duggal, R. (2007). Poverty and health: Criticality of public financing. *Indian Journal of Medical Research 126*:309-317.

Ellis, R.P., M. Alam, and I. Gupta. (2000). Health insurance in India: Prognosis and prospects. *Economic and Political Weekly 35*:207-217.

Goel, P.K., S.K. Garg, J.V. Singh, M. Bhatnagar, H. Chopra, and S.K. Bajpai. (2003). Unmet needs of the elderly in a rural population of Meerut. *Indian Journal of Community Medicine XXVIII*:165-166.

Goldman, N., S. Korenman, and R. Weinstein. (1995). Marital status and health among the elderly. *Social Science and Medicine 40(12)*:1,717-1,730.

Goswami, A., V.P. Reddaiah, S.K. Kapoor, B. Singh, S.N. Dwivedi, and G. Kumar. (2005). Tobacco and alcohol use in rural elderly Indian population. *Indian Journal of Psychiatry 47(4)*:192-197. doi:10.4103/0019-5545.43050.

Government of India. (2011). *National Programme for the Health Care of the Elderly* (NPHCE), Operational guidelines. New Delhi: Government of India.

Gruenberg, E. (1977). The failure of success. *Milbank Memorial Fund Quarterly/Health and Society 55*:3-24.

Gupta, P.C., P.K. Maulik, P.K. Pednekar, and S. Saxena. (2005). Concurrent alcohol and tobacco use among a middle-aged and elderly population in Mumbai. *National Medical Journal of India 18(2)*:88-91.

Gupta I., and D. Sankar. (2002). *Health of the Elderly in India: A Multivariate Analysis* Discussion Paper 46. New Delhi: Institute of Economic Growth. Available: http://iegindia.org/dis_ind_46.pdf.

Harugeri, A., J. Joseph, G. Parthasarathi, M. Ramesh, and S. Guido. (2010). Potentially inappropriate medication use in elderly patients: A study of prevalence and predictors in two teaching hospitals. *Journal of Postgraduate Medicine 56(3)*:186-191.

Highlights of Union Budget, 2011–2012. (2011, February 28). *The Times of India*, p. A1.

Husain, Z., and S. Ghosh. (2010). Is health status of elderly worsening in India?: A comparison of successive rounds of National Sample Survey data. *Munich Personal RePEc Archive*. Report No. 25747. Available: http://mpra.ub.uni-muenchen.de/25747/1/MPRA_paper_25747.pdf.

Indian Institute of Population Sciences. (2007). *NFHS-3. National Family Health Survey, 2005-06*. Mumbai: Indian Institute of Population Sciences. Available: http://www.mohfw.nic.in/nfhs3/index.htm.

Ingle, G.K., and A. Nath. (2008). Geriatric health in India: Concerns and solutions. *Indian Journal of Community Medicine 33*:214-218.

Jha, P., V. Gajalakshmi, P.C. Gupta, et al. (2006). Prospective study of one million deaths in India: Rationale, design, and validation results. *PLoS Medicine 3*:18.

Kodoth, P., and S.I. Rajan. (2008). Property and assets as economic security. Pp. 83-114 in *Institutional Provisions and Care for the Aged: Perspectives from Asia and Europe*, S.I. Rajan, C. Risseeuw, and M. Perera. (Eds.). New Delhi: Anthem Press.

Kosuke, I., and S. Samir. (2004). On the estimation of disability-free life expectancy: Sullivan's method and its extension. *Journal of the American Statistical Association 102*:1,199-1,211.

Kowal, P., K. Kahn, N. Nawi, N. Naidoo, S. Abdullah, A. Bawah, et al. (2010). Ageing and adult health status in eight lower-income countries: The INDEPTH WHO-SAGE Collaboration. INDEPTH WHO-SAGE Supplement. *Global Health Action 3*. Published online doi: 10.3402/gha.v3i0.5302. Available: http://www.globalhealthaction.net/index.php/gha/article/view/5302/6049.

Kumar, V. (2003). Health status and health care services among older persons in India. *Journal of Aging & Social Policy 15(2/3)*:67-83.

Kumari, R.S.S. (2001). *Socio-economic Conditions, Morbidity Pattern and Social Support among Elderly Women in a Rural Area*. Medical College, Thiruvananthapuram, Kerala.

Lena, A., K. Ashok, M. Padma, V. Kamath, and A. Kamath. (2009). Health and social problems of the elderly: A cross-sectional study in Udupi Taluk, Karnataka. *Indian Journal of Community Medicine 34*:131-134.

Lynch, S.M., S.J. Brown, and M.G. Taylor. (2009). The demography of disability. In *International Handbook of Population Aging*, Peter Uhlenberg (Ed.). London: Springer-Verlag.

Mahal, A., P. Berman, and Indicus Analytics. (2002). Estimating Baseline Health Expenditures on the Elderly in India. Draft. Harvard School of Public Health, Department of Population and International Health.

Mathew, E.T., and Rajan, S. I. (2008). Employment as Old Age Security. Pp. 68–82 in *Institutional Provisions and Care for the Aged: Perspectives from Asia and Europe*, S.I. Rajan, C. Risseeuw, and M. Perera (Eds.). New Delhi: Anthem Press.

Mini, G.K. (2008). Socioeconomic and demographic diversity in the health status of elderly people in a transitional society, Kerala, India. Published online in *Journal of Biosocial Science 10*.

Mutharayappa, R., and T.N. Bhat. (2008). Is lifestyle influencing morbidity among elderly? *Journal of Health Management 10(2)*:203-217. doi:10.1177/097206340801000203.

National Sample Survey Organization. (1996). *The Aged in India: A Socio-economic Profile, 1995-96*. National Sample Survey 52nd Round Report. New Delhi: Ministry of Statistics and Programme Implementation, Government of India.

National Sample Survey Organisation. (2006). *Morbidity, Health Care and the Condition of the Aged*. National Sample Survey, 60th Round, Report no. 507 (60/25.0/1). New Delhi: Ministry of Statistics and Programme Implementation, Government of India.

Pal, R. (2010). *Analysing Catastrophic OOP Health Expenditure in India: Concepts, Determinants and Policy Implications*. Mumbai: Indira Gandhi Institute of Development Research.

Patel, V., and M. Prince. (2001). Ageing and mental health in a developing country: Who cares? Qualitative studies from Goa, India. *Psychological Medicine 31*:29-38.

Patel, V., A.K. Kumar, V.K. Paul, K.D. Rao, and K.S. Reddy. (2011). Universal health care in India: The time is right. *The Lancet 377(9764)*: 448-449.

Pope, C., S. Ziebland, and N. Mays. (2000). Qualitative research in health care. Analysing qualitative data. *British Medical Journal 320(7,227)*:114-116.

Radha Devi, D., S. Santhosh, A. Asharaf, and T.K. Roy. (1999). *Aged in a Changing Society: A Case Study of Kerala*. Mumbai: International Institute.

Rajan, R.G., and E.S. Prasad. (2008). A pragmatic approach to capital account liberalization. *Journal of Economic Perspectives 22(3)*:149-172.

Rajan, S.I. (2001). Social assistance for poor elderly: How effective? *Economic and Political Weekly*:613-617.

Rajan, S.I. (2006). *Population Ageing and Health in India*. Mumbai: Centre for Enquiry into Health and Allied Themes.

Rajan, S.I., and S. Aiyar. (2008). Population ageing in India. Pp. 39-54 in *Institutional Provisions and Care for the Aged: Perspectives from Asia and Europe*, S.I. Rajan, C. Risseeuw, and M. Perera (Eds.). New Delhi: Anthem Press.

Rajan, S.I., and S. Kumar. (2003). Living arrangements among Indian elderly: New evidence from National Family Health Survey. *Economic and Political Weekly 38(3)*:75-80.

Rajan, S.I., and Sreerupa. (2008). Disease, disability and healthcare utilization among the aged. Pp. 39-54 in *Institutional Provisions and Care for the Aged: Perspectives from Asia and Europe*, S.I. Rajan, C. Risseeuw, and M. Perera (Eds.). New Delhi: Anthem Press.

Rajan, S.I., U.S. Misra, and P.S. Sharma. (1999). *India's Elderly: Burden or Challenge?* New Delhi: Sage.

Raju, S. (2006). *Ageing in India in the 21st Century: A Research Agenda*. Mumbai: The Harmony Initiative. Available: http://harmonyindia.org/hdownloads/Monograph_FINAL.pdf.

Raju, S. (2000). Ageing in India: An overview. In *Gerontological Social Work in India: Some Issues and Perspectives*, M. Desai and S. Raju (Eds.). New Delhi: B.R. Publishing.

Ranson, M.K., T. Sinha, M. Chatterjee, et al. (2006). Making health insurance work for the poor: Learning from SEWA's community-based health insurance scheme. *Social Science & Medicine 62*:707-720.

Rao, M. (2006). Economic and Financial Aspects of Ageing in India. Paper presented at the UN Regional Workshop on Gender-Responsive Health Security for the Elderly, September 18-19, Seoul, Republic of Korea. Available: http://www.unescap.org/esid/gad/issues/Socialprotection/Report-RegWkshp-HealthSecurity-18-19Sep06-Seoul.pdf.

Rastogi, T., M. Vaz, D. Spiegelman, K.S. Reddy, A.V. Bharathi, M.J. Stampfer, W.C. Willett, and A. Ascherio. (2004). Physical activity and risk of coronary heart disease in India. *International Journal of Epidemiology* 33:759-767. doi:10.1093/ije/dyh042.

Roy, G.S. (1994). Morbidity related epidemiological determinants in Indian aged: An overview. Pp. 114-125 in *Public Health Implications of Ageing in India*, C.R. Ramaachandran and B. Shah (Eds.). New Delhi: Indian Council of Medical Research.

Selvaraj, S., A. Karan, and S. Madheswaran. (2010). Elderly Workforce in India: Labour Market Participation, Wage Differentials and Contribution to Household Income. Unpublished report, Public Health Foundation of India, New Delhi.

Shah, B., and A.K. Prabhakar. (1997). Chronic morbidity profile among elderly. *Indian Journal of Medical Research* 106:265-272.

Shahrawat, R., and K.D. Rao. (2011). Insured yet vulnerable: Out-of-pocket payments and India's poor. Online published in *Health Policy and Planning* (April 21, 2011). doi:10.1093/heapol/czr029.

Shankardass, M. (2009). No one cares about elder abuse in India. *One World South Asia.* Available: http://southasia.oneworld.net/opinioncomment/no-one-cares-about-elder-abuse-in-india.

Shiva Kumar, A.K., C.C. Lincoln, M. Choudhary, G. Shiban, V. Mahajan, A. Sinha, and A. Sen. (2011). Financing health for all: Challenges and opportunities. *The Lancet Special Issue India: Towards Universal Health Coverage*:92-103.

Shrestha, L.B. (2000). Population aging in developing countries. *Health Affairs 19(3)*:204-212.

Sivamurthy, M., and A.R. Wadakannavar. (2001). Care and support for the elderly population in India: Results of a survey rural North Karnataka. Available: http://www.iussp.org/Brazil2001/s50/S55_P04_Sivamurthy.pdf.

Sokolovsky, J. (2001). Living arrangements of older persons and family support in less developed countries. *Population Bulletin of the United Nations, Spl. Issue (Living arrangements of older persons–Critical issues and policy responses)* 42/43:162-192.

Sreerupa (2006). Gender, Ageing and Widowhood: Health Vulnerability and Socio-Economic Influences. M.Phil Dissertation, submitted to Jawaharlal Nehru University, New Delhi.

Sudha, S., C. Suchindran, E.J. Mutran, S.I. Rajan, and P.S. Sarma. (2006). Marital status, family ties and self-rated health among elders in South India. *Journal of Cross-Cultural Gerontology* 21:3-4.

United Nations Department of Economic and Social Affairs, Population Division. (2008). *World Population Prospects (2008 Revision).* Available: http://esa.un.org/unpp/index.asp?panel=2.

Vaz, M., and A.V. Bharathi. (2004). Perceptions of the intensity of specific physical activities in Bangalore, South India: Implications for exercise prescription. *Journal of the Association of Physicians in India* 52:541-544.

Waite, L.J. (2004). Ageing, health, and public policy: Demographic and economic perspectives. *Population and Development Review 30(Suppl.)*:239-265.

World Health Organization. (2002). *Reducing Stigma and Discrimination against Older People with Mental Disorders.* Geneva: World Health Organization and World Psychiatric Association. Available: http://whqlibdoc.who.int/hq/2002/WHO_MSD_MBD_02.3.pdf.

Zaveri, H.G., S.M. Mansuri, and V.J. Patel. (2010). Use of potentially inappropriate medicines in elderly: A prospective study in medicine out-patient department of a tertiary care teaching hospital. *Indian Journal of Pharmacology 42(2)*:95-98.

16

Markers and Drivers: Cardiovascular Health of Middle-Aged and Older Indians[1]

Jinkook Lee, P. Arokiasamy, Amitabh Chandra,
Peifeng Hu, Jenny Liu, and *Kevin Feeney*

With a population of more than 1.2 billion (Census of India, 2011), India is the second most populous country in the world. In the past decade, the country has witnessed accelerated economic growth, emerging as the world's fourth largest economy in purchasing power parity terms (World Bank, 2010). Together with economic development, the country is undergoing a demographic transition: The population is aging rapidly. Currently, the 65+ population in India is roughly 60 million people, accounting for 5% of the population (United Nations Population Division, 2009). By 2050, the 65+ population is projected to climb to more than 13%, or approximately 227 million people. Economic development and population aging have contributed to an emerging trend of noncommunicable diseases, such as cardiovascular diseases and obesity, previously thought to be a concern mostly for affluent or developed countries (Mahal, Karan, and Engelgau, 2009). According to the World Health Organization (World Health Organization, 2009), age-standardized cardiovascular disease mortality among adults 60 years and older was 1,978 per 100,000 persons in India, compared to 800 per 100,000 in the United States.

---

[1]An earlier version of this paper was presented at the International Conference on Policy Research and Data Needs to Meet the Challenges and Opportunities of Population Aging in Asia, organized by the National Academy of Sciences and the Indian National Academy of Science. We thank Drs. David Bloom, James P. Smith, Lisa Berkman, and two anonymous reviewers for their comments and suggestions. This project is funded by NIA/NIH (R21 AG032572-01).

Researchers have documented a strong inverse relation between health and socioeconomic status (SES) in developed countries, such as the United States (Banks et al., 2006; Smith, 2004). However, this relationship is not well established in developing countries like India (Zimmer and Amornsirisomboon, 2001). Further, recent literature suggests that the direction of association between cardiac health and SES in such developing countries may be opposite of what is observed in the developed world; that is, higher SES is associated with increased risk of poor cardiac health (Reddy, 2002; Reddy et al., 2007). As regional and national economies in India continue to expand, the consumption basket of many individuals is changing, leading to dietary changes and increased obesity that pose risks to cardiac health (Subramanian and Smith, 2006). This phenomenon has been documented in other developing countries, such as Brazil, China, and Russia, as well as south Asian countries such as India, Sri Lanka, and Thailand (Monteiro et al., 2004; World Health Organization, 2002).

From recently collected data in the Longitudinal Aging Study in India (LASI) pilot study, we examine SES gradients in cardiovascular health of older Indians across four states using both self-reports and health markers measured at the time of the interview. Self-reports of diagnosed medical conditions are tied to access to healthcare services and, therefore, can mask undiagnosed conditions (Lee and Smith, 2011; Smith, 2007a, 2007b). In countries like India where access to healthcare is limited, the prevalence of undiagnosed conditions is expected to be greater than in developed countries. The use of biomarkers enables us to study health outcomes without self-report biases that may be differentially associated with SES and access to health services. These biomarker measures may also provide additional insights into true disease prevalence as well as the extent of undiagnosis and good management of chronic diseases in India.

METHODS

Data

The study sample is drawn from the pilot survey of LASI. LASI is designed to be a panel survey representing persons at least 45 years of age in India and their spouses. The pilot study was fielded in four states: Karnataka, Kerala, Punjab, and Rajasthan. These four states were chosen to capture not only regional variations, but also socioeconomic and cultural differences. Punjab is an example of a relatively economically developed state located in the north, while Rajasthan, also in the north, is relatively poor. The southern state of Kerala, which is known for its relatively efficient healthcare system and high literacy rate (Shetty and Pakkala,

2010), is included as a harbinger of how other Indian states may develop. Karnataka, located in the south, is used as a reference state.

Data were collected from 1,683 individuals during October through December of 2010. Primary sampling units (PSUs) were stratified across urban and rural districts within each of the four states to capture a variety of socioeconomic conditions. LASI randomly sampled 1,546 households from these stratified PSUs, and among them, households with a member at least 45 years old were interviewed. The household response rate was 88.6%. All age-eligible household members and their spouses regardless of age were asked to be interviewed. The individual response rate was 91.7%, and the response rate for the biomarker component of the survey was 82.5%. We restrict the analysis in this paper to 1,451 respondents who are at least 45 years of age; spouses under age 45 are excluded.

Although the pilot round of LASI only surveyed four states, the overall demographic characteristics of our sample are congruent with the population characteristics of India. However, at the state level, a comparison of sample characteristics of respondents reveals a somewhat greater representation of uneducated individuals in Rajasthan and lesser representation of married individuals, women, and elderly in Karnataka (for more details, see Arokiasamy et al. in Chapter 3 of this volume). While these differences may largely be due to the small sample size of the pilot study, the representatives of our findings should be interpreted with such caveats.

Measures

Hypertension

A binary variable indicating *self-reported diagnosis of hypertension* is created based on the following question: "Has any health professional ever told you that you have high blood pressure or hypertension?" As part of the biomarker module, LASI field investigators measured blood pressure, recording three readings each of systolic and diastolic, using an Omron 712c digital reader. We create a binary variable for *measured hypertension* based on the mean value of the second and third readings and classify respondents as hypertensive if they have systolic blood pressure of at least 140 mm Hg or diastolic blood pressure of at least 90 mm Hg. Because blood pressure tends to stabilize after sitting and resting, the first reading is excluded. For one respondent who had only two measurements for both systolic and diastolic pressure, we calculated the mean of these two readings. The comparison between diagnosed and measured hypertension is critical in differentiating those who are diagnosed and manage their blood pressure well from those who are diagnosed but fail to manage blood pressure, as well as differentiating undiagnosed from diagnosed among those who have high blood pressure readings.

Based on self-reported and measured hypertension, we define *total hypertension* as having ever been diagnosed by a health professional or hypertensive based on blood pressure readings at the time of the interview. Among the hypertensive (defined as total hypertension), we also define a measure of *undiagnosed hypertension* counting respondents who report not having ever been diagnosed with hypertension, but who have high blood pressure based on the field measurements. We then define a measure of *good management* of blood pressure to represent respondents who report having been diagnosed with hypertension but manage to have low blood pressure based on the field measurements.

Obesity

The LASI biomarker module also included anthropometric measures, such as weight, height, and waist and hip circumferences. Based on these measures, we calculate body mass index (BMI) as weight in kilograms divided by height in meters squared and a waist-to-hip ratio (WHR). We create a categorical indicator for obesity if a respondent has a BMI of at least 30 kg/m^2, for overweight if BMI is between 25 and 29.9, and for underweight if BMI is less than 18.5.

Health behaviors

Smoking is constructed as a series of categorical variables for current smokers, former smokers, and those who have never smoked. Here, "smoking" refers to both cigarettes and any sort of chewing tobacco. Drinking is represented by a binary variable indicating whether or not the respondent currently drinks any alcohol. For vigorous physical activities,[2] we construct a categorical variable that indicates the frequency of vigorous physical activities: everyday, sometimes (referring to more than once a week, once a week, or one to three times a month), and never or almost never.

LASI also asked whether or not a respondent has ever visited a private doctor with an Bachelor of Medicine and Bachelor of Surgery (MBBS) degree in his/her lifetime. Respondents' self-report of diagnosis by a health professional is only possible given access to health services, which

---

[2]The question reads, "We would like to know the type and amount of physical activity involved in your daily life. How often do you take part in sports or activities that are vigorous, such as running or jogging, swimming, going to a health center or gym, cycling, or digging with a spade or shovel, heavy lifting, chopping, farm work, fast bicycling, cycling with loads: everyday, more than once a week, once a week, one to three times a month, or hardly ever or never?"

is often determined by socioeconomic standing rather than need. For example, those with higher SES have better access to healthcare and may also be more aware of or more likely to be diagnosed with cardiovascular diseases. We choose to control for having seen a private doctor with an MBBS degree as most respondents who self-reported being diagnosed with a condition reported being diagnosed by a private MBBS doctor. However, this variable provides only limited information about healthcare utilization, not being able to differentiate the extent of healthcare utilization or the use of different healthcare providers. While the current paper is bound by data available from the pilot survey, the baseline instrument of LASI will collect more detailed information about healthcare utilization, addressing this issue.

Socioeconomic status

We use education, per capita household consumption, and caste affiliation as SES measures. In developed countries, education has been found to be the strongest measure of SES in relation to health (Smith, 2007a, 2007b), influencing it through multiple pathways, including health behaviors and access to healthcare (Lee, 2011). We categorize education into three groups: no schooling, primary or middle school education, and high school or more schooling based on a respondent's self-reported highest level of attainment.

Caste is our second measure of socioeconomic standing. Respondents self-report as members of scheduled castes, scheduled tribes, other backward class, and all "others" including "no caste." Scheduled castes and scheduled tribes are particularly disadvantaged due to a historical legacy of inequality; scheduled tribes often represent more geographically isolated, ethnic minority populations while scheduled castes can generally be characterized as socially segregated by traditional Hindu society, often excluded from education, public spaces (such as wells for drinking water and temples), and most other aspects of civil life in India (Subramanian et al., 2008). Many respondents are considered by the Government of India to be a member of an OBC (other backward class). While less marginalized and stigmatized than scheduled castes or tribes, these individuals also face barriers to economic and educational opportunities (Subramanian et al., 2008). Even though much has been done to improve the standing of scheduled tribes and scheduled castes, some of these efforts are relatively recent given the age of our respondents.

As a final measure of SES, we use per capita household consumption. This measure is preferred to income as past studies reveal that consumption is a better indicator of economic status in low-income and rural settings (Strauss et al., 2010). Consumption is measured at the household level, constructed from a sequence of questions that asks about expenses incurred over the previous year in the following categories: food (purchased, home-grown, and meals eaten out), household utilities (e.g., vehicle or home repairs, communications, fuel), fees (taxes, loan repayments, insurance premiums), purchases of durable goods (including clothing), education and health expenditures, discretionary spending items (alcohol and tobacco, entertainment, holiday celebrations, and charitable donations), transit costs, and remittances. The household consumption burden is calculated according to the OECD equivalence scale that differentially weights household members: the household head (1), each additional adult (0.5), and each child (0.3). Total household yearly consumption is then divided by the OECD equivalent household consumption burden to obtain a per capita measure. LASI provides imputed data for missing values using a hot deck method, and we control for imputed consumption in the models to adjust for any systematic bias due to missing data for some components of household consumption. We operationalized this variable as dummy tertile indicators in our analysis. Consumption is more strongly correlated with education than caste. Individuals with at least a high school education have more than two times greater per capita consumption than those without schooling: an average of 53,472 Rupees per capita for those with no schooling, 68,750 for those with primary or middle schooling, and 122,058 for those with high school or more. The differences across castes are less pronounced. Members of scheduled castes and tribes consume less per capita (45,188 and 59,785, respectively) than those of other backward classes and all others (81,403 and 73,800, respectively).

Demographics

We include categorical variables for age (45–54, 55–64, 65–74, and 75 and older) and a dummy indicator for gender.

Analysis

To account for sampling design and non-responses, means and percentages in the descriptive statistics are weighted with individual sample weights designed to be representative within each state. Additionally, we apply an all-state representative weight when pooling individuals across states to look at the sample as a whole. All analyses account for the clustered sample design, which was stratified on state, district, and urban-rural residency.

First, we examine interstate differences in descriptive sample characteristics and socioeconomic status and report a design-corrected Chi-square test (Stata Corporation, 2009).

Second, we examine interstate variations in the prevalence of our cardiovascular health outcomes (i.e., self-reported, measured, total hypertension) and risk factors such as obesity and health behaviors; we again report the design-corrected Chi-square and F-statistics. We compare self-reported with measured hypertension and examine interstate variations in undiagnosed and well-managed blood pressure among the hypertensive (based on total hypertension).

Third, we test the bivariate association between our outcome of interest (i.e., self-reported, measured, and total hypertension as well as percentage of undiagnosed and well managed among the hypertensive) and the demographic, geographic, and socioeconomic risk factors in a pooled sample accounting for stratified, cluster sample design.

We then estimate logistic multivariate models to investigate whether interstate variations and SES gradients hold after accounting for other risk factors, such as obesity and health behaviors. We formally test changes in the odds ratios for interstate and socioeconomic covariates after controlling for obesity and health behaviors. As all our dependent variables are binary variables, we run logistic models and report the odd ratios and confidence interval. Robust standard errors of the regression coefficients are computed to correct for heteroskedasticity.

Of particular interests are obesity and its relationship with socioeconomic status, as it may explain the SES gradients in hypertension we observe. Thus, we estimate multinomial logistic models to estimate body mass index with normal weight as a reference category and ordinary least squares to estimate WHR. We investigate whether SES gradients and state variations in obesity hold after accounting for health behaviors. We formally test the difference in coefficients in states and SES and report F-statistics. All multivariate models are unweighted.

Results

Sample characteristics

Table 16-1 shows the characteristics of our sample. Significant interstate variations reflect patterns in economic development and population growth. While women's representation in the survey does not vary significantly across states, there is an uneven age distribution. Kerala and Rajasthan have greater proportions of elderly; about one-third of the Kerala and Rajasthan populations are aged 65 and older, compared to Karnataka and Punjab where 19% and 25% of respondents, respectively, are of the same age group. Most of our sample are members of an OBC or some "other/none" caste category. However, scheduled tribes and schedule castes are disproportionately represented across states: 35% of

TABLE 16-1 Sample Characteristics: Age 45 and Older

		Unweighted N			
		All states	Karnataka	Kerala	Punjab
All		1,451	315	413	365
Gender	men	706	150	184	188
	women	745	165	229	177
Rural		1,040	206	289	259
Age	45–54	638	156	153	175
	55–64	413	100	129	100
	65–74	256	44	81	53
	75+	144	15	50	37
Caste	scheduled caste	242	53	31	123
	scheduled tribe	152	27	0	0
	other backward class	510	188	177	43
	other/none	546	47	205	199
Education	none	665	135	30	220
	primary/middle school	513	123	249	97
	high school or more	272	57	133	48
Per capita consumption (Rps)	median mean sd				
	at bottom tertile	483	55	139	86
	at middle	469	114	125	135
	at top tertile	480	136	143	144
	total	1,432	305	407	365

NOTES: Consumption tertile calculated on an all-India basis. The cutoff for the middle tertile is 31,672 Indian Rupees, and the cutoff for the top tertile is 57,796 Indian Rupees. The cutoff values, means, medians, and standard deviations are reported with income top-coded at the 95% percentile after imputation. * denotes $p < 0.05$; ** $p < 0.01$; *** $p < 0.001$.
SOURCE: Data from Longitudinal Aging Study in India (LASI) Pilot Wave.

the Rajasthan sample identifies as a scheduled tribe, while the highest proportion of scheduled castes, 33%, is found in Punjab. Punjab also has the higher proportion of respondents who do not belong to a scheduled caste, tribe, or OBC.

The two northern states have relatively lower educational attainment. In Rajasthan, 79% of respondents report having no schooling of any kind, and nearly 60% in Punjab are similarly uneducated. In Kerala, much higher rates of educational attainment are observed—only 7%

Rajasthan	Weighted %					
	All states	Karnataka	Kerala	Punjab	Rajasthan	F-stat
358						
184	48.69%	47.59%	44.87%	51.43%	51.46%	2.04
174	51.31%	52.41%	55.13%	48.57%	48.54%	
286	72.91%	64.33%	75.26%	69.91%	80.77%	9.10***
154	44.30%	49.46%	37.10%	48.06%	43.06%	2.29*
84	28.35%	31.77%	31.10%	27.38%	23.39%	
78	17.84%	14.01%	19.51%	14.43%	21.77%	
42	9.51%	4.76%	12.29%	10.13%	11.78%	
35	14.49%	16.67%	7.04%	33.48%	9.85%	12.63***
125	13.87%	8.57%	0.00%	0.00%	35.40%	
102	39.29%	59.79%	42.93%	11.75%	28.32%	
95	32.34%	14.98%	50.04%	54.77%	26.43%	
280	48.04%	42.59%	7.28%	60.12%	78.65%	37.02***
44	34.06%	38.99%	61.13%	26.67%	12.18%	
34	17.90%	18.41%	31.59%	13.21%	9.17%	
	41,993	55,250	42,387	48,093	28,091	
	55,696	72,431	58,929	58,934	35,979	
	45,103	52,510	45,328	38,811	28,284	
203	34.99%	17.92%	33.41%	23.58%	57.30%	7.35***
95	32.37%	37.30%	31.01%	36.97%	26.71%	
57	32.64%	44.78%	35.58%	39.45%	15.99%	
355	100.00%	100.00%	100.00%	100.00%	100.00%	

report receiving no schooling, and close to one-third of the sample has received some high school education. These socioeconomic differences across states persist when we examine other measures of economic well-being, such as household per capita consumption. Karnataka has the highest amount of per capita consumption, and Rajasthan has the lowest amount: 57% of respondents in Rajasthan fall into the bottom tertile of consumption compared to 18% of respondents in Karnataka and 24% in Punjab.

Interstate variations in health markers

Table 16-2 presents the distribution of self-reports of diagnosed, measured, and total hypertension across the four states. Prevalence of self-reports of diagnosed hypertension differs significantly across states. Kerala has the highest prevalence of self-reported diagnosed hypertension, while Rajasthan has the lowest (33% versus 6%). Interstate variations are also observed in measured blood pressure readings by the interviewer, but

TABLE 16-2 Interstate Variations in Health Markers

Health Markers		Unweighted N			
		All	Karnataka	Kerala	Punjab
Hypertension	diagnosed	274	46	134	73
	measured	544	101	131	167
	total	661	118	201	192
Among hypertensive	undiagnosed	408	78	74	125
	good management	118	17	71	25
Measured BMI	BMI < 18.5	304	84	50	38
	18.5 ≤ BMI < 25.0	669	147	223	144
	25 ≤ BMI < 30	249	47	82	97
	30 ≤ BMI	82	16	20	33
Measured WHR	mean for men				
	Sd for men				
	mean for women				
	Sd for women				
	non missing WHR	1,282	281	361	300
Self-reported smoking	current smoker	219	66	82	14
	Former smoker	69	12	45	2
	never smoked	1,158	237	283	349
Self-reported drinking	current drinker	135	33	50	33
	not a drinker	1,308	281	360	332
Self-reported vigorous physical activity	everyday	296	70	94	49
	1+ per week	93	13	27	33
	once a week	59	7	13	32
	1–3 per month	36	9	7	7
	hardly or never	962	216	269	244
Healthcare utilization	ever visited an MBBS	856	222	293	227

NOTE: * denotes p < 0.05; ** p < 0.01; *** p < 0.001.
SOURCE: Data from Longitudinal Aging Study in India (LASI) Pilot Wave.

much more modestly, ranging from 35% and 36% in Kerala and Karnataka to 52.5% in Punjab. Once accounting for both self-reports of diagnosed hypertension and measured hypertension based on blood pressure readings, the interstate variations in total hypertension are even more modest: The prevalence of total hypertension is the highest in Punjab (60%) and the lowest in Karnataka (42%).

Further investigation of those who are hypertensive illuminates interstate variations in undiagnosis and good management. Rajasthan has the

| Rajasthan | Weighted % | | | | | |
	All	Karnataka	Kerala	Punjab	Rajasthan	F-stat
21	16.96%	14.66%	33.33%	20.03%	5.75%	16.66 ***
145	40.54%	35.64%	34.83%	52.50%	44.82%	5.50 **
150	48.51%	41.60%	53.66%	60.40%	46.46%	4.40 **
131	64.59%	66.14%	36.63%	65.03%	87.60%	17.43 ***
5	16.16%	14.34%	34.54%	13.07%	3.23%	13.44 ***
132	26.74%	28.33%	13.42%	12.16%	41.08%	11.27 ***
155	51.20%	50.02%	59.78%	46.11%	47.95%	
23	16.47%	16.13%	21.63%	31.16%	7.00%	
13	5.59%	5.53%	5.18%	10.57%	3.96%	
	0.960	0.996	0.970	0.966	0.922	4.94 **
	0.145	0.200	0.079	0.111	0.121	
	0.925	0.921	0.957	0.945	0.897	4.78 **
	0.154	0.231	0.080	0.099	0.102	
340						
57	78.38%	20.84%	20.22%	3.85%	16.08%	11.39 ***
10	16.88%	3.79%	10.94%	0.54%	2.82%	
289	4.74%	75.37%	68.83%	95.61%	81.09%	
19	9.12%	10.47%	12.32%	9.06%	5.43%	3.18 *
335	90.88%	89.53%	87.68%	90.94%	94.57%	
83	21.56%	22.17%	23.06%	13.34%	23.35%	2.86 **
20	5.86%	4.07%	6.59%	9.09%	5.68%	
7	3.26%	2.22%	3.23%	8.82%	1.94%	
13	2.68%	2.86%	1.65%	1.89%	3.63%	
233	66.63%	68.68%	65.47%	66.87%	65.39%	
114	57.48%	70.45%	72.16%	62.15%	31.88%	22.17 ***

highest prevalence of undiagnosed with 88% of hypertensive respondents never having received a diagnosis from a health professional, while Kerala has the lowest (37%). Differences in the percentage of respondents who are successfully managing their hypertension follow the same geographic division: One-third of the hypertensive in Kerala have successfully managed their blood pressure, while only 3% of the hypertensive in Rajasthan have managed their blood pressure well.

Significant interstate variations are also observed for obesity measures, such as BMI and WHR. In Punjab, the percentage of the sample with BMIs over 30 (11%) is twice that of any other state. In Rajasthan, 41% of the elderly population is underweight (BMI under 18.5). In terms of WHR, less variation across states is observed, but differences still remain statistically significant: the lowest mean WHR is observed in Rajasthan for both men and women, and greater variance is observed in Karnataka for both men and women.

Health behaviors also differ significantly by states. The southern states of Karnataka and Kerala have notably higher percentages of smokers. Punjab has the lowest percentage of current smokers—only 5% report having used tobacco. The proportion of current drinkers is also low in northern states, with just more than 5% report drinking in Rajasthan. Vigorous physical activities are reported the least frequently by those residing in Punjab. There are significant state variations for healthcare utilization as well. Overall, 57% of respondents report having ever visited a doctor with an MBBS degree, which varies from 32% in Rajasthan to more than 70% in Karnataka and Kerala.

SES gradients in hypertension

In Table 16-3, we present SES gradients for self-reported diagnosis, measured, and total hypertension as well as undiagnosed and good management among the hypertensive. We report sample design-corrected Chi-square test statistics for SES gradients, as well as differences by gender and age.

We observe a significant and positive association between SES and self-reported hypertension diagnosis by a health professional: The prevalence is 7.7% among those with no education compared to 24.5% and 27.2% for those with primary/middle school education and the highest educated group, respectively. That is, more-educated individuals are more likely to report having diagnosed hypertension. However, we do not see such significant education gradients in measured hypertension. Total hypertension, on the other hand, shows a significant difference in prevalence between those with and without formal schooling, but among those with schooling, no prevalence difference is found across different levels of educational attainment.

Among those with hypertension, more-educated individuals are also less likely to have undiagnosed hypertension and more likely to manage their hypertension under control. Among those with measured or self-reported hypertension and no schooling, 82% were undiagnosed compared to 48% among those with high school or more schooling. Similarly, respondents with hypertension and some high school education or more were almost three times more likely to manage their hypertension compared to those with no education.

Per capita household consumption reflects the socioeconomic gradient seen with education. The prevalence of self-reported hypertension among the lowest consumption tertile is almost 10% compared to 23% for the highest per capita consumption group. Similar to education, the association with measured hypertension does not follow that for self-reported; in fact, we do not find statistically significant bivariate associations between per capita consumption and measured and total hypertension. However, we find a very strong per capita consumption gradient in terms of the prevalence of undiagnosed hypertension and the proportion of good management. The undiagnosed prevalence rate is the highest among the low-consumption group (77%) and the lowest among the high-consumption group (52%). Consistent with the education gradients, we find that those at the highest consumption group are more than twice as likely to manage their hypertension under control than those at the lowest consumption group.

Hypertension is also significantly associated with caste. Members of the "other" and "none" caste groups have the highest prevalence of diagnosed hypertension, followed by members of other backward classes, whereas scheduled tribes and castes have the lowest. However, such differences between caste affiliations are no longer statistically significant for measured and total hypertension. Similar to education and per capita income, we observe significant differences by caste for undiagnosed and managed hypertension. More than 90% of all scheduled tribe members were undiagnosed compared to just 54% among those with no scheduled caste or tribe affiliation. Scheduled tribes and scheduled castes were also the least likely to be managing their hypertension; those respondents with no tribe or caste affiliation were more than five times more likely than scheduled tribes to be managing their blood pressure.

Finally, we note some gender and age differences in self-reports of diagnosed hypertension. The prevalence of self-reported diagnosed hypertension is significantly higher among women than men, while we find no significant gender differences in measured or total hypertension

TABLE 16-3 Percentage Self-Reported, Measured, Total, and Undiagnosed Hypertension, and Percentage Good Management

		% Self-Reported		% Measured	
		All	F-stat	All	F-stat
N		1,443		1,309	
All		16.96		40.54	
Gender	men	14.14	6.82*	40.44	0.005
	women	19.64		40.63	
Age	45–54	11.10	4.66**	33.80	3.596*
	55–64	19.52		42.90	
	65–74	24.95		49.71	
	75+	21.70		48.26	
Caste	scheduled caste	9.24	9.76***	34.40	1.168
	scheduled tribe	3.56		47.17	
	OBC	19.28		40.26	
	other/none	23.40		40.62	
Education	none	7.67	30.63***	38.18	1.027
	primary/middle	24.53		44.41	
	high school or more	27.16		39.42	
Per capita consumption tertiles	low	10.06	10.20***	41.76	2.497
	mid	17.57		44.88	
	high	22.87		34.91	
State	Karnataka	14.66	16.66***	35.64	5.499**
	Kerala	33.33		34.83	
	Punjab	20.03		52.50	
	Rajasthan	5.75		44.82	

NOTE: * denotes $p < 0.05$; ** $p < 0.01$; *** $p < 0.001$.
SOURCE: Data from Longitudinal Aging Study in India (LASI) Pilot Wave.

as well as undiagnosed and good management among the hypertensive. Our results also show the evidence of age gradients in the prevalence of hypertension but with different level of undiagnosis. The youngest age group in our sample (aged 45–54) displays the highest prevalence of undiagnosed hypertension, contributing to a steeper age gradient in the prevalence of diagnosed hypertension than that of total hypertension.

Do interstate variations and SES gradients in diagnosed, measured, and total hypertension persist after controlling for obesity and health behavior? Table 16-4 presents the results from three multivariate logis-

% Total Hypertension		% Undiagnosed		% Good Management	
All	F-stat	Hypertensive	F-stat	Hypertensive	F-stat
1,302		661		661	
48.51		64.59		16.16	
46.76	1.23	67.36	1.66	13.09	4.35*
50.14		62.19		18.83	
43.71	5.22**	72.12	1.83	14.31	0.31
51.01		59.24		15.89	
61.97		59.68		19.34	
58.08		64.27		16.47	
38.10	1.99	74.99	9.33***	9.70	6.11**
49.10		92.12		3.25	
49.09		60.81		17.42	
52.23		53.79		22.35	
42.11	5.11**	82.03	20.10***	9.11	8.38***
54.87		54.32		18.75	
53.36		48.25		25.84	
46.88	0.49	76.74	8.29***	10.49	11.95***
51.01		64.27		11.87	
47.12		51.87		25.62	
41.60	4.40**	66.14	17.43**	14.34	13.44**
53.66		36.63		34.54	
60.40		65.03		13.07	
46.46		87.60		3.23	

tic regressions for our pooled sample: for self-reported, measured, and total hypertension. We estimate interstate variations and SES gradients in these health outcomes, controlling for covariates, including age, gender, rural/urban residency, obesity measures (i.e., BMI and WHR), and health behaviors. Logistic models are specified to estimate each of three dependent variables; odds ratios and 95% confidence intervals are presented.

We find that significant interstate differences persist across each of the three models after controlling for all covariates and SES. Respondents living in Punjab have two to three times the risk of hypertension

TABLE 16-4 Logistic Regressions of Self-Reported, Measured, and Total Hypertension

			Self-Reported		
			OR	CI	*
Demo	gender	female	1.773	1.071	2.935	*
	age	55–64	2.474	1.486	4.120	***
		65–74	3.534	2.332	5.357	***
		75+	3.254	1.531	6.915	**
	rural		0.998	0.641	1.553	
State	Punjab		2.747	1.201	6.281	*
	Rajasthan		0.681	0.304	1.526	
	Kerala		2.501	1.461	4.279	**
SES	caste	scheduled caste	0.866	0.500	1.497	
		scheduled tribe	0.801	0.166	3.872	
		OBC	1.117	0.729	1.711	
	education	primary/middle	2.232	1.282	3.885	**
		high school or more	3.135	1.856	5.294	***
	consumption	mid	1.360	0.849	2.177	
		high	1.534	0.858	2.745	
BMI	underweight	BMI < 18.5	0.858	0.466	1.582	
	overweight	25 ≤ BMI < 30	1.817	1.098	3.009	*
	obese	BMI ≥ 30.0	1.335	0.651	2.738	
	WHR		1.952	0.667	5.713	
Health Behaviors	quit smoking		2.006	1.215	3.312	**
	currently smoking		1.612	0.893	2.908	
	currently drinks		0.923	0.491	1.737	
	some exercise		0.883	0.482	1.615	
	daily exercise		0.866	0.481	1.561	
	MBBS visit		1.691	1.122	2.550	*
N			1,251			
F-stat			6.64	***		

NOTES: * denotes $p < 0.05$; ** $p < 0.01$; *** $p < 0.001$. OR = odds ratios, CI = confidence intervals.
SOURCE: Data from Longitudinal Aging Study in India (LASI) Pilot Wave.

than those residing in Karnataka across all measures of hypertension (self-reports, measured, and total). Respondents in Kerala, on the other hands, are 250% more likely to self-report hypertension, but no statistical difference was observed for measure and total hypertension. Respondents in Rajasthan have increased odds of measured hypertension than

Measured				Total (self-reported or measured)			
OR	CI			OR	CI		
1.154	0.868	1.535		1.320	0.944	1.846	
1.638	1.184	2.266	**	1.849	1.296	2.638	**
2.028	1.363	3.018	***	2.977	1.913	4.633	***
2.284	1.303	4.002	**	2.740	1.571	4.780	***
1.022	0.730	1.432		0.956	0.681	1.343	
2.360	1.540	3.617	***	2.895	1.736	4.829	***
1.849	1.007	3.392	*	1.716	0.987	2.985	
0.682	0.464	1.002		1.292	0.897	1.860	
1.007	0.649	1.564		0.967	0.619	1.509	
1.784	0.948	3.354		1.785	0.957	3.329	
1.196	0.843	1.698		1.185	0.837	1.677	
2.326	1.542	3.508	***	1.985	1.307	3.014	**
1.966	1.090	3.546	*	2.132	1.233	3.687	**
1.320	0.902	1.933		1.313	0.899	1.916	
0.722	0.496	1.050		0.955	0.655	1.393	
0.715	0.495	1.033		0.786	0.538	1.148	
1.340	0.893	2.010		1.878	1.320	2.671	***
1.317	0.709	2.444		1.138	0.597	2.168	
1.992	0.760	5.220		1.689	0.672	4.245	
0.718	0.344	1.499		0.768	0.444	1.328	
0.730	0.470	1.134		0.907	0.585	1.407	
1.329	0.780	2.263		1.152	0.742	1.787	
1.142	0.752	1.735		0.968	0.617	1.517	
1.458	1.037	2.050	*	1.464	1.008	2.127	*
1.016	0.770	1.339		1.191	0.909	1.561	
1,201				1,198			
3.11	**			3.95	**		

respondents in Karnataka, while no significant difference is observed in self-reported hypertension.

We also find significant education gradients in all three measures of hypertension. Respondents who have completed some schooling are twice more likely to have hypertension than those without any schooling (total hypertension). It is also interesting to note that education gradients are more pronounced when we examined diagnosed hypertension than the prevalence based on measured or total hypertension. However, per capita consumption and caste are no longer significantly associated with hypertension once we control for other covariates.

In addition, and consistent with bivariate findings, we find significant gender difference in self-reports of hypertension diagnosis, but no gender difference in measured or total hypertension. We find significant age gradients across all measures, reflecting a well-documented association with cardiovascular health. We also find that overweight is a significant determinant of self-reported and total hypertension, but not statistically significant for measured hypertension. Smoking in the past is also found to be a significant risk factor for diagnosed hypertension, but not for measured or total hypertension. Although counterintuitive, we find that physical exercise every day is positively associated with measured and total hypertension. Notably, we find significant associations between healthcare utilization (i.e., having ever visited an MBBS doctor) and having been diagnosed with hypertension. Those who have ever visited an MBBS doctor are 1.6 times more likely to answer affirmatively than those who have never visited an MBBS doctor.

Do obesity and health behaviors explain interstate variations and SES gradients in total hypertension? We further investigate whether obesity and health behaviors may explain some of the interstate differences and the SES gradients in our measure of total hypertension, and the results are presented in Table 16-5. Obesity significantly reduced the interstate variations, as well as the education gradients, though we stress that interstate variations and SES gradients still persist after controlling for obesity. That is, obesity explains some of the interstate variations and education gradients, but not all of the variances. Accounting for health behaviors, however, does not additionally reduce the socioeconomic gradient or geographic differences we observe.

SES gradients in obesity

We first present the bivariate association between SES and two obesity measures, BMI and WHR, in Table 16-6. We observe significant association with each measure of SES: caste, education, and consumption for obesity. Scheduled tribes had the largest percentage underweight (54%), while respondents who were not of a scheduled tribe or caste had the highest prevalence of obesity at 7% for OBC and respondents with other or no caste. Additionally, about one-quarter of other or no-caste respondents were overweight, so that 35% of respondents in this group were overweight or

TABLE 16-5 Do Obesity and Health Behaviors Explain Interstate Variations and SES Gradients in Total Hypertension? Results from Logistic Regression Models

		Model A	Model B	Model C	A vs. B	B vs. C
State	Punjab	3.082***	2.670***	2.895***	4.74**	1.59
	Rajasthan	1.511	1.519	1.716		
	Kerala	1.232	1.175	1.292		
SES	caste				2.38	0.13
	scheduled caste	0.882	0.936	0.967		
	scheduled tribe	1.623	1.815	1.785		
	OBC	1.163	1.189	1.185		
	education				4.72*	1.98
	primary/middle	2.196***	2.080**	1.985**		
	high school or more	2.234**	1.978**	2.132**		
	consumption				2.72	0.08
	mid	1.315	1.287	1.313		
	high	1.039	0.950	0.955		

NOTES: Model A includes only covariates in the table, as well as rural, female, and age. Model B includes all covariates of Model A plus obesity measures; Model C includes all covariates in Model B plus those for health behaviors. Table presents odds ratios for the three models and the F-statistics when testing coefficients across models. * denotes $p < 0.05$; ** $p < 0.01$; *** $p < 0.001$.

SOURCE: Data from Longitudinal Aging Study in India (LASI) Pilot Wave.

TABLE 16-6 SES Gradients in Obesity

		BMI		
		% Underweight	% Normal	% Overweight
N	1,304	304	669	249
All	100.00%	26.74	51.20	16.47
Caste	scheduled caste	30.67	53.81	10.22
	scheduled tribe	53.56	42.12	3.58
	OBC	23.49	52.49	17.51
	other/none	16.49	52.67	24.03
Education	none	38.03	49.19	9.31
	primary/middle	20.64	52.57	19.69
	high school or more	8.27	53.92	29.43
Per capita	low	38.54	48.30	11.19
consumption	mid	26.76	51.56	14.63
tertiles	high	13.65	53.90	24.66

NOTE: * denotes $p < 0.05$; ** $p < 0.01$; *** $p < 0.001$.
SOURCE: Data from Longitudinal Aging Study in India (LASI) Pilot Wave.

obese. Education and per capita consumption showed a similar gradient. Those without education or in the bottom expenditure tertile had the highest percentage of respondents underweight (38–39%), while those with some high school education or in the top tertile for per capita consumption were about 32–38% overweight or obese. Across both men and women, we see smaller waist-to-hip (WTH) ratios for consumption, but the association between WTH ratio and caste and education are only significant for men.

Do interstate variations and SES gradients in obesity persist after controlling for health behavior? Table 16-7 displays the results of our multinomial logistic regression for BMI. We find persistent interstate variations in BMI even after controlling for other covariates. The residents of Punjab are less likely to be underweight and more likely to be overweight and obese than the residents of Karnataka. The residents of Kerala are less likely to be underweight than those in Karnataka but no more likely to be overweight or obese.

Similarly, we find that higher SES as measured by education also increased the odds of being overweight or obese and decreased the odds of being underweight. Consumption also increased the odds of being obese and decreased the odds of being underweight, but did not show significant association with the odds of being overweight. Caste affiliation, another measure of SES, also showed significant association with obesity.

| % Obese | Chi-sq | * | WHR | | | |
			Men	F-stat	Women	F-stat
82			626		656	
5.59			0.961		0.923	
5.31	8.67	***	0.964	4.34**	0.923	2.69
0.74			0.905		0.887	
6.50			0.981		0.931	
6.82			0.963		0.930	
3.47	16.02	***	0.932	4.62*	0.914	1.37
7.10			0.980		0.934	
8.38			0.982		0.935	
1.98	10.84	***	0.939	3.46*	0.924	6.41**
7.05			0.957		0.902	
7.80			0.989		0.948	

We also find that respondents aged 75 and older significantly increased the odds of being underweight compared to normal BMI. Women also increased the odds of being overweight and obese. Among health behaviors, currently smoking showed significant relationships with BMI. Current smoking increased the multinomial odds of being underweight and decreased the odds of being overweight compared to respondents in a healthy BMI range. Table 16-8 shows that health behaviors did not account for any interstate variations or SES gradients.

Table 16-9 presents the results of OLS regression of WHR. Once we control for basic demographic characteristics, interstate variations and SES gradients in WHR are no longer statistically significant.

DISCUSSION

Our analysis examines several markers and potential drivers of cardiovascular health of middle-aged and older adults in India using data from representative samples of four states: Karnataka, Kerala, Punjab, and Rajasthan. Using both self-reported and measured health outcomes, we find that there are significant socioeconomic and interstate variations in the prevalence of hypertension. Notably, such variations are more evident in self-reports of hypertension diagnosis than measured hypertension, suggesting self-report bias associated with the access to healthcare. Based

TABLE 16-7 Multinomial Logistic Regression Results of Obesity: BMI

Reference = Normal			Underweight			
			RRR	CI		*
Demo	gender	female	0.798	0.564	1.129	
	age	55–64	0.895	0.618	1.296	
		65–74	1.307	0.855	1.997	
		75+	2.100	1.271	3.472	**
	rural		1.409	0.959	2.070	
State	Punjab		0.439	0.260	0.742	**
	Rajasthan		0.855	0.540	1.355	
	Kerala		0.420	0.258	0.686	**
SES	caste	scheduled caste	1.221	0.757	1.969	
		scheduled tribe	1.816	1.060	3.111	*
		OBC	1.187	0.794	1.776	
	education	primary/middle	0.935	0.618	1.413	
		high or more	0.456	0.243	0.857	*
	consumption	mid	0.797	0.557	1.140	
		high	0.451	0.294	0.690	***
Health Behaviors	quit smoking		0.939	0.459	1.921	
	currently smoking		1.710	1.104	2.649	*
	currently drinks		0.962	0.548	1.688	
	some exercise		0.901	0.561	1.447	
	daily exercise		0.830	0.566	1.217	
	MBBS visit		0.741	0.530	1.036	
N			1,278			
Wald chi2			7,089.82***			

NOTE: * denotes $p < 0.05$; ** $p < 0.01$; *** $p < 0.001$.
SOURCE: Data from Longitudinal Aging Study in India (LASI) Pilot Wave.

on blood pressure readings, our estimate of hypertension prevalence of Indians aged 55–64 (43%) are comparable to those in the same age group in the United States (40%) and United Kingdom (39%) (Banks et al., 2006). Our results are in line with other previous studies in India. Gupta (2004) observes significant interstate variations, ranging from 4.5% in rural Haryana to 44–45% in urban Mumbai. Hypertension, accounting for both self-reported and directly assessed blood pressure readings taken during the interview, is estimated to affect 49% of Indians aged 45 and older and exhibits similar interstate variation, ranging from 42% in Karnataka to 60% in Punjab.

Changing lifestyle factors have been cited as a contributing cause

Overweight				Obese			
RRR	CI			RRR	CI		
1.672	1.156	2.419	**	5.889	2.896	11.972	***
1.018	0.701	1.477		1.913	1.076	3.399	*
0.960	0.609	1.514		2.226	1.132	4.379	*
0.756	0.397	1.439		0.396	0.088	1.785	
0.782	0.553	1.106		0.710	0.431	1.170	
2.678	1.627	4.407	***	4.234	1.800	9.963	**
0.725	0.385	1.363		2.083	0.855	5.077	
0.915	0.561	1.493		0.669	0.309	1.446	
0.550	0.331	0.913	*	0.895	0.389	2.058	
0.496	0.176	1.392		0.000	0.000	0.000	***
0.893	0.619	1.288		1.220	0.658	2.261	
1.999	1.285	3.110	**	3.137	1.585	6.208	**
2.532	1.506	4.259	***	3.266	1.506	7.084	**
1.005	0.651	1.550		2.442	1.145	5.211	*
1.353	0.885	2.069		2.675	1.233	5.804	*
0.967	0.470	1.991		1.551	0.426	5.648	
0.494	0.257	0.950	*	0.635	0.206	1.951	
1.313	0.676	2.551		2.635	0.932	7.454	
0.844	0.514	1.386		0.972	0.436	2.167	
0.705	0.461	1.080		0.914	0.443	1.882	
1.052	0.748	1.480		0.844	0.491	1.449	

of these trends. For example, obesity is particularly prevalent in Punjab compared to other states. We found the supporting evidence that obesity explains some of the interstate variations and SES gradients in hypertension prevalence, but obesity and health behavior do not account for all of the interstate variations and SES gradients. After controlling for these lifestyle factors, we find that interstate variations and SES gradients in hypertension persist. Identifying what contributes to such interstate variations and SES gradients calls for further research.

The results of our analyses also suggest significant interstate variations in diagnosis and management of such diseases and the role that the healthcare system plays. Respondents in Kerala had significantly lower

TABLE 16-8 Do Health Behaviors Explain Interstate Variations and SES Gradients in Obesity? Results from Multinomial Logistic Regression Models

		Model A (Demo)		
		Underweight	Overweight	Obese
State	Punjab	0.403**	2.861***	4.359***
	Rajasthan	0.866	0.707	2.038
	Kerala	0.421***	0.863	0.676
Caste	scheduled caste	1.219	0.534*	0.890
	scheduled tribe	1.870*	0.492	0.005***
	OBC	1.171	0.839	1.187
Education	primary/middle	0.901	2.003**	3.075**
	high school or more	0.411**	2.765***	3.291**
Consumption	mid	0.792	0.997	2.361*
	high	0.451**	1.369	2.630*

NOTE: * denotes p < 0.05; ** p < 0.01; *** p < 0.001.
SOURCE: Data from Longitudinal Aging Study in India (LASI) Pilot Wave.

likelihoods of undiagnosed hypertension than all other states. Coupled with the highest percentage of respondents having ever seen a licensed private doctor and a high proportion of respondents diagnosed with hypertension keeping their blood pressure under control, the development of the health infrastructure may play a critical role in shaping the course of disease management as such chronic conditions become more prevalent. In fact, having ever seen a licensed doctor was significantly related to self-reported diagnoses of hypertension.

We find significant SES gradients in hypertension—particularly with education—suggesting that those individuals with higher SES are at increased risk for hypertension when compared to those lower on the socioeconomic ladder. Education remains significant even after adjusting for obesity and health behaviors. Once we control for education, per capita household consumption and caste are no longer significantly associated with hypertension, suggesting that the historical disadvantages associated with caste membership as well as differences in consumption levels are predominantly mediated by education.

Our analyses also illustrate that individuals at the lowest SES are the most vulnerable to undiagnosed hypertension. This result is not surprising given that these individuals may also be less likely to be diagnosed due to more limited access to healthcare services. We also find that among

Model B (Demo + health behavior)			Model A vs. B		
Underweight	Overweight	Obese	Underweight	Overweight	Obese
0.439**	2.678***	4.234**	2.41	3.73	0.45
0.855	0.725	2.083			
0.420**	0.915	0.669			
1.221	0.550*	0.895	1.00	5.93	2.02
1.816*	0.496	0.006***			
1.187	0.893	1.220			
0.935	1.999**	3.137**	4.34	5.53	0.68
0.456*	2.532***	3.266**			
0.797	1.005	2.442*	0.05	0.63	1.18
0.451***	1.353	2.675*			

those who are hypertensive, the more educated are more likely to keep their blood pressure under control. This finding is consistent with what has been found in other studies (Reddy et al., 2007).

The results of this study focus on the increasingly complex dynamic between health and its socioeconomic determinants, though it is not without limitations. Given the cross-sectional design of the LASI pilot survey, we cannot speak to causality of lower SES influencing health outcomes and highlight our findings only in the context of associations. Furthermore, due to small sample size, we cannot further examine SES gradients within states. We also do not have individual-level consumption data and acknowledge the limitation of our healthcare utilization measure.

Particularly in India, access to healthcare is closely tied to the same determinants of health outcomes, such as SES, caste, gender, and geography (Balarajan, Selvaraj, and Subramanian, 2011; De Costa et al., 2009). Furthermore, one of the most striking features of healthcare in India is its heterogeneity, ranging from the best possible evidence-based care to health-threatening practices by unqualified care providers (Banerjee, Deaton, and Duflo, 2003; Das and Hammer, 2007; Ramaraj and Alpert, 2008). Therefore, further research attention and analyses of how access to and quality of healthcare influences health outcomes are needed to deepen our understanding of the relationship between health and SES.

TABLE 16-9 OLS Regression Results of WHR

			Estimates	SE	*
Demo	gender	female	−0.032	0.009	**
	age	55–64	0.001	0.012	
		65–74	0.002	0.012	
		75+	0.004	0.015	
	rural		0.000	0.012	
State	Punjab		−0.001	0.022	
	Rajasthan		−0.032	0.022	
	Kerala		0.001	0.019	
SES	caste	scheduled caste	−0.004	0.014	
		scheduled tribe	−0.022	0.017	
		OBC	0.004	0.009	
	education	primary/middle	0.004	0.012	
		high school or more	0.004	0.014	
	consumption	mid	−0.008	0.010	
		high	0.014	0.013	
Health Behaviors	quit smoking		−0.003	0.016	
	currently smoking		−0.008	0.013	
	currently drinks		0.032	0.014	*
	some exercise		−0.022	0.011	*
	daily exercise		−0.016	0.011	
	MBBS visit		0.011	0.009	
N		1,255			
F-stat		4.24		***	

NOTE: * denotes $p < 0.05$; ** $p < 0.01$; *** $p < 0.001$.
SOURCE: Data from Longitudinal Aging Study in India (LASI) Pilot Wave.

CONCLUSIONS AND IMPLICATIONS

Our study contributes to a better understanding of the associations between higher socioeconomic status and increased risk of hypertension. Data from the pilot study of the Longitudinal Aging Study in India show two-fold increases in the risk of these conditions for individuals of older ages, those who have higher education, and those who are overweight. Our comparison between self-reports and directly assessed measures of hypertension reiterates the significance of bias associated with self-reported medical conditions. The prevalence estimates based on a doctor's diagnosis will seriously underestimate the true disease prevalence. As access to healthcare services increases, the prevalence of undiagnosed diseases will decline, but such declines will reach the socioeconomically disadvantaged group last. These findings are consistent with the inter-pretation that a rapid epidemiological transition in India is taking place due to changes in diet and lifestyle (Popkin et al. 2001; Yusuf et al., 2001) associated with economic development. Balancing economic growth with population health, perhaps through strengthening the healthcare system, should be considered in tandem to tackle the rapidly changing etiology of noncommunicable diseases in India.

REFERENCES

Balarajan, Y., S. Selvaraj, and S.V. Subramanian. (2011). Health care and equity in India. *The Lancet* 377:505-515.

Banerjee, A., A. Deaton, and E. Duflo. (2003). Health care delivery in rural Rajasthan. *Economic & Political Weekly* 39:944-949.

Banks, J., M. Marmot, Z. Oldfeld, and J.P. Smith. (2006). Disease and disadvantage in the United States and in England. *Journal of American Medical Association* 295:2,037-2,045.

Census of India. (2011). *2011 Census of India*. New Delhi: Government of India Office of the Registrar General and Census Commissioner.

Chatterjee, S. (2011). The Health and Well-being of Older Indians—Results from WHO's Study on Global AGEing and Adult Health (SAGE). Presented at the National Academies Conference on Aging in Asia, Delhi, India, March 14-15.

Das, J., and J. Hammer. (2007). Location, location, location: Residence, wealth, and the quality of medical care in Delhi, India. *Health Affairs* 26:338-351.

De Costa, A., A. Al-Muniri, V.K. Dirwan, and B. Eriksson. (2009). Where are healthcare providers? Exploring relationships between context and human resources for health Madhya Pradesh province, India. *Health Policy* 93:41-47.

Gupta, R. (2004). Trends in hypertension epidemiology in India. *Journal of Human Hypertension* 18:73-78.

Gupta, R., V.P. Gupta, and N.S. Ahluwalia. (1994). Education status, coronary heart disease, and coronary risk factor prevalence in a rural population in India. *British Medical Journal* 309:1,332.

Lee, J. (2011). Pathways from education to depression. *Journal of Cross-Cultural Gerontology* 26:121-135.

Lee, J., and J. Smith. (2011). The effect of health promotion on diagnosis and management of diabetes. *Journal of Epidemiology and Community Health*. doi:10.1136/jech.2009.087304.

Longitudinal Aging Study in India, Pilot Wave (2011). Harvard School of Public Health; International Institute of Population Sciences, Mumbai; and RAND Corporation. Available: https://mmicdata.rand.org/megametadata/?section=study&studyid=36.

Mahal, A., A. Karan, and M. Engelgau. (2010). *The Economic Implications of Non-Communicable Disease for India*. Washington, DC: World Bank.

Monteiro, C.A., E.X. Moura, W.L. Conde, and B.M. Popkin. (2004). Socioeconomic status and obesity in adult population in developing countries: A review. *Bulletin of the World Health Organization* 82:940-946.

Popkin, B., S. Horton, S. Kim, A. Mahal, and J. Shuigao. (2001). Trends in diet, nutritional status, and diet-related non-communicable diseases in China and India: The economic costs of the nutrition transition. *Nutrition Reviews* 59:379-390.

Ramaraj, R., and J.S. Alpert. (2008). Indian poverty and cardiovascular disease. *The American Journal of Cardiology* 102:102-166.

Reddy, K.S. (2002). Cardiovascular diseases in the developing countries: Dimension, determinants, dynamics and directions for public health action. *Public Health Nutrition 5(1A)*:231-237.

Reddy, S.R., D. Prabhakaran, P. Jeemon, K.R. Thankappan, P. Joshi, V. Chaturvedi, L. Ramakrishnan, and F. Ahmed. (2007). Education status and cardiovascular risk profile in Indians. *Proceedings of the National Academy of Sciences of the USA 104(41)*:1,623-1,628.

Shetty, U., and T.M.P. Pakkala. (2010). Technical efficiencies of healthcare system in major states of India: An application of NP-RDM of DEA formulation. *Journal of Health Management 12*:501.

Smith, J.P. (2004). Unraveling the SES-health connection *Population Development Review 30*:133-150.

Smith, J.P. (2007a). The impact of socioeconomic status on health over the life course. *The Journal of Human Resources 42(4)*:739-764.

Smith J.P. (2007b). Nature and causes of trends in male diabetes prevalence, undiagnosed diabetes, and the socioeconomic status health gradient. *Proceedings of National Academy of Sciences USA 104*:13225e31.

Stata Corporation. (2009). *Stata: Release 11. Statistical Software.* College Station, TX: StataCorp LP.

Strauss, J., X. Lei, A. Park, Y. Shen, J.P. Smith, Z. Yang, and Y. Zhao. (2010). *Health Outcomes and Socio-Economic Status Among the Elderly in China: Evidence from the CHARLS Pilot.* RAND Working Paper #WR-774. Santa Monica, CA: RAND Corporation.

Subramanian, S.V., and G.D. Smith. (2006). Patterns, distribution, and determinants of under- and over-nutrition: A population based study of women in India. *American Journal of Clinical Nutrition 84*:633-640.

Subramanian, S.V., L.K. Ackerson, M.A. Subramanyam, and K. Sivaramakrishnan. (2008). Health inequalities in India: The axes of stratification. *The Brown Journal of World Affairs 14(2)*:127-138.

United Nations Population Division (UNPD). (2009). *World Population Prospects: The 2008 Revision.* New York: United Nations.

World Bank (2010). India: Country Overview September 2010. Available: http://www.worldbank.org.in/.

World Health Organization. (2002). *Globalization, Diets and Non-communicable Diseases.* Geneva: World Health Organization.

World Health Organization. (2009). Disease and Injury Country Estimates, Health Statistics and Health Information System. Available: http://www.who.int/healthinfo/global_burden_disease/estimates_country/en/index.html.

Yusuf, S., S. Reddy, S. Ounpuu, and S. Anand. (2001). Global burden of cardiovascular diseases: Part I (general considerations, the epidemiologic transition, risk factors and the impact of urbanization). *Circulation 104*:2,746-2,753.

Zimmer, Z.N., and P. Amornsirisomboon. (2001). Socioeconomic status and health among older adults in Thailand: An examination using multiple indicators. *Social Science and Medicine 52*:1,297-1,311.

17

Aging, Health, and Chronic Conditions in China and India: Results from the Multinational Study on Global AGEing and Adult Health (SAGE)[1]

Paul Kowal, Sharon Williams, Yong Jiang, Wu Fan,
P. Arokiasamy, and *Somnath Chatterji*

China and India are the two most populous countries in the world. Combined, they were home to more than 34% of the world's 784 million people aged 60 and older in 2011. China's proportion of older people will grow from over 12% of its total population currently to 34% in 2050. Meanwhile, India's older population will grow from close to 8% to almost 20% over the same time period. The proportion of people aged 60 and older will exceed that of people aged 0–14 years by 2019 in China and by 2050 in India (United Nations, 2011a). In 2050, more than three-quarters of 1 billion people aged 60 and older will live in China and India, constituting 38% of the world's 60-plus population.

Population aging in China and India will likely be accompanied by an increase in chronic disease burden. An estimated 66% of the Chinese health burden and 45% of the Indian health burden are expected to be in older adults by 2030 (Chatterji et al., 2008). Furthermore, population aging will result in an estimated 200% increase in deaths from cardio-

[1]The World Health Organization's Study on Global AGEing and Adult Health (SAGE) is supported by the U.S. National Institute on Aging through Interagency Agreements (OGHA 04034785; YA1323-08-CN-0020; Y1-AG-1005-01) and through an NIH research grant (R01-AG034479). The National Institute on Aging's Division of Behavioral and Social Research, under the directorship of Dr. Richard Suzman, has been instrumental in providing continuous intellectual and other technical support to SAGE and has made the entire endeavor possible. The Chinese government and the Shanghai Metropolitan Center for Disease Control and Prevention contributed financial and in-kind support for SAGE China. The China and India SAGE teams conducted the interviews and produced high-quality results. We would like to acknowledge Jesse Cramer, who assisted with the literature search for this chapter.

vascular disease in China between 2000 and 2040 (Leeder et al., 2005). In addition, the rapid economic growth in these countries accompanied by rapid urbanization may also contribute to the increase of noncommunicable diseases. Urbanization is associated with unhealthy nutrition and physical inactivity, leading to obesity and increases in the prevalence of chronic diseases such as diabetes (Wang et al., 2005, 2007). The number of people with diabetes in China is estimated to be more than 92 million, with another 148 million pre-diabetic (Yang et al., 2010). India has the second largest estimated number of people with diabetes currently, at 51 million (International Diabetes Federation, 2009).

Mean life expectancies at birth and age 60 were higher in China (74 years and 20 years) than India (65 years and 17 years) in 2010, with the differences between the countries projected to shrink over the next two decades (see Table 17-1). The most recent healthy life expectancy (HALE) at birth estimates for China were 65.0 years for men and 67.8 years for women in 2007 (World Health Organization, 2008). At age 60, HALE is 13.7 years for Chinese men and 15.5 years for women. HALE at birth in India is 55.9 years for men and 56.7 years for women. The difference in HALE between the genders at age 60 in India is small, with 11.1 years for men and 11.9 years for women. In comparison to HALE at 60 years for both sexes combined of 14.6 years in China and 11.5 years in India, older people living in Indonesia can expect 11.9 years of healthy life remaining at age 60; in the United States, 17.3 years; and in Japan, 20.2 years.

Recent Global Burden of Disease estimates show a higher age-standardized overall disease burden in India than China, but with a higher proportion of noncommunicable disease (NCD) burden to overall burden in China than India (Abegunde et al., 2007; World Health Organization, 2008) (see Figure 17-1). The composition of NCDs across the countries is also notable, with considerable differences in cerebrovascular and ischemic heart diseases and unipolar depressive disorders. It is estimated that 44% of the total burden of disease in China in 2004 was from adults aged 45 and older (Chatterji, 2008), which is expected to increase to more than 65% by 2030. In India, the figure was 26% in 2004, rising to 46% by 2030.

In light of the demographic and health changes occurring in China and India, and in response to conferences in 2010 and 2011 to address population aging in Asia hosted by five national science academies, including the Chinese Academy of Social Sciences and Indian National Science Academy, this chapter summarizes selected health results from the World Health Organization's (WHO) Study on Global AGEing and Adult Health (SAGE) Wave 1 for the two nations with the largest numbers of older persons. Health state and chronic condition patterns are compared and contrasted across the two countries to further improve the understanding

TABLE 17-1 Population Aged 60 and Older, Life Expectancy (LE) at Birth and Age 60, China and India, 2010 and 2030

Country	2010					2030				
	Total, N*	Median Age	60+, N* (%)	LE at birth (yrs)	LE at 60 (yrs)	Total, N*	Median Age	60+, N* (%)	LE at birth (yrs)	LE at 60 (yrs)
World	6 895	29.2	759.0 (11.0)	68.9	20.1	8 321	34.1	1 378 (16.6)	73.1	21.6
China	1 341	34.5	165.2 (12.3)	74.0	19.9	1 393	42.5	340 (24.4)	77.4	21.6
India	1 224	25.1	92.7 (7.6)	65.2	17.4	1 523	31.2	188 (12.3)	70.5	19.0

NOTE: * in millions (000,000).
SOURCES: Data from United Nations (2011a) and World Health Organization (2008).

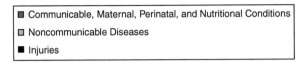

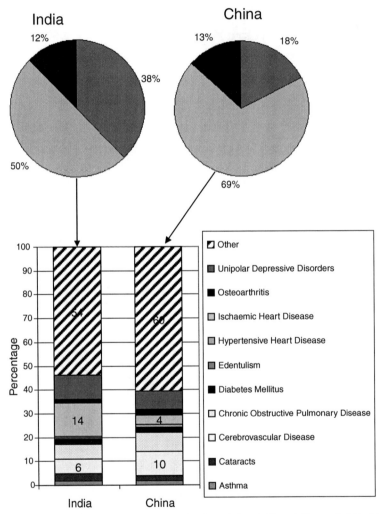

FIGURE 17-1 Percentage of age-standardized Disability-Adjusted Life Years (DALY) by Global Burden of Disease cause categories and percentage of overall noncommunicable disease burden contributed by selected health conditions in China and India, 2004.

NOTE: DALY is a health gap measure that combines the time lived with disability and the time lost due to premature mortality.

SOURCE: Data from World Health Organization (2008).

of age gradients and gender differences in health outcomes in China and India. The results also describe the approach to measurement of health and chronic diseases used by WHO, to highlight differences in reporting bias across countries and the methods SAGE employs to account for these biases.

STUDY METHODS

SAGE Wave 1

SAGE is a longitudinal study with nationally representative cohorts of persons aged 50 and older in China, Ghana, India, Mexico, the Russian Federation, and South Africa, with comparison samples of younger adults aged 18–49 years in each country. The study focuses on health and health-related outcomes and their determinants.

SAGE was implemented as a face-to-face household interview in China (2008–2010) and India (2007–2008). The samples were drawn from a current frame using a stratified, multistage cluster design so as to allow each household and individual respondent to be assigned a known non-zero probability of selection. Half the interviews in China were completed using a computer-assisted personal interview. In both China and India, the samples were selected to be nationally representative, using multi-stage sampling plans. In China, the survey was carried out in Guandong, Hubei, Jilin, Shaanxi, Shandong, Shanghai, Yunnan, and Zhejiang, covering four regions. The entire sample of India was followed up from households included in SAGE Wave 0 conducted in 2003, and was collected in the states of Assam, Karnataka, Maharashtra, Rajasthan, Uttar Pradesh, and West Bengal.

The SAGE survey instruments cover a broad range of topics, including health and its determinants, disability, subjective well-being, emotional and financial well-being, health care utilization, and health systems responsiveness. SAGE has included methodologies to improve cross-population comparability of self-reported health and well-being data through the inclusion of biomarkers, performance tests, anchoring vignettes, and additional validation studies. The anchoring vignettes approach included a short story that describes a concrete level of health in a given health domain, such as mobility (King et al., 2004; Salomon, Tandon, and Murray, 2004). Respondents are asked to rate the vignettes using the same questions and response categories that they use to describe their own health state along the same domain.

SAGE[2] has also worked to harmonize methods and results with a number of studies, including the U.S. Health and Retirement Study, Chinese Health and Retirement Longitudinal Study, and Longitudinal Aging Study in India.

Variables

Gender and age were collected, as well as area of residence, education, marital status, and income and consumption information. Four age groups were used for the analyses, 18–49, 50–59, 60–69, and 70-plus years. Education variables were mapped to an international standard classification in each country to improve comparability (United Nations Educational, Scientific and Cultural Organization, 2006). Income or wealth quintiles were derived from the household ownership of durable goods, dwelling characteristics (type of floors, walls, and cooking stove), and access to services for the dwelling, such as improved water, sanitation, and type of cooking fuel used. Durable goods included number of chairs, tables, or cars, and if, for example, the household has electricity, a television, fixed line or mobile phone, and a bucket or washing machine. A total of 21 assets and wealth indicators were included with overlaps and differences in the asset lists by country.

The income and wealth data were recoded into dichotomous variables, with the resulting data set being reshaped, as though each household had multiple observations for wealth (each item being one observation). A pure random effect model was fit based on the multiple items per household. The result provides indicator-specific thresholds on the latent income scale such that a household is more likely to respond affirmatively than not when its permanent income exceeds this threshold (Ferguson et al., 2003). This "asset ladder" was generated and is country-specific. Using a Bayesian post-estimation (empirical Bayes) method, households were arranged on the asset ladder, where the raw continuous income estimates are transformed in the final step into quintiles.

The survey instrument asked about difficulties in functioning in eight domains of health (mobility, self-care, pain/discomfort, cognition, interpersonal activities, vision, sleep/energy, and affect) and related vignettes, behavioral risk factors (tobacco use, alcohol use, physical inactivity, diet), disability, happiness, chronic conditions (asthma, angina, arthritis, depression, and diabetes), and healthcare utilization. In addition, objectively observed performance tests (including grip strength and a four-meter timed walk) and anthropometric measurements (including weight,

---

[2]More information, survey materials and results for SAGE are available at http://www.who.int/healthinfo/systems/sage/en/index.html.

height, and waist circumference) were conducted. However, the latter results are not reported in this chapter.

OVERALL SELF-REPORTED GENERAL HEALTH

A single overall self-rated general health question is used in SAGE: "In general, how would you rate your health today?" with a five-point response scale from very good to very bad. A single general health question has been shown to be a good predictor of numerous health outcomes, but raises concerns about comparability and inconsistency of results, which is why a multidimensional approach to measuring health state, combined with vignette methodologies, is also used in SAGE (Bowling, 2005; Fayers and Sprangers, 2002; Salomon et al., 2009; Sen, 2002; Subramanian et al., 2009).

Health State

The 16 questions asked about difficulties in functioning across multiple health domains. In this approach to measuring health, an individual's health state is considered a vector of capacities to function across a parsimonious set of domains in day-to-day life. As noted above, these domains included mobility, self-care, pain/discomfort, cognition, interpersonal activities, vision, sleep/energy, and affect. Examples of the questions asked about one domain (mobility) are below:

Q2002: Overall in the last 30 days, how much difficulty did you have moving around?

Q2003: Overall in the last 30 days, how much difficulty did you have in vigorous activities ("vigorous activities" require hard physical effort and cause large increases in breathing or heart rate)?

Respondents could answer using a five-point scale: 1 = None; 2 = Mild; 3 = Moderate; 4 = Severe; 5 = Extreme/Cannot do. A single health state score is generated using the Binormal Hierarchical Ordered Probit (BiHOPIT) method. Vignette adjustments of the composite health state scores were used to improve comparability of results across the two countries. The anchoring vignette technique used the same questions and response categories as used for self-assessment. The vignettes are used to fix the level of ability on a given health domain so that when analyzing the results, the variation in categorical responses can be attributed to variation in response category cut-points: that is, at what point a respondent moves from mild to moderate, or severe to extreme on the categorical response scales (Hopkins and King, 2010; Salomon et al., 2004). The additional information provided by the vignette ratings helps to describe the effects of different covariates on two important issues: (1) the level of the underlying latent variable and (2) the cut-points on the latent variable scale. Scores were normalized and then transformed to a scale of 0 to 100, with zero representing worst health and 100, best health.

Chronic Conditions

In this chapter, five chronic conditions are summarized. Respondents were asked if they had been diagnosed with any of the following chronic medical conditions: angina, arthritis, asthma, diabetes, or depression. The question format used was, "Have you ever been told by a health professional that you have . . . ?", or "Have you ever been diagnosed with . . . ?" for each health condition.

In addition to self-reported diagnosis, a set of symptomatic questions based on each condition was also asked, except for diabetes where a validated set of symptomatic questions are not currently available. The set of symptoms for each condition was derived from standard instruments, such as the World Mental Health Survey version of the Composite International Diagnostic Interview for the diagnosis of depression (Kessler and Ustun, 2004) or the Rose questionnaire for angina (Rose, 1962). The pattern of responses to the symptom questions for the four conditions (angina, arthritis, asthma, and depression) was combined with results from a separate diagnostic item probability study implemented in 2003 by WHO (Moussavi et al., 2007). This study used Receiver Operating Characteristic (ROC) analysis to create the symptom-reporting algorithm-based estimates. The method describes the sensitivity and specificity of an instrument, in this case an algorithm combining responses to different symptomatic questions. The ROC curve combines the true-positive rate and the false-positive rate of each algorithm, and the one with the highest area under the curve ("AUC statistic") is ultimately selected to derive the estimated rates.

Respondents were also asked if they were ever treated for each chronic condition they reported, if they had received treatment in the past one year (an estimate of being on longer-term regular therapy for the chronic condition), and if they were currently on treatment at the time of the interview. These two combined give an estimate of healthcare coverage and disease chronicity.

Statistical Analyses

The analyses focused on sex and age differences in health and chronic conditions. For the single overall general health question, an ordered logistic regression produced proportional odds ratios. A composite health state score in SAGE was generated using the 16 questions asked in eight health domains. A BiHOPIT model, a modification of the Compound Hierarchical Ordered Probit (CHOPIT) (Tandon et al., 2003), was used to take into account the responses to the vignettes that adjusted for response biases across the countries. BiHOPIT and CHOPIT are both generalizations of the ordered probit model, and allow the model cut-points to vary by the same covariates that the ordinal health response variables do. This means that the covariates have a two-way effect, one from the model and one from the cut-points. The latter is driven by the vignette responses. This more analytically intensive approach enables modeling to account for different health expectations, for example based on wealth, and corresponding health. BiHOPIT is computationally more efficient than CHOPIT, but provides similar results.

The prevalence of each condition was estimated separately and was generated using probability weights based on WHO's World Standard Population and the UN Statistical Division (Ahmad et al., 2001; United Nations, 2009). Results were age-standardized to improve the validity of comparisons across the two countries. Cases with age, gender, or residence variables missing were dropped from the analyses. STATA 11.2 was used for all analyses.

RESULTS

The samples included 14,793 respondents in China and 11,230 respondents in India (see Table 17-2). The Indian sample included a large number of younger (18–49) women from SAGE Wave 0 added to the Wave 1 sample as part of a nested study to meet the add-on sampling targets and study objectives. Otherwise, the percentages of men and women at older ages were similar in the two countries. A higher percentage of respondents in India resided in rural areas as compared to China; the India sample also had a slightly lower percentage in the lowest wealth quintile and slightly higher percentage in the highest wealth quintile.

The weighted results are also included in Table 17-2, with more men than women and more than 80% currently married/cohabiting in both countries. China had more older and wealthier adults than India.

Overall Health

Using the single overall self-rated general health question, male sex, younger age, urban residence, higher wealth, and living in China had significantly higher log odds of better health (see Table 17-3). Differences in the odds of good health categories, as compared to the lowest level health category, were statistically significant between the countries, as well as

TABLE 17-2 Demographic Characteristics, Weighted and Unweighted Sample Sizes[a] with Percentage, SAGE China and India, 2007–2010.

Gender	China Unweighted N^b (%)	China Weighted N^b (%)	India Unweighted N^b (%)	India Weighted N^b (%)
Men	6 883 (46.5)	7 525 (50.9)	4 349 (38.7)	5 714 (50.9)
Women	7 910 (53.5)	7 268 (49.1)	6 881 (61.3)	5 516 (49.1)
Age Group				
18-49	1 636 (11.1)	10 980 (74.2)	4 670 (41.6)	8 448 (75.2)
50–59	5 701 (38.5)	1 713 (11.6)	2 939 (26.2)	1 353 (12.0)
60–69	3 919 (26.5)	1 215 (8.2)	2 235 (19.9)	860 (7.7)
70–79	2 770 (18.7)	709 (4.8)	1 058 (9.4)	445 (4.0)
80+	773 (5.2)	176 (1.2)	328 (2.9)	126 (1.1)
Residence				
Urban	7 205 (48.7)	7 172 (48.5)	2 845 (25.3)	2 861 (25.5)
Rural	7 588 (51.3)	7 621 (51.5)	8 385 (74.7)	8 369 (74.5)
Marital Status				
Never married	279 (1.9)	849 (5.7)	621 (5.5)	1 057 (9.4)
Currently married	12 295 (83.1)	13 116 (88.7)	8 715 (77.6)	9 194 (81.9)
Cohabiting	27 (0.2)	36 (0.2)	—	—
Separated or divorced	267 (1.8)	225 (1.5)	79 (0.7)	60 (0.5)
Widowed	1 911 (12.8)	554 (3.7)	1 814 (16.2)	917 (8.2)
Missing	14 (0.1)	15 (0.1)	1 (0.0)	2 (0.0)
Wealth Quintile				
Lowest	2 948 (19.9)	1 531 (10.4))	2 232 (19.9)	2 565 (22.8)
Second	2 949 (19.9)	2 477 (16.8)	2 232 (19.9)	2 431 (21.7)
Middle	2 948 (19.9)	2 672 (18.1)	2 232 (19.9)	2 269 (20.2)
Fourth	2 947 (19.9)	3 290 (22.2)	2 234 (19.9)	1 887 (16.8)
Highest	2 948 (19.9)	4 764 (32.2)	2 229 (19.9)	2 028 (18.1)
Missing	53 (0.4)	59 (0.4)	71 (0.6)	50 (0.4)
Total	14 793 (100)	14 793 (100)	11 230 (100)	11 230 (100)

[a]SAGE samples are representative of the 50+ population, with a smaller group of younger adults selected for comparison purposes. In India, the sample of 18- to 49-year-old women was supplemented to meet the objectives of a nested study.
[b]In millions (000,000).
SOURCE: Data from SAGE Wave 1.

clear differences by gender and gradients by age and income quintiles. Marital status did not significantly impact health reporting.

Using the continuous composite health state measure, a decline in health state with increasing age is seen in both countries; however, the level of health is higher at all age points in China as compared to India (see Figure 17-2). The differences were more pronounced between the countries in the ages from about 40 to 60 years, possibly indicating a cohort effect.

TABLE 17-3 Ordered Logistic Regression Results for Overall Self-Rated General Health

Independent Variables (referent group)	Ordered Logit Coefficient	Standard Error
Gender (male)	1.45*	0.04
Age Group (18–49)		
50–59	2.59*	0.09
60–69	3.90*	0.14
70+	5.97*	0.25
Residence (urban)	1.10*	0.03
Marital Status (married/cohabiting)	1.05	0.03
Wealth Quintile (lowest)		
Second	0.75*	0.03
Middle	0.65*	0.03
Fourth	0.56*	0.02
Highest	0.40*	0.02
Country (China)	1.25*	0.03

NOTE: * denotes $p = 0.00$. $N = 25640$; chi-square ($df = 11$) = 3169; pseudo R-squared = 0.05.
SOURCE: Data from SAGE Wave 1.

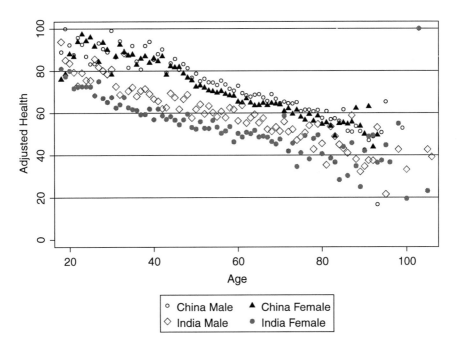

FIGURE 17-2 Vignette-adjusted health scores by age, gender, and country.
SOURCE: Data from SAGE Wave 1.

Health was better (higher health scores) in men than women in both countries, with greater differences between the genders in the health scores in India than China. An analysis of the contributions of the different domains to the overall health state score may help to better understand the determinants and drivers of health between the genders and at different ages.

Chronic Conditions

Overall, 33% of Chinese and 49% of Indian respondents aged 50 and older reported at least one chronic condition. The percentage of people with a chronic condition increased with increasing age in both countries. At each age group, Chinese men and women had lower levels of reported chronic conditions than their Indian counterparts. Comparing the youngest (18–49) to oldest (70+) age groups, women had a 33 percentage-point difference in both countries (52% versus 85% in China and 41% versus 74% in India). The age-group difference between younger and older men was 28 percentage points in China, but 36 percentage points in India, which was the largest difference in rates of reported health conditions.

In general, men reported lower levels of chronic conditions than women in both China and India, with some differences between the sexes by age. For those with no chronic conditions, the largest differences between the genders were seen in the 50–59 and 60–69 age groups in China, and the 60–69 age group in India (see Figure 17-3). For those with one condition, the largest differences were in the 50- to 59-year-old men versus women in China and the 60- to 69-year-old men and women in India. For those with two or more chronic conditions, the biggest differences between the gendrs were seen in the older two cohorts in China and the 50–59 age group in India.

Angina

The percentage of Indians (19.6%) reporting angina through the Rose questionnaire was double that in China (10%) for the 50-plus population. However, Indians were far less likely to have received recent (in the two weeks prior to interview) or longer-term (over the past 12 months) treatment.

China

Angina increased with age in both genders in China. The percentages with angina by self-report and symptom-reporting were not dissimilar by age group but with larger differences between the two methods of assessment in women than men. For instance, 3.0% of men aged 50–59 had angina

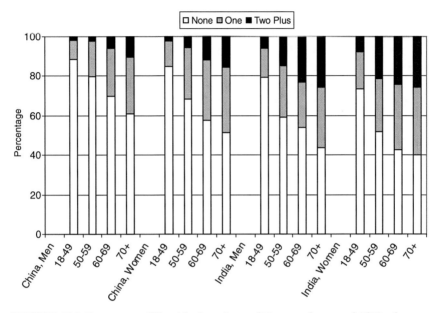

FIGURE 17-3 Percentage (%) with chronic conditions and co-morbidities by age, gender, and country.
SOURCE: Data from SAGE Wave 1.

by self-report and 3.6% by symptom reporting, compared to 5.9% and 7.9%, respectively, for women. Women had higher rates of angina than men at all age groups. Current and longer-term treatment levels were similar in men and women and increased with age.

India

The percentages of men with angina increased with increasing age in both men and women in India. Angina self-report versus symptom-reporting in India resulted in significantly different rates for men and women. Using the 50–59 age group as an example, the differences by method of ascertainment between men (5.9% by self-report and 12.3% by symptom-reporting) and women (4.0% and 20.4%) in India were large. Using self-report, men had higher rates of angina than women; however, using symptom-reporting, a larger percentage of women had angina than men. In addition, men were more likely to be on longer-term and current (in past two weeks) therapy than women.

Arthritis

Twenty-two percent of Chinese and 25% of Indians aged 50 and older had arthritis based on symptom-reporting. Using this method, rates of arthritis were slightly higher in India than China but lower in India than China using self-report. Percentages receiving current or ongoing therapies for arthritis were higher in China than India.

China

Arthritis increased steadily with age in China for men and women. Both methods of assessing arthritis prevalence produced similar results in both men and women. Rates of arthritis were higher in women (30.3%) than men (20.6%) for the 70-plus age group, but similar in the 18–49 age group (10.3% in women and 8.3% in men). Levels of treatment were again similar for the genders across the different age groups, with slightly more men receiving longer-term treatments in the 70-plus age group.

India

Levels of arthritis increased with age in men in India, but remained at about 28% across the older three age groups (50–59, 60–69, and 70-plus) in women. The percentage with arthritis for both genders was slightly higher using the symptom-reporting method as compared to self-report. The differences between men and women were similar using either method. The percentage of men aged 50–59 with arthritis was 19.5%; it was 28.4% for women. Women reported higher levels of ongoing treatment over the past year compared to men. Younger men were more likely to be on current therapy (in the two weeks prior to interview) than younger women.

Asthma

The percentage with asthma in the 50-plus population was lower in China (3.9%) than in India (11.0%). Asthma increased with age in both countries, and higher levels were reported in India than China at all age groups using either method. Longer-term and current treatment levels were typically higher in India than China for asthma.

China

Younger (18–49) and older (70-plus) women in China reported lower levels of asthma compared to men in the same age groups. Less than 1%

(0.6%) of younger women and 6.0% of older women had asthma as compared to 1.4% of younger men and 7.7% of older men. The middle-age groups had similar percentages for both genders. Levels were higher in the symptom-reporting method than the self-report at all ages and in both sexes. The percentages receiving current (more than 20%) and longer-term (more than 30%) treatment were similar in men and women.

India

The percentage with asthma increased from 4.9% in younger men to 16.9% in older men in India, and from 3.5% in younger women to 11.1% in older women. Men in India reported higher levels of asthma than women across all age groups, based on either self-report or symptom-reporting. Levels of current (close to 30%) and longer-term (over 40%) treatment of asthma were similar in both genders.

Diabetes

The percentage reporting diabetes was similar in China (6.6%) and India (6.9%) in the 50-plus population. The patterns of diabetes by age and gender between the two countries were more mixed than for any of the other conditions. Diabetes rates increased with age in China but showed somewhat variable patterns in India. Rates are higher in the younger two age groups for Indian men (2.9% in the 18–49 age group and 8.8% in the 50–59 group) compared to Chinese men (1.4% and 3.3%, respectively), but the percentages were similar for older Indians (7.2% in the 60–69 and 8.2% in the 70-plus age groups) and Chinese men (7.5% and 8.4%, respectively). A higher percentage of women than men in China had diabetes, but a lower percentage of women than men in India had diabetes. Current and longer-term treatment rates for diabetes are higher in China than in India.

China

The percentage with diabetes increased with age for Chinese men and women: from 1.4% of younger men to 8.4% of older men, and from 1.8% of younger women to 10.0% of older women. The percentage of younger men receiving current (94.2%) or longer-term (86.4%) treatment was higher than in younger women (75.7% and 67.6%, respectively); otherwise, the treatment rates were high (more than 80%) and comparable between the genders.

India

The age pattern for diabetes was less clear for both men and women in India, with a higher percentage reporting diabetes in the 50–59 age group for men (8.8%) and women (5.5%) than the 60–69 age group for men (7.2%) and women (5.1%). As with asthma, a higher percentage of Indian men reported diabetes as compared to Indian women. Longer-term treatment rates were typically above 70% for men and women and current treatment rates above 50%.

Depression

Compared with the other conditions, depression showed the largest differences in reporting by country, with much lower reported levels in China than in India. Just 2.0% of Chinese people aged 50-plus reported depression using the CIDI questions, while 19.3% of Indians had depression. The differences in depression by age were small in both countries. Not surprisingly, the levels of depression by symptom-reporting were much higher than by self-report. Undertreatment of depression was rife: the percentage on current or longer-term therapy was less than 20% in each age group for men and women in China and India.

China

The percentage of women reporting depression was slightly higher than men, with only slight differences in depression by age group. Treatment levels were low overall, with higher rates in younger age groups than older age groups.

India

Depression increased with increasing age in India, with slightly higher percentages in women than men in each age group. For example, 15.8% of men aged 50–59 and 21.2% of men aged 70 and older had depression, as compared to 18.9% and 25.3% of women. Current and ongoing treatment levels were low at all ages and in men and women.

Co-Morbidity

A substantially larger proportion of Indian respondents reported multiple morbidities than Chinese respondents at each age group for both men and women. For example, 5.7% of Chinese men and 11.9% of Chinese women aged 60–69 reported multiple chronic diseases, compared to 23.3%

of Indian men and 24.3% of Indian women in the same age group. The two countries had similar percentages of persons reporting one chronic condition at each age group, for both males and females.

DISCUSSION

WHO's SAGE, Wave 1 data provide cross-country comparable health results. Differences in levels of health states are evident when comparing China and India, even after correcting for possible reporting biases using vignette methodologies. A striking result is that health state scores for women aged 50–59 were similar to men aged 60–69, and women aged 60—69 similar to men aged 70+ in both countries. This finding suggests a decade difference in health levels for women as compared to men. This difference may shrink drastically because of highly skewed gender ratios in both countries and the positive impact of women on men's longevity and health (Economist, 2010a, 2010b). Given the difference in morbidity, women still live longer than men in both countries.

Differences in self-reported health levels between the genders have been well documented but inconsistent (Bath, 2003; Benyamini et al., 2003; Fang et al., 2003; Hairi et al., 2010). Here the differences were significant within the countries, as well as between China and India. Some of this could be due to the differences in composition of the sample in each country, with a higher proportion of rural dwellers in the India sample, more people in the wealthier income quintiles in China, and more people in the poorer income quintiles in India. The reporting of health conditions was also different by gender and country, with the biggest difference seen for the reporting of depression. Despite the measures taken in SAGE to overcome reporting biases, the well-documented low reporting of depression in China was also found here, and will prompt a revisit of the measurement technique used for depression for Wave 2 in China in 2012 (Bromet et al., 2011).

The declines in overall self-reported health with increasing age were clear using either the single overall general health question or the multidimensional approach to measuring health. A more consistent gradient was clearly shown using the continuous measure, and can be deconstructed to identify the determinants driving the differences at different ages, levels of income, and between the two countries. The health status of respondents in China, for both males and females, was consistently better across all ages as compared to respondents in India. The vignette adjustment narrows this difference somewhat as compared to the unadjusted results. Respondents in China report fewer difficulties in health domains as compared to respondents in India; however, respondents in India have vignette-rating patterns suggesting that they identify health problems at lower thresholds, that is, they have stricter standards (detailed results not shown, available from authors). Nonetheless, the differences in health status between China and India are validated by the levels and differences in healthy life expectancy (HALE) at age 60 in China (14.6 years) and India (11.5 years). With increasing longevity in China and India, and the rise in obesity and NCDs so striking that even large multinational corporations are taking note (JWT Intelligence, 2010), the steady decline in health using the health state measures has implications for disability in older age and the compression or expansion of morbidity in these middle-income countries (Gu et al., 2009; Tyagi and Kapoor, 2010). Longitudinal data and improved measurement methods are needed to provide valid measures of health and to disentangle the complexities of health in older age (National Research Council, 2001). SAGE is providing the data and methodologies to address aging and health across a number of countries, including health measures, modifiable risk factors, and health-related outcomes that will form the basis of future studies.

It is estimated that 80% of cardiovascular disease deaths occur in lower- and middle-income countries, including China and India (Bonow et al., 2002). Considerable underreporting of the five chronic diseases presented here was demonstrated through comparing self-reports and symptom-reporting. For example, the low levels and under-reporting of mental health conditions and depression in China, through a variety of measurement techniques, is noted (Lee et al., 2006; Parker, Gladstone, and Chee, 2001; Shen et al., 2006). The rate of major depressive disorder in SAGE (2.0%) matches that found in a study in metropolitan China (Shen et al., 2006). The technique used in SAGE to measure this affective disorder was informed by the World Mental Health Survey Initiative (http://www.hcp.med.harvard.edu/wmh/). Understanding the limitations of the current estimates and employing methods to improve measurement have further implications for the true burden of NCDs in China and India, and the health systems' response to chronic conditions.

Furthermore, co-morbidity has a large impact on health and well-being (Haagsma et al., 2011; Moussavi, 2007), yet complexities of multiple chronic conditions are understudied and not well understood (Tinetti and Studenski, 2011). In an effort to improve the evidence base for planning and policymaking, SAGE measures are attempting to reduce well-known reporting biases for chronic conditions in epidemiological health studies to improve the understanding about impacts of co-morbidity on health. India currently has much higher levels of people with multiple chronic conditions than China; however, China's underreporting of conditions, particularly mental health conditions, is well documented.

China's levels of treatment for the different chronic health conditions were generally higher than India, with the highest levels of treatment for angina and diabetes. Overall though, and in particular for depression, the healthcare coverage for patients with these NCDs is strikingly low. The levels and treatment of NCDs will need to be tracked over time to assess the burden on governments, the labor force, and healthcare systems. SAGE has incorporated biomarker measurements to independently assess risks for and levels of chronic disease (from height, weight and waist circumference, to glycosylated hemoglobin and C-reactive protein from dried blood spots) and will be reported separately.

The concern over NCDs in lower- and middle-income countries was raised in WHO's Moscow Declaration (World Health Organization, 2011) in April 2011 with specific statements about the huge burden in developing countries. Moving towards universal health coverage (Gwatkin and Ergo, 2010; World Health Organization, 2010a), especially targeting poorer and vulnerable population groups at the outset, and addressing the burden of increasing urbanization (Dobbs and Sankhe, 2010; WHO, 2010b) and the social determinants of health (Marmot, 2009) are mechanisms to shift the ongoing health transitions. The topics raised in this chapter are also a timely follow-up to the United Nations General Assembly High-level Meeting on Non-communicable Diseases (United Nations, 2011b) held in September 2011.

SAGE has many strengths, including nationally representative samples with large numbers in different older age groups, a method for measuring health and related techniques for improving cross-national comparability, and assessment of angina, arthritis, asthma, and depression through self-report and validated symptom-reporting methods (Moussavi et al., 2007; Tandon, Murray, and Shengalia, 2004). While the accuracy of self-reported health conditions is robust in high-income countries and wealthier populations, the same is not true in situations where low access to healthcare and low literacy levels reduce the reliability of self-report (Sen, 2002). In low- and middle-income countries, validated algorithms of disease symptoms offer a method to generate reliable prevalence estimates (Rose, 1962; Sembajwe et al., 2010). SAGE has also included biomarker and anthropometric measurements to help minimize biases in prevalence rates based on self-report and will complement these results in future studies. Increasingly, objective health outcomes, such as grip strength, timed walk, and results from collected blood samples, are used to improve our understanding of subjective or perceived health, although they may also mirror or deviate from the self-reported measures (Cooper et al., 2011). In this case, the results from the blood tests and performance tests are forthcoming from each country team. The need for improved data collection has been noted as an issue for healthcare equity even in high-income countries (Weissman and Hasnain-Wynia, 2011). SAGE provides one such data collection platform across a number of countries, including China and India.

REFERENCES

Abegunde, D.O., C.D. Mathers, T. Adam, and M. Ortegon. (2007). The burden and costs of chronic diseases in low-income and middle-income countries. *The Lancet* 370:1,929-1,938.

Ahmad, O.B., C. Boschi-Pint, A.D. Lopez, C.J.L. Murray, R. Lozano, and M. Inoue. (2001). *Age Standardization of Rates: A New WHO Standard*. Geneva: World Health Organization.

Bath, P.A. (2003). Differences between older men and women in the self-rated health-mortality relationship. *The Gerontologist* 43(3):387-395.

Benyamini, Y., T. Blumstein, A. Lusky, and B. Modan. (2003). Gender differences in the self-rated health-mortality association: Is it poor self-rated health that predicts mortality or excellent self-rated health that predicts survival? *Gerontology* 43(3):396-405.

Bonow, R.O., L.A. Smaha, S.C. Smith, G.A. Mensah, and C. Lenfant. (2002). The international burden of cardiovascular disease: Responding to the emerging global epidemic. *Circulation* 106:1,602-1,605.

Bowling, A. (2005). Just one question: If one question works, why ask several? *Journal of Epidemiology & Community Health* 59:342-345. doi:10.1136/jech.2004.021204.

Bromet, E., L.H. Andrade, I. Hwang, N.A. Sampson, J. Alonso, G. de Girolamo, R. de Graaf, K. Demyttenaere, C. Hu, N. Iwata, A.N. Karam, J. Kaur, S. Kostyuchenko, J.P. Lépine, D. Levinson, H. Matschinger, M.E. Mora, M.O. Browne, J. Posada-Villa, M.C. Viana, D.R. Williams, and R.C. Kessler. (2011). Cross-national epidemiology of DSM-IV major depressive episode. *BMC Medicine* 26(9):90.

Chatterji, S., P. Kowal, C. Mathers, N. Naidoon, J.P. Smith, and R. Suzman. (2008). The health of aging populations in China and India. *Health Affairs* 27(4):1,052-1,063.

Cooper, R., D. Kuh, C. Cooper, C.R. Gale, D.A. Lawlor, F. Matthews, R. Hardy, and the FALCon and HALCyon Study Teams. (2011). Objective measures of physical capability and subsequent health: A systematic review. *Age Ageing* 40:14-23.

Dobbs, R., and S. Sankhe. (2010, July). Comparing urbanization in China and India. *McKinsey Quarterly*.

Economist. (2010a, 4 May). Gendercide. The worldwide war on baby girls: Technology, declining fertility and ancient prejudice are combining to unbalance societies. Available: http://www.economist.com/node/15636231.

Economist. (2010b, 11 August). Health and the sex ratio. A healthy relationship: The mere presence of women seems to bring health benefits to men. Available: http://www.economist.com/node/16789152.

Fang, X.H., C. Meng, X.H. Liu, X.G. Wu, H.J. Liu, L.J. Diao, and Z. Tang. (2003). Study on the relationship between self-rated health situation and health status in the elderly—an 8-year follow-up study from the Multidimensional Longitudinal Study of Aging in Beijing. *Zhonghua Liu Xing Bing Xue Za Zhi* 24(3):184-188.

Fayers, P.M., and M.A.G. Sprangers. (2002). Understanding self-rated health. *The Lancet* 359:187-188.

Ferguson, B., A. Tandon, E. Gakidou, and C.J.L. Murray. (2003). Estimating permanent income using indicator variables. In *Health Systems Performance Assessment: Debates, Methods and Empiricism*, C.J.L. Murray and D.B. Evans (Eds.). Geneva: World Health Organization.

Gu, D., M.E. Dupre, D.F. Warner, and Y. Zeng. (2009). Changing health status and health expectancies among older adults in China: Gender differences from 1992-2002. *Social Science & Medicine 68(12)*:2,170-2,179.

Gwatkin, D.R., and A. Ergo. (2010). Universal health coverage: Friend or foe of health equity? *The Lancet 377(9,784)*:2,160-2,162.

Haagsma, J.A., E.F. van Beeck, S. Polinder, H. Toet, M. Panneman, and G.J. Bonsel. (2011). The effect of comorbidity on health-related quality of life for injury patients in the first three years following injury: Comparison of three comorbidity adjustment approaches. *Population Health Metrics 9*:10.

Hairi, N.N., A. Bulgiba, R.G. Cumming, V. Naganathan, and I. Mudla. (2010). Prevalence and correlates of physical disability and functional limitation among community dwelling older people in rural Malaysia, a middle income country. *BMC Public Health 10*:492.

Hopkins, D.J., and G. King. (2010). Improving anchoring vignettes: Designing surveys to correct interpersonal incomparability. *Public Opinion Quarterly*:1-26. doi: 10.1093/poq/nfq011.

International Diabetes Federation. (2009). *Diabetes Atlas, 4th Edition*. Available: http://www.idf.org/diabetesatlas.

JWT Intelligence. (2010). *Spotlight on marketers as obesity rises in China and India*. Available: http://www.jwtintelligence.com/2010/08/spotlight-on-marketers-as-obesity-rises-in-china-and-india/.

Kessler, R.C., and T.B. Ustun. (2004). The World Mental Health (WMH) Survey initiative version of the World Health Organization (WHO) Composite International Diagnostic Interview (CIDI). *International Journal of Methods in Psychiatric Research 13*:93-121.

King, G., C.J.L. Murray, J.A. Salomon, and A. Tandon. (2004). Enhancing the validity and cross-cultural comparability of measurement in survey research. *American Political Science Review 98(1)*:191-207.

Lee, A., M.Y.L. Chiu, A. Tsang, H. Chui, and A. Kleinman. (2006). Stigmatizing experience and structural discrimination associated with the treatment of schizophrenia in Hong Kong. *Social Science & Medicine 62*:1,685-1,696.

Leeder, S., S. Raymond, H. Greenberg, H. Liu, and K. Esson. (2005). *A Race Against Time: The Challenge of Cardiovascular Disease in Developing Economies*. New York: Columbia University.

Marmot, M. (2009). Closing the health gap in a generation: The work of the Commission on Social Determinants of Health and its recommendations. *Global Health Promotion 16*:23-27.

Moussavi, S., S. Chatterji, A. Tandon, V. Patel, and B. Ustun. (2007). Depression, chronic diseases, and decrements in health: Results from the World Health Surveys. *The Lancet 370(9590)*:851-858.

National Research Council. (2001). *Preparing for an Aging World: The Case for Cross-National Research*. Panel on a Research Agenda and New Data for an Aging World. Committee on Population and Committee on National Statistics, Division of Behavioral and Social Sciences and Education. Washington, DC: National Academy Press.

Parker, G., G. Gladstone, and K.T. Chee. (2001). Depression in the planet's largest ethnic group: The Chinese. *American Journal of Psychiatry 158*:857-864.

Rose, G.A. (1962). The diagnosis of ischemic heart pain and intermittent claudication in field surveys. *Bulletin of the World Health Organization 27*:645-658.

Salomon, J.A., A. Tandon, and C.J.L. Murray for the World Health Survey Pilot Study Collaborating Group. (2004). Comparability of self-rated health: Cross sectional multi-country survey using anchoring vignettes. *British Medical Journal 328*:258-261.

Salomon, J.A., S. Nordhagen, S. Oza, and C.J.L. Murray. (2009). Are Americans feeling less healthy? The puzzle of trends in self-rated health. *American Journal of Epidemiology* 170:343-351.

Sembajwe, G., M. Cifuentes, S.W. Tak, D. Kriebel, R. Gore, and L. Punnett. (2010). National income, self-reported wheezing and asthma diagnosis from the World Health Survey. *European Respiratory Journal* 35:279-286.

Sen, A. (2002). Health: Perception versus observation. *British Medical Journal* 324:860-861.

Shen, Y.C., M.Y. Zhang, Y.Q. Huang, Y.L. He, Z.R. Liu, H. Cheng, A. Tsang, S. Lee, and R. Kessler. (2006). Twelve-month prevalence, severity, and unmet need for treatment of mental disorders in metropolitan China. *Psychological Medicine* 26:257-267.

Study on Global AGEing and Adult Health, Wave 1. (2010). World Health Organization. Available: http://www.who.int/healthinfo/systems/sage/en/index1.html.

Subramanian, S.V., M.A. Subramanyam, S. Selvaraj, and I. Kawachi, I. (2009). Are self-reports of health and morbidities in developing countries misleading? Evidence from India. *Social Science Medicine* 68(2):260-265.

Tandon, A., C.J.L. Murray, J.A. Salomon, and G. King. (2003). Statistical models for enhancing cross-population comparability. In *Health Systems Performance Assessment. Debates, Methods and Empiricism*, C.J.L. Murray and D.B. Evans (Eds.). Geneva: World Health Organization.

Tandon, A., C.J.L. Murray, and B. Shengalia. (2004). Measuring health care need and coverage on a probabilistic scale in population surveys. Population Association of America. Available: http://paa2004.princeton.edu/download.asp?submissionId=41208.

Tinetti, M.E., and S.A. Studenski. (2011). Comparative effectiveness research and patients with multiple chronic conditions. *New England Journal of Medicine* 364(26):2,478-2,481.

Tyagi, R., and S. Kapoor. (2010). Functional ability and nutritional status of Indian elderly. *Open Anthropology Journal* 3:200-205.

United Nations. (2009). *World Population Prospects: The 2008 Revision*. New York: United Nations, Department for Economic and Social Information, Population Division.

United Nations. (2011a). *World Population Prospects: The 2010 Revision* (medium variant). New York: United Nations, Department for Economic and Social Information, Population Division.

United Nations. (2011b). General Assembly resolution A/RES/65/238. New York, USA. United Nations Educational, Scientific and Cultural Organization. International Standard Classification of Education, 1997. (1997). Available: http://www.unesco.org/education/information/nfsunesco/doc/isced_1997.htm.

United Nations Educational, Scientific and Cultural Organization. (2006). *ISCED 1997: International Standard Classification of Education* (May 2006 re-edition). New York: United Nations. Available: http://www.uis.unesco.org/Library/Documents/isced97-en.pdf.

Wang, H., S. Du, F. Zhai, and B.M. Popkin. (2007). Trends in the distribution of body mass index among Chinese adults, aged 20-45 years (1989-2000). *International Journal of Obesity* 31(2):272-278.

Wang, L., L. Kong, F. Wu, Y. Bai, and R. Burton. (2005). Preventing chronic diseases in China. *The Lancet* 366(9,499):1,821-1,824.

Weissman, J.S., and R. Hasnain-Wynia. (2011). Advancing health care equity through improved data collection. *New England Journal of Medicine* 364:2,276-2,277.

World Health Organization. (2008). *Global Burden of Disease: 2004 Update*. Geneva: World Health Organization.

World Health Organization. (2010a). *World Health Report 2010. Health Systems Financing: The Path to Universal Coverage*. Geneva: World Health Organization.

World Health Organization. (2010b). *World Health Day 2010. Why Urban Health Matters*. Geneva: World Health Organization. Available: http://www.who.int/world-health-day/2010/media/whd2010background.pdf.

World Health Organization. (2011, 29 April). *Moscow Declaration. First Global Ministerial Conference on Healthy Lifestyles and Noncommunicable Disease Control.* Available: http://www.who.int/nmh/events/moscow_ncds_2011/conference_documents/moscow_declaration_en.pdf.

Yang, W., J. Lu, J. Weng, W. Jia, L. Ji, J. Xiao, Z. Shan, J. Liu, H. Tian, Q. Ji, D. Zhu, J. Ge, L. Lin, L. Chen, X. Guo, Z. Zhao, Q. Li, Z. Zhou, G. Shan, and J. He. (2010). China National Diabetes and Metabolic Disorders Study Group. Prevalence of diabetes among men and women in China. *New England Journal of Medicine* 362:1,090-1,101.

18

Life Satisfaction of the Older Thai: Findings from the Pilot HART[1]

Dararatt Anantanasuwong and *Udomsak Seenprachawong*

Thailand has become an aging society. In 2007, 11% or approximately 7 million people of the total population was aged 60 and older. In 2030, one-fourth of the population (approximately 17.7 million people) will be aged 60 and older. In preparing for the transition to an aging society, the Thai government has developed public policy and strategies to create national long-term plans for the elderly[2] since 1986, and included language on the issue in the 2007 Constitution.[3] Internationally, the Ministry of Social Development and Human Security has been authorized to take responsibility for protecting and improving the quality of life of the Thai elderly in compliance with the Madrid International Plan of Action on Ageing (MIPAA) 2002–2010. The center of this public commitment is the development of an aging society that advances health and well-being into old age and ensures an enabling and supportive environment.

In formulating plans and strategies under this commitment, the government and the relevant agencies have relied mainly on a national database on aging provided by the central survey agency, the National Statistical Office (NSO), i.e., a bi-annual national cross-section survey

---

[1]The authors acknowledge the kind support from the Research Development Committee of the National Institute of Development Administration in writing this chapter.

[2]The First National Long-term Plan for the Thai Elderly, 1986–2001, and the Second Long-term Plan for the Thai Elderly, 2002–2021.

[3]Sections 30, 40, 53, 80, and 84 in the Constitution of Thailand 2007 include statements to protect and improve the quality of life of the Thai elderly.

on aging.[4] The cross-section data from the household surveys have contributed significantly in understanding the current status and situation of the older population in Thailand, both by researchers and policymakers. However, to understand the aging process of the population is a life-course study that involves specialists in multi- and interdisciplinary fields, such as demography, epidemiology, health, psychology, economics, sociology, and survey methodology. An intensive database from each round of the survey and from the same sample households and individuals in each dimension will enhance knowledge about the process of aging biologically, psychologically, sociologically, and economically.

A national longitudinal study using panel data to formulate scientific knowledge on aging and to inform public policy, such as the Health and Retirement Study (HRS) conducted by the University of Michigan, has not been carried out nor has it been an interest of Thai researchers. Such a survey would be complicated, time-consuming, and costly to collect, maintain, and disclose the data, which may be the main reason preventing NSO or other research organizations in Thailand from conducting a large-scale longitudinal panel survey on the older population. Yet, longitudinal studies using panel data like the HRS have contributed significantly to advances in knowledge about demography, economics, sociology, and epidemiology of aging. Currently, HRS has become the pathbreaker for longitudinal and panel studies on aging around the globe[5] (Hauser and Willis, 2004, 2011).

During 2006–2007, a group of researchers at the National Institute of Development Administration saw the value of a large-scale longitudinal study of aging like the HRS and attempted to establish a similar study in Thailand. A proposal for a pilot project, titled the Panel Survey and Study on Health, Aging, and Retirement in Thailand (HART), was developed in 2008 and received a one-year research grant from the National

---

[4]The national cross-section survey on aging was conducted bi-annually with a sample size of 79,500 households by interviewing each member aged 50 and older. The questionnaire is composed of various dimensions: demography, living conditions, employment and income, health and healthcare, social activities, information access, transfer and visit, knowledge in elderly care, and household asset ownership.

[5]HRS' contribution to the scientific knowledge of aging has influenced the development of large-scale longitudinal studies in many countries. These include the Mexican Health and Ageing Study (MHAS), English Longitudinal Study of Ageing (ELSA), Korean Longitudinal Study of Ageing (KLoSA), Japanese Study of Aging and Retirement (JSTAR), China Aging and Retirement Longitudinal Study (CHARLS), and Longitudinal Aging Study for India (LASI) (Hauser and Weir, 2011).

Research Council of Thailand (NRCT) in 2009.[6] The pilot baseline survey of 1,500 household samples[7] was conducted during August–October 2009 by interviewing, face-to-face, one member aged 45 and older from each household.[8] In 2011, a second pilot HART project received a one-year research grant from the National Higher Education Commission (NHEC). A national-scale panel survey and study on aging in Thailand is expected to follow after the learning experiences from the pilot HART projects are digested.[9]

This chapter is one of several research studies[10] using the baseline data collected from the pilot survey. It focuses on the life satisfaction dimension of the older Thai.[11] Life satisfaction has a long research history. A considerable amount of research has been devoted to explain life satisfaction of the older population (Elwell and Maltbie-Crannell, 1981; George, Okun, and Landerman, 1985; Liang et al., 1980; McClelland, 1982; Mutran and Reitzes, 1981). Among the socioeconomic characteristics, several factors have been pointed out as explanatory variables of life satisfaction: age, gender, income, educational level, physical status, emotional health, social support, and locus of control. Many studies have reported a negative relationship between happiness and age (Campbell, 1981; Ferring et al., 2004). However, a significant positive relationship was reported by several other studies (Jason and Mueller, 1983; Witt et al.,

---

[6]The pilot HART proposal was mentored by Dr. James P. Smith from RAND and received personal support from Dr. Richard M. Suzman from the U.S. National Institute on Aging (NIA). The pilot HART proposal was submitted for research funding from NIA and from NRCT. With the funding approval from NRCT, the NIA funding application has been withdrawn. However, Dr. Smith kindly agreed to mentor the pilot project as an international advisor. The survey instrument was an adoption of that of KLoSA with some adjustments to fit local conditions. Because of funding constraints, paper questionnaires, not computer-assisted personal interviewing, were used for conducting face-to-face interviews.

[7]The household samples were drawn from the NSO sampling frame from the "2004 Household Surveys in Bangkok, Nonthaburi, Pathumthani, Samuthprakarn, and Khonkaen" by using a two-stage stratified sampling method.

[8]The individual respondents were chosen by the following rule: first from the eligible head of the household; if the head of the household is not eligible, then the most eligible volunteer household members. The project acknowledges the possibility of sampling bias in the individual sampling process in the pilot survey, which can raise concerns about the representativeness of the data. However, the learning experience from the pilot survey will lead to the quality improvement of the future national-scale panel survey.

[9]It is hopeful that NRCT will grant research funding for the national longitudinal study on aging with the baseline survey in 2012.

[10]The researchers from the pilot HART project are developing four papers for publication, including this one, using the baseline data from the pilot survey. The other papers will concern aging of the population in Thailand, family structure and intergenerational transfers, and financial and social capital of the Thai elderly.

[11]As a leading study on life satisfaction of the aging in Thailand based on data from the pilot HART project, the authors include the data from respondents aged 45 and older.

1980). Delhey (2004) found only a slight effect of income on life satisfaction. Diener (1984, 2000) found no relationship between income and life satisfaction. Nonetheless, Veenhoven (2000) related income to life satisfaction at the national level and found a larger effect of income, and the same positive relationship was found by Inglehart (1997) at a country level. A study done by Fernandez-Ballesteros, Zammaron, and Ruiz (2001) found moderate positive effects of socioeconomic variables, including income and education, on life satisfaction. With regard to physical health, a substantial body of evidence positively relates health with life satisfaction (Fernandez-Ballesteros, Zammaron, and Ruiz, 2001; Lehr, 1982; Mannell and Dupuis, 1996).

In sum, life satisfaction has been considered the subjective expression of quality of life (Abu-Bader, Rogers, and Barusch, 2002; Fernandez-Ballesteros, Zammaron, and Ruiz, 2001). There is a link between advancing age and decreased subjective well-being in social, physical, and economic domains (Dolyer and Forehand, 1984; George et al., 1985; Jason and Mueller, 1983). In other words, the major life events experienced in the aging process are expected to have a profound impact on the aging population's life satisfaction. As people get older, life satisfaction may decrease sharply year by year as they are affected by major life events such as retirement and physical health deterioration. Therefore, an examination of differences in the aging population's life satisfaction becomes critical for social welfare programs. This is especially relevant for Thailand as an aging society. Subgroups of the population perceive satisfaction with life domains differently. Individuals have different lifestyles and behaviors, which determine their perceptions of their satisfaction with life domains. In order to design adequate welfare programs, policies, and regulations for the aging population, an understanding of the relationships between people's individual characteristics and their perceptions of satisfaction with life is needed.

With the availability of data on life satisfaction from the pilot HART survey, this chapter is an attempt to lay the groundwork for a study on life satisfaction of the older Thai. Its main purpose is to explain life satisfaction of older Thai respondents in three respects: (1) whether differences in life satisfaction in general exist between those in the urban and rural areas in Bangkok and vicinity and in Khonkaen, (2) which factors are associated with life satisfaction in general, and (3) the degree of association of specific life satisfaction domains with life satisfaction in general.

The chapter is organized into five parts. First, the significance of the longitudinal study on aging and the life satisfaction of the older population are introduced. We then elaborate on the characteristics of older Thai respondents from the pilot HART baseline data and describe the differences in life satisfaction in different domains between respondents in urban and rural areas. We next present the analytical models used, followed by an explanation of the empirical findings. The chapter closes with our conclusion.

BASELINE DATA AND LIFE SATISFACTION DOMAINS OF OLDER THAI RESPONDENTS

In the 2009 pilot baseline survey of the HART project, the collected data consisted of seven dimensions: population characteristics, family and transfer, health, employment, income and expenditures, assets and debts, and life expectancy and life satisfaction.[12] Life satisfaction perception and other relevant data were selected from the rich database according to the scope of the study. This present analysis is, thus, necessary cross-sectional because only one series of the survey has been completed.

The socioeconomic factors selected include the respondent's age, marital status, gender, educational level, membership in social clubs, employment status, and household characteristics such as income and assets. The data on perceived life satisfaction consist of five domains: physical health, economic status, relationship with children, relationship with spouse, and life in general. The sample size drawn from the database is 1,468 observations from Bangkok and its vicinity and Khonkaen province.[13]

The descriptive statistics for the 2009 survey are presented in Table 18-1 through Table 18-4. Of the total, 66.7% of the respondents were female and 33.3% were male. Sixty-three percent of the respondents reported having no income from work, while 25% of those who work reported incomes of less than 100,000 baht per year.[14] The majority of respondents (70%) had a primary level of education. More than half of the respondents were between 45 and 59 years old.

Table 18-5 summarizes responses obtained from the urban and rural samples for the domains of health, income, and family life. The last panel presents responses to the question regarding life satisfaction in general. For all domains and for general satisfaction, the distributions in the urban and rural respondents are significantly different (see the Chi-squared tests reported at the bottom of each panel).

Before turning to between-location differences, it is useful to highlight some differences across the domains of life. Both urban and rural people appear to be more unsatisfied with their spousal relationship

---

[12]A homepage on the HART project with the data archive is under construction. The baseline data from the pilot project will be accessible by the public when construction is completed.

[13]The complete data from the 1,500 respondents (observations) resulted in 1,468 after all the missing values were rejected.

[14]Approximately equivalent to US$3,330 (US$1 = 30 Baht).

TABLE 18-1 Distribution of Respondents by Province and Gender (in percentage)

Province	Female	Male	Total
Bangkok	20.7	9.7	30.4
Vicinity	18.1	9.4	27.5
Khonkaen	27.9	14.2	42.1
Total	66.7	33.3	100.0

SOURCE: Data from HART pilot (2009).

TABLE 18-2 Distribution of Respondents by Province and Age Group (in percentage)

	Age				
Province	45–59	60–69	70–79	Over 80	Total
Bangkok	15.3	8.8	5.0	1.4	30.4
Vicinity	15.1	7.7	3.9	0.8	27.5
Khonkaen	21.5	10.8	6.9	2.8	42.0
Total	51.8	27.3	15.8	5.0	100.0

SOURCE: Data from HART pilot (2009).

than with other domains. Approximately 30% of respondents are not happy with their relationship with their spouses. The economic status domain is next, followed by the physical health domain. Finally, a small proportion of both urban and rural respondents appear to be dissatisfied with their relationship with their children.

We first considered how satisfied respondents in the two locations are with their physical health. Rural respondents (65%) tend to be more satisfied with their physical health than urban respondents (57%). Similarly, a larger fraction of rural respondents (46%) said that they are satisfied with their economic status compared to 34% among urban respondents. A slightly larger fraction of rural respondents (63%) are happy with their relationship with their spouse, compared to 59% among urban respondents. Regarding relationship with their children, rural respondents (80%) appear to be more satisfied than urban respondents (76%). The majority of both urban and rural respondents appear to be satisfied with their lives when answering a question about life satisfaction in general. However, rural respondents (80%) are much more satisfied with their lives in general than urban respondents (69%).

TABLE 18-3 Distribution of Respondents by Province and Income from Work (in percentage)

Province	No Income from Work	<100,000 baht/year	100,000–200,000 baht/year	200,001–300,000 baht/year	300,001–400,000 baht/year	400,001–500,000 baht/year	More than 500,000 baht/year	Total
Bangkok	20.3	6.3	2.7	0.7	0.1	0.1	0.3	30.4
Vicinity	16.8	6.7	2.7	0.5	0.3	0.4	0.1	27.5
Khonkaen	26.4	12.1	2.2	0.7	0.4	0.2	0.1	42.0
Total	63.4	25.1	7.5	2.0	0.9	0.7	0.5	100.0

SOURCE: Data from HART pilot (2009).

TABLE 18-4 Distribution of Respondents by Province and Education (in percentage)

Province	No Schooling	Primary	Secondary	High School	Diploma	Undergraduate	Graduate	Doctoral	Other	Total
Bangkok	2.5	19.7	2.1	3.0	0.5	1.2	0.1	0.0	1.4	30.4
Vicinity	1.3	18.0	2.5	2.2	0.6	1.3	0.0	0.0	1.6	27.5
Khonkaen	1.7	32.2	2.2	2.3	0.8	2.1	0.2	0.1	0.4	42.0
Total	5.4	69.9	6.9	7.5	1.9	4.6	0.3	0.1	3.5	100.0

SOURCE: Data from HART pilot (2009).

TABLE 18-5 Perceived Satisfaction with Domain of Life (in percentage)

	Rural	Urban
1. How satisfied are you with your physical health?		
Very dissatisfied	5.89	6.26
Not satisfied	9.86	10.92
Neither satisfied nor not satisfied	18.31	24.89
Satisfied	27.14	39.59
Very satisfied	38.80	18.34
Pearson Chi-Square =	77.3884	p-value = 0.0000
2. How satisfied are you with your economic status?		
Very dissatisfied	7.94	6.84
Not satisfied	13.96	18.20
Neither satisfied nor not satisfied	32.01	40.32
Satisfied	23.43	24.75
Very satisfied	22.66	9.90
Pearson Chi-Square =	47.6906	p-value = 0.0000
3. How satisfied are you with your spouse relationship?		
Very dissatisfied	24.71	28.53
Not satisfied	3.71	2.04
Neither satisfied nor not satisfied	7.94	10.04
Satisfied	16.39	27.80
Very satisfied	47.25	31.59
Pearson Chi-Square =	51.6912	p-value = 0.0000
4. How satisfied are you with your children relationship?		
Very dissatisfied	6.66	9.61
Not satisfied	1.92	2.18
Neither satisfied nor not satisfied	10.50	11.50
Satisfied	20.23	35.66
Very satisfied	60.69	41.05
Pearson Chi-Square =	63.5018	p-value = 0.0000
5. How satisfied are you with your life in general?		
Very dissatisfied	2.18	2.33
Not satisfied	3.33	4.08
Neither satisfied nor not satisfied	13.70	24.45
Satisfied	26.76	42.94
Very satisfied	54.03	26.20
Pearson Chi-Square =	120.0655	p-value = 0.0000

SOURCE: Data from HART pilot (2009).

EMPIRICAL FINDINGS

In order to understand how socioeconomic and demographic factors are associated with life satisfaction in general, we employed an ordered probit estimation method. In this analysis, the dependent variable is the ranking the respondent gave for his perceived life satisfaction in general. The respondent was asked to rate life satisfaction in general: very dissatisfied ($y = 0$); not satisfied ($y = 1$); neither satisfied nor dissatisfied ($y = 2$); satisfied ($y = 3$); and very satisfied ($y = 4$). The respondents rate the level of life satisfaction as a discrete ordinal number (0, 1, 2, 3, 4). In addition, standardized regression coefficients were computed from a multiple regression method in order to investigate the degree of influence each domain of life has on life satisfaction in general.

The results of the factors associated with life satisfaction in general of the older Thai respondents are summarized in Table 18-6. All statistically significant coefficients, based on a two-tailed test at the 0.05 significant levels, are marked. As indicated in Table 18-6, level of education (EDU), age (AGE), income from work (INCOME), ownership of house (OWN), and gender (MALE) are related to level of satisfaction with life in general. The higher a respondent's level of education, the happier with quality of life he or she indicates. Older respondents tend to be happier with their life in general, and high-income respondents tend to be happier with their lives than the low-income respondents. Similarly, the respondents who are house owners indicate higher satisfaction with their life than the ones who are not. Regarding the gender variable, male respondents appear to be more satisfied with their lives than their female counterparts. Respondents who are actively involved in social clubs (MEMBER) and meet with friends (FRIEND) tend to be happier with their lives compared to those who are not. In addition, the respondents who are in urban areas (URBAN) appear to be happier with their life in general than those who live in rural areas.[15]

The investigation of the degree of association of each domain of life on life satisfaction in general is shown in Table 18-7.[16] As expected, the results show that satisfaction with life in general is positively associated with satisfaction within each of the four domains. Life satisfaction in general is a function of physical health (standardized beta = 0.322), economic status (standardized beta = 0.239), relationship with spouse (standardized beta = 0.115), and relationship with children (standardized beta = 0.238). The results indicate that physical health has the strongest association with life satisfaction in general. Relationship with spouse is least associ-

---

[15]This result, which was tested statistically using an econometric model, is different from the descriptive result described earlier.

[16]The respondents who have no children were excluded from the analysis.

TABLE 18-6 Satisfaction with Life in General

	Coefficient	t-ratio	P-value
SINGLE	−0.1602	−1.1047	0.2693
EDU	0.1802	7.3310	0.0000
FRIEND	0.3988	5.6000	0.0000
MEMBER	0.4270	5.1650	0.0000
OWN	0.3697	5.9970	0.0000
WORK	0.8677	12.3837	0.0000
AGE	0.0939	3.1335	0.0017
INCOME	0.0825	2.5014	0.0124
MALE	0.1260	2.0627	0.0391
URBAN	0.1590	2.3419	0.0192

SOURCE: Data from HART pilot (2009).

TABLE 18-7 Ranking of Four Domains of Life Affecting Life Satisfaction

Domains	Standardized Coefficient	t-ratio	P-value
(Constant)		15.401	0.0000
Physical health	0.322	13.430	0.0000
Economic status	0.239	10.111	0.0000
Relationship with spouse	0.115	5.089	0.0000
Relationship with children	0.238	10.433	0.0000
Dependent variable: Life satisfaction			

SOURCE: Data from HART pilot (2009).

ated with life satisfaction. A 1-point change in perceived physical health satisfaction is associated with increased life satisfaction by 0.322 point, whereas a 1-point change in perceived spouse relationship satisfaction is associated with increased life satisfaction by only 0.115 point, holding other things constant. Economic status and relationship with children are moderately related to life satisfaction.

CONCLUSIONS

Employing the baseline data from the pilot HART project, this study focused on three main questions about life satisfaction of Thai respondents aged 45 and older in Bangkok and the vicinity and Khonkaen. We looked at whether perceived life satisfaction of respondents in the rural and urban areas is different, what factors are related to their life satisfaction in general, and the degree of association of specific domains of satisfaction with their life satisfaction in general. The results indicate that the perceived life satisfaction of respondents in rural and urban areas in five domains—physical health, economic status, spouse relationship, children relationship, and life in general—are significantly different. Level of education, age, income from work, ownership of house, and being male are positively and significantly associated with life satisfaction in general. Other factors that are significantly associated with life satisfaction in general include being involved in social activities, meeting friends, and living in an urban area. The degree of association of each domain with life satisfaction in general indicates that physical health has the strongest association with life satisfaction in general, while relationship with spouse is least associated.

The study indicates clearly that the aging process in Thailand is just beginning. Older Thai respondents perceived their life satisfaction positively or optimistically. However, the finding that the highest proportion of them, both in rural and urban areas, are not satisfied with their relationship with their spouse implies that the marriage dimension of the older Thai may become an important policy issue to address.

Related to the factors associated with life satisfaction, building a good environment with facilities where the Thai elderly can participate in social activities and meet friends, creating economic security (e.g., financial literacy, employment, and asset ownership), and gaining and maintaining good physical health are also important public policies for the aging society.

REFERENCES

Abu-Bader, S.H., A. Rogers, and A.S. Barusch. (2002). Predictors of life satisfaction in frail elderly. *Journal of Gerontological Social Work 38(3)*:3-17.

Campbell, A. (1981). *The Sense of Well-Being in America*. New York: McGraw-Hill.

Delhey, J. (2004). *Life Satisfaction in an Enlarged Europe*. Luxembourg: Office for Official Publications of the European Communities.

Diener, E. (1984). Subjective well being. *Psychology Bulletin 95*:542-575.

Diener, E. (2000). Subjective well being. *American Psychologist 55*:34-43.

Dolyer, D., and M.J. Forehand. (1984). Life satisfaction and old age. *Research on Aging 6*:432-448.

Elwell, F., and A.D. Maltbie-Crannell. (1981). The impact of role loss upon coping resources and life satisfaction of the elderly. *Journal of Gerontology 36*:223-232.

Fernandez-Ballesteros, R., M.D. Zammaron, and M.A. Ruiz. (2001). The contribution of socio-demographic and psychological factors to life satisfaction. *Aging Society 21*:25-43.

Ferring, F.D., C. Balducci, V. Burholt, C. Wenger, F. Thissen, G. Weber, and I. Hallberg. (2004). Life satisfaction of older people in six European countries: Findings from the European Study on Adult Well-being. *European Journal of Ageing* 1:15-25.

George, L.K., M.O. Okun, and R. Landerman. (1985). Age as a moderator of the determinants of life satisfaction. *Research on Aging* 7:209-233.

Hauser, R.M., and D. Weir. (2011). Longitudinal studies of aging in the United States. *EURAMERICA 41(1)*:87-179.

Hauser, R.M., and R.J. Willis. (2004). Survey design and methodology in the Health and Retirement Study and the Wisconsin Longitudinal Study. Pp. 209-235 in *Aging, Health, and Public Policy: Demographic and Economic Perspectives*, L.J. Waite (Ed.). New York: The Population Council.

Inglehart, R. (1997). *Modernization and Postmodernization: Cultural, Economic, and Political Change in Societies*. Princeton, NJ: Princeton University Press.

Jason, P., and K.F. Mueller. (1983). Age, ethnicity and well-being: A comparative study of Anglos, Blacks and Mexican Americans. *Research on Aging* 5:353-368.

Lehr, U. (1982). Socio-psychological correlates of longevity. *Annual Review of Gerontology and Geriatrics* 3:102-147.

Liang, J., L. Dvorkin, E. Kahana, and F. Mazian. (1980). Social integration and morale: A re-examination. *Journal of Gerontology* 35:746-757.

Mannell, R.C., and S. Dupuis. (1996). Life satisfaction. In *Encyclopedia of Gerontology, Second Edition*, J.E. Birren (Ed.). San Diego, CA: Pergamon Press.

McClelland, K.A. (1982). Self-conception and life satisfaction: Integrating and subculture and activity theory. *Journal of Gerontology* 37:723-732.

Mutran, E., and D.C. Reitzes. (1981). Retirement, identity and well-being: Realignment of role relationships. *Journal of Gerontology* 36:741-749.

Panel Survey and Study on Health, Aging, and Retirement in Thailand. (2009). Bangkok: National Research Council of Thailand.

Veenhoven, R. (2000). The four qualities of life: Ordering concepts and measures of the good life. *Journal of Happiness Studies* 1:1-39.

Witt, D.P., G.D. Lowe, C.W. Peek, and E. Curry. (1980). The changing association between age and happiness: Emerging trend or methodological artifact. *Social Forces* 58:1,302-1,307.

Biographical Sketches of Contributors

DARARATT ANANTANASUWONG is senior researcher in economics in the Research Center and School of Development Economics of the National Institute of Development Administration (NIDA) in Bangkok, Thailand. Her research interests have been in sustainable development and environmental economics. Recently she has extended her interests into the sustainability of Thai society with an aging population. She is program director of the Health, Aging, and Retirement Study (HART) in Thailand. In 2009, with her research colleagues from NIDA, she conducted the baseline pilot HART project with funding from the National Research Council of Thailand; in 2011, the second pilot project was in progress with funding from the National Higher Education Commission. She completed the Ph.D. program in economics at Kyoto University and also has a Ph.D. in economics from the University of Tennessee, Knoxville.

PERIANAYAGAM AROKIASAMY is professor in the Department of Development Studies at the International Institute for Population Sciences in Mumbai, India. He has more than two decades of teaching and research experience in demography, development, and health studies. A Wellcome Trust postdoctoral fellow in population studies at the London School of Economics from 1999–2000, he has been a consultant to the World Health Organization (WHO) and the Harvard School of Public Health. His research experience also includes coordinating and conducting three major national research projects: the National Family Health Survey India-3 in 2005–2007, the WHO–World Health Survey India in

2003–2005, and the Study on Global AGEing and Adult Health in 2006–2007. He is currently involved in initiating a major nationally representative longitudinal aging study, the Longitudinal Ageing Study in India, in collaboration with the Harvard School of Public Health and the U.S. National Institute on Aging. He has a Ph.D. in population studies from Annamalai University in India.

LISA BERKMAN is director of the Harvard Center for Population and Development Studies. A social epidemiologist whose work focuses extensively on psychosocial influences on health outcomes, her research has been oriented toward understanding social inequalities in health related to socioeconomic status, different racial and ethnic groups, and social networks, support, and social isolation. The majority of her work is devoted to identifying the role of social networks and support in predicting declines in physical and cognitive functioning and the onset of disease and mortality, especially related to cardiovascular or cerebrovascular disease. She has been an innovator in linking social experiences with physical and mental health outcomes and coedited the first textbook on social epidemiology, *Social Epidemiology*. She is a member of the Institute of Medicine and past president of the Society for Epidemiologic Research. She has M.A. and Ph.D. degrees in epidemiology from the University of California, Berkeley.

DAVID E. BLOOM is Clarence James Gamble professor of economics and demography at the Harvard School of Public Health, director of Harvard University's Program on the Global Demography of Aging, and principal investigator of the Longitudinal Aging Study in India. Previously, he served on the faculty at Carnegie Mellon University and Columbia University. Bloom is an elected fellow of the American Academy of Arts and Sciences, a faculty research associate of the National Bureau of Economic Research (Programs in Labor Economics, Health Care, and Aging), and a member of the book review board of *Science* magazine. He chairs the World Economic Forum's Global Agenda Council on Ageing and Society. He has written extensively on education and health in developing countries, labor and employment issues in the United States and globally, and environmental quality. His current interests include the effects of population health and population dynamics on economic growth and development, the value of vaccination, and population aging in India and other countries. He has a B.S. in industrial and labor relations from Cornell University and an M.A. in economics and a Ph.D. in economics and demography from Princeton University.

WEI CAI is a consultant working in the Development Research Group at the World Bank in Washington, DC. Her research interests include

China's internal and external migration and population aging. She has an M.A. in development economics and China studies from Oxford University.

BENJAMIN CAPISTRANT is a doctoral candidate in the Department of Society, Human Development, and Health at the Harvard School of Public Health. His research focuses on the social epidemiology of aging in global health, in particular how health in older age affects one's family, especially the health effects of caregiving. His other work investigates social gradients in health, including disability, mental health, and cardiovascular disease among middle and older age adults in the United States and globally.

AMITABH CHANDRA is an economist and professor of public policy at the Harvard Kennedy School of Government. He is also a research fellow at the IZA Institute for the Study of Labor in Bonn, Germany, and at the National Bureau of Economic Research. His research focuses on productivity, cost growth, and racial disparities in healthcare. In 2011, he served on the Special Commission on Provider Price Reform in Massachusetts. He is an editor of the *Review of Economics and Statistics, Economics Letters*, and the *American Economic Journal*. He is the recipient of an Outstanding Teacher Award, the Upjohn Institute's International Dissertation Research Award, the Kenneth Arrow Award for best paper in health economics, and the Eugene Garfield Award for the impact of medical research. He has been a consultant to the RAND Corporation, Microsoft, and the Blue Cross Blue Shield Foundation of Massachusetts. He has a Ph.D. in economics from the University of Kentucky.

SOMNATH CHATTERJI leads the multicountry studies program in the Department of Health Statistics and Information Systems at the World Health Organization (WHO) in Geneva, Switzerland. In that position, he coordinates the Study on Global AGEing and Adult Health (SAGE), which is supported by the U.S. National Institute on Aging. SAGE also is being implemented at eight Health and Demographic Surveillance sites as part of the International Network for the Demographic Evaluation of Populations and Their Health in Developing Countries. Building on SAGE, studies are also being carried out in three European countries. The measurement of health and health-related outcomes, their trends and determinants, with an emphasis on older adults, is the main focus of the international studies of the team. Chatterji leads the World Mental Health surveys on the epidemiology of mental disorders in 30 countries. He also coordinates work on the WHO Quality of Life measure, which is used internationally in clinical and population studies. He was closely involved with the development of the International Classification of Functioning, Disability and Health and the WHO Disability Assessment Schedule. He trained as a psychiatrist in Bangalore, India.

SUBHOJIT DEY is assistant professor at the Indian Institute of Public Health in Delhi, India, which is a part of the Public Health Foundation of India. He has worked extensively in Africa and India—in collaboration with the U.S. National Cancer Institute and the International Agency for Research on Cancer in Lyon, France—and has continued interests in the health of populations in developing countries. His particular focus is chronic diseases, particularly cancer, and also environmental exposures, such as those related to xenoestrogens and industrial agents. He teaches quantitative research methods, including epidemiology and biostatistics. He has an M.B.B.S. from the Jawaharlal Institute of Postgraduate Medical Education and Research in Pondicherry; an M.D. in alternative medicine from the Indian Institute of Alternative Medicine in Kolkata; and an M.P.H. in international health epidemiology and a Ph.D. in epidemiology from the University of Michigan's School of Public Health.

WU FAN is director general of the Shanghai Municipal Center for Disease Control and Prevention in Shanghai, China. Previously, she was the first director of the National Center for Chronic and Noncommunicable Disease Control and Prevention, Chinese Center for Disease Control and Prevention, and executive director of the World Health Organization's Collaborating Centre on Community-based Integrated Noncommunicable Disease Control and Prevention. Her areas of expertise include public health, especially noncommunicable disease control. She contributed to the establishment of the noncommunicable disease control network across the country, from the national to the county level; assisted the Ministry of Health to determine the responsibilities and tasks of each level in the network; and has worked to effectively control both communicable and noncommunicable diseases in Shanghai. She leads Shanghai's program Building the Public Health Capacity and is responsible for the Shanghai Field Epidemiology Training Program in collaboration with the U.S. Centers for Disease Control and Prevention. She is also the principal investigator for the Study on Global AGEing and Adult Health in China. She has a B.S. in preventive medicine from the Shanghai Medical University and an M.S. in social medicine and public health management from Fu Dan University in Shanghai.

KEVIN FEENEY is a research assistant at the RAND Corporation and technical advisor for the Longitudinal Aging Study in India pilot. His work focuses on cross-national studies related to the economics of aging and health economics in the United States, Europe, and Asia. He graduated from the University of Chicago with a B.A. in economics.

JOHN GILES is senior labor economist in the Development Research Group at the World Bank in Washington, DC. He is also a research fellow at the IZA Institute for the Study of Labor in Bonn, Germany. His current research interests include the movement of labor from agricultural to non-agricultural employment, internal migration and its effects on households and communities, poverty traps, household risk-coping and risk management behavior, population aging and retirement decisions in developing countries, and the relationship between social protection systems and labor supply decisions. Prior to joining the World Bank in 2007, he was associate professor of economics at Michigan State University. His work has appeared in *Economic Development and Cultural Change, Economic Journal*, the *Journal of Comparative Economics*, the *Journal of Development Economics*, the *Journal of Public Economics*, the *Review of Economics and Statistics*, and *World Development*, among others. He has a Ph.D. in economics from the University of California, Berkeley.

HAO HONG is a Ph.D. candidate in the Department of Economics of Pennsylvania State University. His research interests include political economy, economic development, and experimental economics. He has a B.A. in automation from Tsinghua University in Beijing and an M.S. in economics from the China Center for Economic Research at Peking University.

PEIFENG (PERRY) HU is associate professor in the Division of Geriatric Medicine of the School of Medicine at the University of California, Los Angeles. His primary research focus has been on biomarkers, psychosocial factors, and their relations with health outcomes in older adults. He has extensive research experience working with large population-based surveys in multiple countries examining the relations between socioeconomic factors and health, including the Longitudinal Aging Study in India, the China Health and Retirement Longitudinal Study, the Indonesia Family Life Survey, the Midlife in the United States Study, and the Internal Migration and Health in China Project. In addition to his clinical training in internal medicine and geriatric medicine, he has a Ph.D. in epidemiology from the University of California, Los Angeles.

YUQING HU is a first-year master's student in the Economics Department of Duke University, where she also serves as a committee member of the Economics Masters Council. Her research interests include market design, labor economics, health economics, and the economics of education and development. Her current study focuses on family inter-generational transfers in China and the United States and the matching markets of the Chinese college admission system. She is the recipient of the Duke Leadership in an Aging Society Program Award. During her undergraduate years, she did research on the China Health and Retirement Longitudinal Study and was a survey team member of the Environmental Economics Program in China. She also explored leadership roles in several organizations, including the global youth organization AIESEC and Junior Achievement in China. In 2011, she received a B.S in information management and information systems from Beijing Language and Culture University and a B.A in economics from Peking University as a double degree.

HIDEHIKO ICHIMURA is professor of economics in the Graduate School of Economics at the University of Tokyo. Previously, he was professor in the Department of Economics at the University College London. His areas of expertise include semiparametric analysis and econometric program evaluation. He is a co-principal investigator of the Japanese Study of Aging and Retirement. He is a fellow of the Econometric Society and a past co-editor of *Review of Economic Studies*. He has a Ph.D. in economics from the Massachusetts Institute of Technology.

YONG JIANG is deputy director of the Surveillance Division of the National Center for Chronic and Noncommunicable Disease Control and Prevention, China Center for Disease Control and Prevention. His work has been dedicated to noncommunicable disease risk factor surveillance and death cause surveillance in China since 2004. He was the key national coordinator of noncommunicable disease risk factor surveillance in 2004, 2007, and 2010, and he was key investigator in the World Health Organization's Study on Global AGEing and Adult Health in China. He has conducted original research in aging health, health informatics, geographic epidemiology, and surveillance of chronic diseases and risk factors. He has a B.S. in clinical medicine and an M.S. in epidemiology and statistics from North China Coal Medical College.

PAUL KOWAL is a scientist in the Multi-Country Studies Unit of the Department of Health Statistics and Information Systems at the World Health Organization (WHO) in Geneva, Switzerland. He is also senior research fellow at the University of Newcastle's Research Centre on Gender, Health and Ageing. He has 14 years of experience with WHO working on multicountry studies on aging, health, and well-being. He is co-principal investigator for the WHO Study on Global AGEing and Adult Health. He has a B.S. in pharmacy practice from the University of

Wisconsin–Madison, an M.S. in pharmacoepidemiology from the University of Minnesota, and a doctor of pharmacy from the University of Washington.

J.K. LAKSHMI is assistant professor at the Indian Institute of Public Health in Hyderabad, India (Public Health Foundation of India), where she teaches health promotion, health communication, and environmental health. She is also involved in research on road safety and the engagement of traditional, alternative, and complementary healthcare providers. She has worked as a consultant homoeopath, program assistant (drug and alcohol rehabilitation), research assistant (dairy calcium and physical activity studies), and course instructor (women's health) during and between academic courses. Her research and teaching interests are traditional, complementary, and alternative medicine; cultural influences on health; environmental health; physical activity; aging; the health of disadvantaged populations; and health communication. She has a bachelor's degree in homoeopathic medicine and surgery from the University of Health Sciences in Andhra Pradesh, India, and an M.S. in health promotion and a Ph.D. in health promotion, disease prevention, and gerontology from Purdue University.

JINKOOK LEE is senior economist at RAND Corporation and professor at the Pardee RAND Graduate School. Before joining RAND, she was a professor at the Ohio State University and has held visiting positions at the Federal Reserve Board and the University of Wisconsin–Madison. Her research interests include the economics of aging, family economics, and consumer finances, with particular interest in interdisciplinary research on the health and well-being of the elderly. Her recent work includes education gradients in health and their potential pathways in various policy environments and cultures, dyadic analyses of spousal influences on health and well-being, and health disparities across subpopulations in both developed and developing countries. She has developed several large-scale, multidisciplinary longitudinal studies and has been a co-principal investigator of the Longitudinal Aging Study in India since its inception. She leads the research network of the Health and Retirement Studies around the world and has developed the Survey Meta Data Repository with her colleagues at RAND. She has a Ph.D. in family economics from Ohio State University.

RONALD LEE is professor of demography and Jordan family professor of economics at the University of California, Berkeley, where he also is director of the Center for the Economics and Demography of Aging. His research interests include the economic demography of intergenerational transfers, the design of public pension programs, and evolutionary theories of aging. He co-directs the National Transfer Accounts project, which integrates age into the national accounts. He has developed methods for probabilistic population forecasting, combining approaches from statistics and demography, including the Lee-Carter method for forecasting mortality and life expectancy, and used these methods to develop probabilistic public budget forecasts. He is an elected member of the National Academy of Sciences, the American Association for the Advancement of Science, the American Academy of Arts and Sciences, and the American Philosophical Society and a corresponding member of the British Academy. He has an M.A. in demography from the University of California, Berkeley, and a Ph.D. in economics from Harvard University.

XIAOYAN LEI is assistant professor of economics at the China Center for Economic Research in the National School of Development at Peking University in China. Her research spans the areas of labor economics, health economics, and the economics of aging. Her earlier studies used U.S. data to investigate the relationships among health, labor supply, transfer, and public health insurance programs. Her most recent research focuses on health, aging, and labor issues in China. She is also an active member of the research team for designing and conducting the China Health and Retirement Longitudinal Study. She has a Ph.D. in economics from the University of California, Los Angeles.

LIN LI is associate chief physician and a researcher in the Institute of Hospital Management Research at the People's Liberation Army General Hospital in Beijing, China, and a research fellow in the China Center for Health Economics Research at Peking University. He has extensive experience in hospital management and was an administrative assistant in a military hospital. He is a member of the scientific team for the China Health and Retirement Longitudinal Study project and contributed to the pilot survey, serving as an enumerator, trainer, and director of the fieldwork. Currently he focuses on healthcare policy research, including hospital size in China, and the relationship between health and socioeconomic status among the Chinese people. He has an M.D. in health economics from the Second Military Medical University in Shanghai.

JENNY LIU is an economist at the University of California, San Francisco, and also an adjunct member of the research staff at the RAND Corporation. Her research interests include studying the relationship between health, aging, and the labor supply in China and India, as well as examining issues related to child health, the burden of malaria, and malaria interventions in various countries in Sub-Saharan Africa. She conducts policy-oriented research on malaria control programs in partnership with the Global Malaria Programme of the World Health Organization. She has a B.A. in molecular and cell biology, M.A. degrees in international affairs and public policy, and a Ph.D. in health policy from the University of California, Berkeley.

MALAY MAJMUNDAR is a program officer at the National Research Council of the U.S. National Academies. He has worked on studies on federal budget policy, immigration enforcement and statistics, criminal justice, and demography and aging. He has a B.A. in political science from Duke University, a J.D. from Yale University, and a Ph.D. in public policy from the University of Chicago.

ANDREW MASON is professor of economics at the University of Hawaii at Manoa and senior fellow at the East-West Center in Honolulu, Hawaii. He is also a member of the Center for the Economics and Demography of Aging at the University of California, Berkeley. He codirects the National Transfer Accounts (http://www.ntaccounts. org) network, an international project involving researchers from more than 35 countries who are developing a comprehensive approach to measuring and studying the changes in population age structure and the generational economy in both rich and poor countries. His current research is concerned with the macroeconomic effects of population aging, including the effects on standards of living, capital accumulation, and economic growth as well as the effects on public programs, their sustainability, and their impact on generational equity. He has a Ph.D. in economics from the University of Michigan.

DEVAKI NAMBIAR is a postdoctoral fellow at the Public Health Foundation of India and adjunct faculty member in the Indian Institute of Public Health–Delhi. A former Fulbright scholar and U.S. National Institutes of Health predoctoral and postdoctoral fellow, her research applies critical theory and mixed-method evaluations to the understanding of policy-making on health and its social determinants, focusing in particular on the role of the private nonprofit sector and civil society in health promotion across the life span. She has conducted research and has ongoing research collaborations in Australia, Bangladesh, Pakistan, Tanzania, Vietnam, the United Kingdom, and the United States. She is a member of the People's Health Movement, the Medico Friend Circle, and the American Public Health Association. She has been a peer reviewer for *Global Public Health* and was a core member of the technical secretariat for India's High-Level Expert Group on Universal Health Coverage. She has a Ph.D. in public health from the Johns Hopkins Bloomberg School of Public Health.

MARIJA OZOLINS is a law student studying international refugee law at Boston College Law School. At the Harvard School of Public Health, she was technical adviser for the Longitudinal Aging Study in India pilot and contributed to projects ranging from measuring the social and physical determinants of community health to strategizing about more efficient mechanisms of global health governance. She has a B.A. in international studies from the University of Mary Washington.

ALBERT PARK is chair, professor of social science, and professor of economics at the Hong Kong University of Science and Technology. He is also a research fellow at the Center for Economic Policy Research and the Institute for the Study of Labor. Previously, he held faculty positions at the University of Michigan and Oxford University. Park is a development and labor economist whose research focuses on the Chinese economy. In recent years, he has published articles on poverty and inequality, migration and employment, health and education, and the economics of aging in China. He has co-directed numerous survey research projects in China and currently serves as a co-principal investigator for the China Health and Retirement Longitudinal Study and principal investigator for the Gansu Survey of Children and Families. He has consulted frequently for the World Bank and was lead international consultant on its most recent China poverty assessment report (2009). He has a Ph.D. from Stanford University.

K. SRINATH REDDY is president of the Public Health Foundation of India, which was established to strengthen the capacity for training, research, and policy development in the area of public health in India. Formerly head of the Department of Cardiology at the All India Institute of Medical Sciences, Reddy is a global leader in preventive cardiology and has worked to promote cardiovascular health, tobacco control, chronic disease prevention, and healthy living across the life span. He has served on many expert panels of the World Health Organization and chairs the Science and Policy Initiatives Committee of the World Heart Federation. He currently chairs India's High-Level Expert Group on Universal Health Coverage. He chairs the Core Advisory Group on Health and Human Rights for the National Human Rights Commission of India and is also a member of the National Science and Engineering Research Board of government of India. Appointed in 2009 as the first Bernard Lown visiting professor of cardiovascular health at the Harvard School of Public Health, he is also an adjunct professor of the Rollins School of Public Health and Emory University and an honorary professor of the Sydney Medical School. He is a foreign associate member of the Institute of Medicine (U.S. National Academies). He has an M.B.B.S. from Osmania Medical College in Hyderabad, India, an M.D. and a D.M. (cardiology) from the All India

Institute of Medical Sciences in Delhi, and an M.Sc. in clinical epidemiology from McMaster University in Hamilton, Canada.

UDOMSAK SEENPRACHAWONG is associate professor of economics in the School of Development Economics of the National Institute of Development Administration in Bangkok, Thailand. He has a broad range of interests in applied economics, especially in health economics, environmental economics, and tourism economics. He has a Ph.D. in business administration (economics) from the University of Memphis. He also has a certificate in environmental economics from the University of Gothenburg, Sweden.

T.V. SEKHER is associate professor in the Department of Population Policies and Programs at the International Institute for Population Sciences (IIPS) in Mumbai, India. His areas of research interest are social demography, gender issues, public health, and population aging. He has been a visiting fellow at the Wellcome Trust Centre for the History of Medicine of the University College London, Fondation Maison des Sciences de l'Homme in Paris, and Lund University in Sweden. He also served as a consultant to the United Nations Population Fund–India. He is one of the national coordinators of demographic and health surveys undertaken by IIPS, such as the District Level Household and Facility Survey for the India Ministry of Health and Family Welfare, the Study on Global AGEing and Adult Health, and the Longitudinal Aging Study in India. He is the editor of the journal *Demography India*. He has a Ph.D. in sociology and demography from the Institute for Social and Economic Change through Bangalore University.

KABIR SHEIKH is research scientist and director of the Health Governance Research Hub at the Public Health Foundation of India. He has 10 years of experience in health policy and systems research, teaching and training, health systems strengthening, and policy development in 15 states of India, Sub-Saharan Africa, the Asia-Pacific, Bangladesh, Brazil, and globally with the World Health Organization. His current interests focus on health systems governance in low- and middle-income settings, ethics in health systems, and health policy and systems research methodology. He was a Bellagio scholar-in-residence in 2011 and an Aga Khan Foundation international scholar in 2003–2006. He has a doctorate in health policy from the London School of Hygiene and Tropical Medicine and training in medicine and infectious disease epidemiology.

YAN SHEN is professor of economics at the China Center for Economic Research of Peking University in China. Her research interests include applied and theoretical econometrics. Her current empirical studies focus on economic development and institutional arrangements in China, particularly in rural finance, and the economic behaviors of Chinese elderly. Her publications appear in the *Journal of Applied Econometrics, Economic Development and Cultural Change*, the *Asia Pacific Journal of Accounting and Economics*, and the *China Journal of Economics*, among others. She is a reviewer for the *China Economic Review, Economic Development and Cultural Change, World Development*, the *International Economic Journal*, the *China Economic Quarterly*, the *Journal of Econometrics*, and the *China Journal of Economics*. She has a bachelor's degree in economics from Peking University and a Ph.D. in economics from the University of Southern California.

SATOSHI SHIMIZUTANI is senior research fellow at the Institute for International Policy Studies. Previously, he worked in the Economic Planning Agency (now called the Cabinet Office) of the Japanese government and also served in a variety of positions, including as associate professor of economics at Hitotsubashi University. His research has focused on the Japanese economy, on which he has written numerous journal articles and published two books in Japanese. He was a principal investigator of the Japanese Study of Retirement and Aging from its inception. He has a B.A. in law from the University of Tokyo and a Ph.D. in economics from the University of Michigan.

BONDAN SIKOKI is director of SurveyMeter, a nongovernment research organization based in Yogyakarta, Indonesia, that carries out large panel surveys. She was the field director for the Indonesian Fertility Survey, the Indonesian Resource Mobilization Study (1993), and the Indonesian Family Life Study (1997–1998) and the co-principal investigator of the Indonesian Family Life Study. She was also field director of the Work and Iron Status Evaluation, a large-scale iron supplementation experiment in part of central Java. She directed a longitudinal household and community survey in Aceh to study the impacts and recovery in the aftermath of the 2004 tsunami. Sikoki is co-author of a book on changing Indonesian living standards. Prior to her engagement at SurveyMeter, she held various positions in universities in Nigeria; her last position was assistant director of research and training of the Consultancy Research and Development Centre at the University of Port Harcourt. She has an M.A. in sociology/population studies from the University of Michigan.

JAMES P. SMITH holds the RAND chair in labor markets and demographic studies and was the director of RAND's Labor and Population Studies Program from 1977 to 1994. He has led numerous projects, including studies of the economics of immigration, the economics of aging, wealth accumulation and savings behavior, the relation of health and economic status, and the causes and consequences of economic growth. For 30 years Smith has worked extensively in Europe and Asia. He currently serves as chair of the National Institute on Aging Data Monitoring's Committee for the Health and Retirement Survey and was chair of the National Science Foundation's Advisory Committee for the Panel Study of Income Dynamics. He has served as an international adviser on implementing health and retirement surveys in China, India, Korea, Thailand, Indonesia, continental Europe, and England. He has twice received the National Institutes of Health MERIT Award, the most distinguished honor it grants to a researcher. In 2011, he was elected to the Institute of Medicine. He has a Ph.D. in economics from the University of Chicago.

JOHN STRAUSS is professor of economics at the University of Southern California. He has more than 30 years of research and survey experience in the developing world, focusing in particular on health, nutrition, and their interactions with various aspects of economic development. His earlier work on nutrition and labor productivity in Sierra Leone pioneered the application of methods that can disentangle causality between health and income and led to a large literature on this topic. He is editor-in-chief of *Economic Development and Cultural Change* and, in 2008, co-edited a major survey and syntheses of scientific research in economic development, *Handbook of Development Economics, Volume 4*. He has been the principal investigator of the Indonesia Family Life Survey for Waves 3 and 4 and is co-principal investigator of the China Health and Retirement Longitudinal Study. He has held academic positions at Michigan State University, Yale University, and the University of Virginia. He is also affiliated with the RAND Corporation and has an honorary professorship (Chang Jiang scholar) with the National School of Development at Peking University. He has a Ph.D. in economics and agricultural economics from Michigan State University.

DEWEN WANG is social protection economist in the World Bank's Beijing office. His work focuses on China's social insurance and social assistance programs, labor market dynamics, population aging, and economic reform and growth. For his work in the Guangdong Province of China, he received a Vice Presidential Unit Team Award from the World Bank in 2009. Prior to joining the World Bank, he was professor and division chief of the Institute of Population and Labor Economics at the Chinese Academy of Social Sciences. He has also served as a deputy division director of China's Ministry of Agriculture and was a research fellow at the Research Center for Rural Economy. He has a Ph.D. in economics from Nanjing Agricultural University.

SHARON R. WILLIAMS is assistant professor of anthropology and a faculty fellow in the Center on Aging and the Life Course at Purdue University. Her research interests include understanding how biology, culture, and the environment impact the process of aging and health across the life span and the development of field-based methods for the assessment of biological markers of chronic disease or risk for chronic disease. She has a B.S. in molecular genetics and a Ph.D. in anthropology from Ohio State University.

DAVID A. WISE is the Stambaugh professor of political economy at the John F. Kennedy School of Government at Harvard University. He is also the area director of Health and Retirement Programs and director of the Program on the Economics of Aging at the National Bureau of Economic Research and a senior fellow at the Hoover Institution at Stanford University. He has written extensively on the determinants of retirement in the United States, in particular the retirement incentives of defined benefit pension plans. For some time, he has been directing an international comparative project analyzing the effect of public pension program provisions that often induce early retirement from the labor force. He has also written extensively about the saving effect of personal retirement programs, the market risk of personal accounts compared with the job-change risk of defined benefit pension plans, and the future accumulation of pension assets associated with the conversion from retirement saving through defined benefit plans to saving through 401(k) and other personal retirement plans. His current research emphasizes the financial circumstances of retirees with particular reference to the importance of health. He has a B.A. from the University of Washington and an M.A. in statistics and a Ph.D. in economics from the University of California, Berkeley.

FIRMAN WITOELAR is a research economist at the Development Economics Research unit of the World Bank in Washington, DC. His research interest is in the area of microeconomics of development and includes such topics as risk sharing, family formation and dissolution, health behavior and outcomes, education, labor market outcomes, and household surveys. Witoelar was involved in the Indonesia Family Life Survey Wave 3 (2000) and was a co-principal investigator of the Indonesia Family Life Survey Wave 4 (2007). He has used this experience to help set up tracking operations and provide training for tracking respondents in other longitudinal household surveys in other countries. He has a B.A. in economics and development studies from the University of Indonesia, an M.A. in economics from Brown University, and a Ph.D. in economics from Michigan State University.

LI YANG is associate professor of health economics in the Department of Health Policy and Management of the School of Public Health of Peking University in China. She also serves as a member of the Asia Executive Committee of the International Society for Pharmacoeconomics and Outcomes Research. Her research interests include pharmaceutical policy and pharmacoeconomics, the economic impact of chronic diseases, and aging issues. She has a Ph.D. in health economics from Fudan University in China and has been a postdoctoral researcher at the University of Vienna and a visiting scholar at the Harvard Medical School.

YAOHUI ZHAO is professor of economics at the China Center for Economic Research of Peking University in China and a research fellow at the IZA Institute for the Study of Labor in Bonn, Germany. She is deputy director of the Institute for Social Science Surveys of Peking University. Since 2007, she has been directing the China Health and Retirement Longitudinal Study, a nationally representative sample of Chinese residents aged 45 and older. Her research interests include labor and demographic economics, social security systems pertaining to the elderly, and health economics. She has B.A. and M.A. degrees in economics from Peking University and a Ph.D. in economics from the University of Chicago.

YUHUI ZHENG is a Bell research fellow at the Harvard Center for Population and Development Studies. Her research interests include the economics of aging, economic incentives and health behaviors, social and economic status and health, and applied econometrics. She has published papers on topics related to food prices and obesity, the impact of accelerated medical technology advance on aging in America, the economics of disease prevention, the effects of pharmacy benefit design, and how neighborhood design impacts walking. She has a B.S. in engineering from Tsinghua University in Beijing, China, and a Ph.D. in policy analysis from the Pardee RAND Graduate School.

COMMITTEE ON POPULATION

The Committee on Population was established by the National Research Council in 1983 to bring the knowledge and methods of the population sciences to bear on major issues of science and public policy. Primarily, the committee deals with questions concerning the determinants and consequences of changes in population size, structure, and distribution, and their implications for policy makers and researchers in both developed and developing countries. The committee also fosters communication between policy makers and researchers in different disciplines and countries. In recent years, the committee has been concerned with a range of issues related to national and international population policy, including studies on population aging; urbanization; the transition to adulthood; population projections; and changing patterns of fertility, marriage, mortality, and migration. The committee's activities include consensus studies, workshops, and conferences.